Contents

Ezdine Bouhlel and Roy J Shephard

OPTIMIZING PHYSICAL PERFORMANCE DURING FASTING AND DIETARY RESTRICTION

Implications for Athletes and Sports Medicine

OPTIMIZING PHYSICAL PERFORMANCE DURING FASTING

AND DIETARY RESTRICTION

Implications for Athletes and Sports Medicine

Ezdine Bouhlel
University of Manouba, Tunisia

Roy J Shephard
University of Toronto, Canada

CRC Press
Taylor & Francis Group
Boca Raton   London   New York

CRC Press is an imprint of the
Taylor & Francis Group, an **informa** business

6   Hydration and Fluid Restriction in Athletes. 117
Roy J Shephard

Preface

This book examines the effects of Ramadan observance, sustained fasting and food restrictions upon the metabolism and physical performance in healthy well-trained subjects. The text is based upon recent findings, as cited in peer-reviewed literature and presented at international congresses, as well as original experiments conducted by the authors in the Laboratory of Physiology of the Faculty of Medicine of Sousse (Tunisia). The overall aim is to present these findings simply and clearly, beginning from fundamental principles, so that the material can be understood not only by sports physicians and graduate students in exercise science but also by coaches, trainers, nutritionists and the athletes themselves. The chapters are written by authors who have had long experience in the supervision of athletes during fasting. Each chapter offers a critical review of 30–100 recent investigations, together with relevant citations, but also includes clearly stated teaching objectives, definitions of key terms, a succinct summary of key points, summaries of practical implications for the athlete and questions for discussion, either in class or between athletes and their coaches.

The metabolic responses to physical activity with a normal *ad libitum* diet are well established. However, until recently, relatively few studies have assessed the effects of Ramadan observance or sustained fasting upon the physiological responses to exercise and resulting changes in physical performance. This topic is now of concern, as ever more people engage in fasting, not only in the traditional Muslim nations of the Middle East and the Arab world (Ramadan observance) but also in the developed countries of Europe and North America (therapeutic fasting, 'making weight' and Greek Orthodox fasting). Coaches, trainers and sports physicians are increasingly confronted by competitors who have chosen to engage in one of these various forms of fasting while training or participating in international competitions.

An introductory chapter defines the characteristics and requirements of fasting or food restrictions, including the daily intermittent fasting of Ramadan. The text then goes on to address the metabolic responses observed during continuous total fasting or dietary restriction, and Ramadan intermittent fasting. Potential changes are considered in regard to overall body composition and energy balance, followed by a detailed evaluation of the impact in turn upon carbohydrate, lipid and protein metabolism and body hydration. The book later considers the impact of fasting upon various aspects of body physiology and athletic performance in healthy competitors. Issues range from displaced circadian rhythms and an altered secretion of various hormones to oxidative stress, with impairments of cognitive performance and vigilance. Finally, the text makes nutritional recommendations and considers the most effective tactics to maintain training schedules, conserve competitive abilities and speed recovery processes for athletes who seek to engage in their habitual patterns of training and/or competitive sports while observing the requirements of fasting or dietary restriction.

We hope that this book will provide some definitive answers to the many questions that persist about the physiology of fasting and that it will be helpful to both athletes and their mentors as they face the challenge of combining fasting with the continuation of a successful international athletic career.

Ezdine Bouhlel
Roy J Shephard

Contributors

Ezdine Bouhlel
Faculty of Medicine of Sousse
Research Unit of Physiology
University of Sousse
Sousse, Tunisia

and

Higher Institute of Sport and Physical
    Education of Tunis
University of Manouba
Manouba, Tunisia

Mohamed Dogui
Faculty of Medicine of Monastir
Laboratory of Physiology of Alertness,
    Attention and Performance
Hospital of Sahloul Sousse
Sousse, Tunisia

Roy J Shephard
Faculty of Kinesiology and Physical
    Education
University of Toronto
Toronto, Ontario, Canada

Zouhair Tabka
Faculty of Medicine of Sousse
Research Unit of Physiology
Sousse, Tunisia

1

Introduction
Characteristics of Fasting

Ezdine Bouhlel and Roy J Shephard

Learning Objectives

1. To define notions of total fasting, dietary or food restrictions
2. To understand the model of Ramadan intermittent fasting
3. To examine the requirements of Ramadan observance as specified by the Qu'ran
4. To consider the implications of Ramadan observance for sedentary individuals
5. To evaluate the situation of athletes during Ramadan

Total Fasting and Dietary Restrictions

Fasting is defined as a voluntary or involuntary abstention from food, accompanied or not by water consumption. From a medical point of view, the fasting period starts from the sixth hour after the last meal. Fasting has been known since antiquity, and it has been practised for both medical and spiritual reasons. In the classical era, good health was thought to depend upon an appropriate balance of four body humors, and dieting, along with purging and leeching, was a frequent element in the physician's advice. Thus Hippocrates said [11]:

> Our food should be our medicine. Our medicine should be our food. But to eat when you are sick is to feed your sickness.

And Plutarch advised [10]:

> Instead of using medicine, rather, fast a day.

In our modern society, various forms of dietary restriction are frequently encountered. Physicians classify their patients in terms of their body mass index (BMI; the ratio M/H^2, where M is the body mass in kg and H is the standing height in meters). A large proportion of sedentary individuals are overweight (BMI > 25 kg/m²) or obese (BMI > 30 kg/m²). Those who are overweight or obese are at an increased risk of various chronic diseases, and physicians will attempt to restore an optimal BMI (20–25 kg/m²) by a combination of increased physical activity and a decreased food intake sufficient to create a negative energy balance of 2–4 MJ/day. Physicians also impose short periods of fasting as a prelude to anesthesia.

Fasting is a common component of many spiritual practices. In Catholic and Orthodox Churches, voluntary total starvation may continue for a day or more, but an *ad libitum* intake of water is in general allowed. It is highly recommended to adherents during certain seasons such as Lent, but it may also be adopted at other times of the year to meet personal spiritual needs. Fasting is seen as an act that not only is likely to improve health, but also as a means of learning self-control and strengthening spirituality. Prayer is often combined with the fasting. Fasting is not generally required of young children or people in delicate health. Parents may gradually introduce the practice to their children by shifting mealtime in a way that causes a few hours of fasting until they reach an age of religious maturity (often 12 or 13 years of age).

Quite long periods of fasting, usually with a normal intake of water, are a common component of political protests and can occur during famines or wartime sieges. In a few instances (as in the Minnesota starvation trial of Ancel Keys and colleagues), there have been deliberate laboratory studies of prolonged starvation.

Athletes may engage in fasting or severe dietary restriction in sports such as gymnastics or figure skating that are judged in part on physical appearance. Those participating in weight-classified sports such as wrestling may also engage in short-term (7-day) restriction of food and fluid intake in an attempt to compete in a lower weight category than what their body build should actually require. Dietary restriction or total starvation may also occur by misadventure, if a party of mountaineers, arctic explorers or shipwrecked mariners find themselves in a situation where rigorous exercise is needed to escape from a dangerous situation but supplies of food and/or water have been exhausted. Finally, food intake may be restricted by gastrointestinal disorders, and some patients with a condition known such as *anorexia nervosa* may engage in a combination of obsessive exercise and rigorous limitation of food intake until their body mass is reduced to a dangerously low level.

Food deprivation can thus be total or partial, with or without provision of water. Variables to be considered include the following:

- The degree of food deficit (usually expressed as a percentage of the daily energy requirement)
- The composition of any food provided (percentages of carbohydrates, lipid and protein)
- The timing of any food intake that is allowed
- The extent of fluid restriction
- The duration of the fast
- The nature of the fast: partial or total, short or long term, continuous or intermittent

- The individual's initial food reserves
- The patterns of training and activity required during the fast
- The initial health of the individual
- The environment in which the fasting occurs (particularly heat and humidity)

We will discuss in more specific detail the intermittent fasting of Ramadan, the fasts required by the Greek Orthodox Church, and Daniel fasting.

Intermittent Fasting during Ramadan

Ramadan is a Muslim celebration that lasts about 29 days, occupying the ninth month of the Islamic lunar calendar, the recording of which began with the *Hijra*. Ramadan begins a day or more after appearance of the crescent moon (Hilāl). Ramadan is thought to be the month when Mohammed received his first revelations. Thus, in chapter 2 of the Qu'ran we read:

> The month of Ramadan is that in which was revealed the Qu'ran; a guidance for mankind, and clear proofs of the guidance, and the criterion (of right and wrong). And whosoever of you is present, let him fast the month, and whosoever of you is sick or on a journey, a number of other days. Allah desires for you ease; He desires not hardship for you; and that you should complete the period, and that you should magnify Allah for having guided you, and that perhaps you may be thankful.

(Chapter Al-Baqra 2, verse 185)

شَهْرُ رَمَضَانَ الَّذِىٓ اُنْزِلَ فِيْهِ الْقُرْاٰنُ

هُدًى لِّلنَّاسِ وَبَيِّنٰتٍ مِّنَ الْهُدٰى

وَالْفُرْقَانِ ۚ فَمَنْ شَهِدَ مِنْكُمُ الشَّهْرَ

فَلْيَصُمْهُ ۚ وَمَنْ كَانَ مَرِيْضًا اَوْ عَلٰى سَفَرٍ

فَعِدَّةٌ مِّنْ اَيَّامٍ اُخَرَ ۗ يُرِيْدُ اللّٰهُ بِكُمُ

الْيُسْرَ وَلَا يُرِيْدُ بِكُمُ الْعُسْرَ

وَلِتُكْمِلُوا الْعِدَّةَ وَلِتُكَبِّرُوا اللّٰهَ عَلٰى مَا

هَدٰىكُمْ وَلَعَلَّكُمْ تَشْكُرُوْنَ ۝

For a Muslim, Ramadan is the most sacred month of the year, and its observance is one of the 'Five Pillars of Islam', practised by believers throughout the world.

The first day of Ramadan advances by 11 days each year relative to the Gregorian calendar. In consequence, Ramadan rotates through differing seasons, over a 33-year cycle. This affects both the duration of the daily fast and the climatic conditions to which fasters are exposed, thus modifying the extent of effects upon the individual's metabolism, fluid needs and/or physical performance [9].

Overall Requirements for Observant Muslims

The celebration of Ramadan imposes many requirements upon the devout Muslim, including daytime abstinence from food and fluids, smoking, sexual relations and swearing. Greater amounts of time are devoted to prayers (*salat*) and a reading of part or all of the Qu'ran (often with nightly attendance at mosques). Many Muslims also choose to give much of their normal annual charitable donations (*zakat*) as well as undertaking supplementary good deeds (*sadaqa*) at this season, in the belief that judgment day rewards for such actions are greater if performed during Ramadan. This is particularly true of the Night of Power (*Laylat al-Qadr*), when Mohammed was thought to receive his first revelation. This night was 'better than one thousand months' [of proper worship] (Qu'ran, Chapter 97:3).

Fasting

Muslims find value in fasting at all times of the year, but this is especially true during Ramadan. The Qu'ran specifies:

> And whosoever of you is present (at his home), let him fast the month, and whosoever of you is sick or on a journey, a number of other days.

(Chapter Al-Baqarah 2, verse 185)

The fasting and abstinence from fluid (*sawm*) extends from sunrise to sunset on each day of the holy month, from the pre-dawn meal or *suhoor* to the post-sunset meal of *iftar*; the latter is often celebrated communally. Fasting is obligatory (*fardh*) from the age of puberty; all Muslims are required to observe the fast throughout the month, with the exception of individuals who are sick, pregnant, breast-feeding, menstruating or debilitated. Islamic law has also been flexible in regard to travelers and those whose only source of income might be affected by the observance of Ramadan. They have been allowed to fast at another time, or to make a charitable donation instead.

The average duration of the daily fast is 12 hours, but it can continue for as long as 22 hours in the polar regions during summertime. Muslims living or competing in such regions are permitted (and usually choose) to adopt the fast period of either Mecca or the nearest temperate location.

Implications for Sedentary Individuals

Ramadan has major implications for the behaviour of all citizens in Muslim countries, often affecting the behaviour not only of believers but also of those who do not observe the fast (complicating experimental studies where comparisons are made between observant and non-observant individuals). The frequency and timing of food intake are inevitably changed for those who are fasting, and there may be changes in the quantity of food ingested; some who are obese see Ramadan as an opportunity to lose weight, while others who attend many communal celebrations may actually gain weight. However, it is generally possible for a sedentary person to meet their daily food and fluid requirements during the hours of darkness. From the qualitative point of view, a greater variety of foods may also be ingested during Ramadan than at other times during the year. For example, we have observed increases in the proportion and/or the absolute amounts of carbohydrate and fat intake during Ramadan [2]; some observers have also commented on a greater intake of fruits and thus possibly of micronutrients.

In general, only two meals are taken during Ramadan. The main meal is eaten soon after sunset, and a second smaller one is taken just before the sun rises. Many celebrants of Ramadan also follow the tradition of Mohammed of eating dates at *iftar*. Some people drink repeatedly during the night to make good fluid losses incurred during the hours of daylight.

The combination of nighttime eating and drinking, nightly attendance at mosque prayers, and performance of various good deeds may lead to a substantial shortening in the total nocturnal sleep time during Ramadan [1,5]. Roky et al. [5] found a reduction of nocturnal sleep time by 40 minutes, accompanied by increased sleep latency, and a decrease in slow-wave sleep. However, in countries where the majority of the population are Muslim, employees may be allowed to start work later or to take a daytime nap. Plainly, behavioural changes to facilitate the observance of Ramadan are much more difficult in countries where most of the population are non-Muslim and have little interest in accommodating those who engage in this celebration.

Implications for Athletes

Since athletes have a much higher daily consumption of energy than most sedentary people and also lose much more water from the body in sweating and the humidification of expired air, the observance of Ramadan presents a much greater challenge to those who are active than to those who are sedentary. Given also that most athletic events are won or lost by small margins, the disturbance of sleep and the progressive depletion of glycogen and fluid reserves over a long day of fasting are likely to have a negative impact upon competitive performance. When competitions are held in Muslim countries, it may be possible to modify the timing of competition to accommodate those who are fasting, and in any event, most of their rivals will be performing with a similar handicap. However, this is not the case in most international competitions. Nevertheless, many Muslim athletes choose to fast despite the need to maintain training schedules and/or to compete against non-fasting athletes during the afternoon and early evening.

Conflict between Religion and Sport?

The Olympic Games of ancient Greece were conceived in a religious setting, with the festival concluding as the successful competitors made solemn vows to Zeus and other Gods. The early fathers of the Christian church were opposed both to the worship of pagan gods associated with the classical Olympic Games and the brutality of Roman spectator sport [7]. Tertullian (160–220 CE), a prolific early Christian author from Carthage, condemned Christian attendance at circuses, stadiums and amphitheatre spectacles in *De spectaculis,* a treatise he wrote for young catechumens [4]. On the other hand, the words 'ascetic' and 'athletic' were initially almost interchangeable, and the athlete became a symbol in much early Christian teaching. In his *Epistle to Polycarp*, Ignatius of Antioch (c. 35–117 CE) wrote:

> Be sober, as an athlete of God. The prize is incorruptibleness and eternal life, whereof you also are convinced.... athletes are wont to be skinned and yet to be victorious... fight together, run you all at the same pace.

Similarly, Tertullian compared the martyr's training to that of the athlete [4]:

> The agonothete, ...who presided over Greek games and bestowed the prize "is God Himself"; the Xystarch, who played the role of judge, is the Holy Spirit; the spectators are the angels and the trainer Jesus Christ.

But attitudes changed, particularly in England, under Cromwell and the Puritans, with opposition not only to Sunday sport, but also to any involvement in sport and games. The influence of the Sunday Observance Act, passed in 1625, had a major influence upon the behaviour of Protestant Christians for the next 300 years. The film *Chariots of Fire* (1981) portrayed a dramatic incident from the Paris Olympic Games of 1924, when Eric Liddell, an outstanding British sprinter and Evangelical Christian, refused to participate in the 100 m heats because these events were scheduled on a Sunday. Fortunately, Harold Abrahams, a Jewish compatriot, was able to win the race for Britain.

Some 90 years later, neither personal sabbatarianism nor the restrictions of the Lord's Day Observance Act have any great influence upon athletic competitions. On the other hand, a growing contingent of Muslim contestants from both traditionally Muslim countries and the western world face the question 'how far is my athletic performance going to be compromised if I observe the requirements of Ramadan intermittent fasting?' Over 3000 Muslim competitors and officials attended the London Olympics in August of 2012, the first

Summer Olympic Games to coincide with Ramadan since 1980, and such concerns will be faced once again as the FIFA World Cup competitions are held in Brasil during Ramadan (June/July 2014).

Imams in some countries have interpreted the second part of Al-Baqarah 2, verse 185, as a justification for athletes postponing their observance of Ramadan until after they have completed their competition. Just prior to the London Olympics, a committee of senior Imams met in Egypt, at Al Azhar University, to consider this issue. They issued a *fatwā* that stated that athletes were not *required* to fast during their participation in the Olympic Games. However, the observance of Ramadan has remained a personal decision. An Imam who served as chaplain to the Athlete's Village at the London Olympics commented [8]:

> Most of the athletes I've met are delaying fasting for a later date. But some are fasting on all the days except on the day they have to compete.

However, a survey of Moroccan participants in the soccer competition found 9 players who were observing Ramadan and 13 (all of whom were Muslim) who were not fasting.

The extent to which Ramadan observance compromises performance and endangers safety is still debated, although this present text may help in clarifying these questions. The International Olympic Committee established a workshop in 2009 to examine the effects of Ramadan on athletes [3]. After reviewing some 400 published articles, it concluded: 'Fasting of short duration or intermittent nature has little or no effect on the health or performance of most athletes … Ramadan observance has only limited adverse consequences for either training or competitive performance'.

Fasting in the Greek Orthodox Church

Much of the fasting in the Greek Orthodox Church affects the quality of the food ingested rather than the total energy intake [9]. During the 40 days of the Nativity, devout Orthodox Christians abstain from meat, eggs and dairy products every day; on Wednesdays and Fridays, they also abstain from fish and olive oil. During the 48 days of Lent, they again abstain from meat, eggs and dairy products and avoid olive oil on weekdays; they also abstain from fish on every day except March 25 and Palm Sunday. A third 15-day fast marks the Assumption, with daily avoidance of meat, eggs and dairy products, abstinence from olive oil on weekdays and abstinence from fish except on August 6. During the remainder of the year, cheese, eggs, fish, meat, milk and olive oil are proscribed on Wednesdays and Fridays, with the exceptions of the weeks following Christmas, Easter and Pentecost. The diet is thus restricted for 180–200 days per year, and during these periods the diet of the devout person consists mainly of bread, fruits, legumes, nuts, seafood, snails and vegetables [6]. In some, but not all individuals, the total energy intake is reduced during the periods of fasting, and there is usually a decreased intake of protein and fat; there may also be a reduced intake of calcium and riboflavin [8]. However, there do not seem to have been any specific studies on Orthodox fasting and athletic performance.

Daniel Fasting

The Daniel fast has its origins in the biblical story of Daniel, who asked not to defile himself by royal food and wine, eating a diet restricted to pulses and water for 10 or 21 days. The modern Daniel fast varies in length from 10 to 40 days and is often practised in January. The diet typically involves an *ad libitum* intake of a diet restricted to fruits, vegetables, whole grains, legumes, nuts, seeds and oil. It is, in essence, a vegan diet, with proscription of refined foods, white flour, preservatives, additives, sweeteners, flavorings, caffeine and alcohol. Again, there is a decreased intake of total energy, protein and fat during the period of the fast [8].

Focus of the Present Text

The aim of the present text is to summarize current knowledge about the various types of complete and partial fast in relation to the competitive athlete, commenting on issues of experimental design and information regarding changes in sleep patterns and cognition, disturbances of nutrition and hydration, problems in maintaining training schedules, likely effects upon performance in various events, medical issues including the danger of heat stress in endurance events, questions of injury prevention and doping control, potential methods of minimizing adverse effects and potential directions for future research.

Conclusions

Continuous or total fasting is commonly practised for religious or medical reasons and can continue for long periods. This kind of fasting can have major effects upon body composition and performance and should be supervised by a nutrition specialist to ensure an adequate intake of micronutrients and avoid health complications. Athletes may undergo severe dieting in an attempt to enhance physical appearance, and this can lead to the potentially dangerous 'female athletic triad'. Competitors in weight-classified sports may also seek a major decrease of body mass in the week prior to competition, with adverse effects upon performance. Although the fasting of Ramadan is confined to daylight hours, it is perhaps the most severe challenge for the athlete, since it requires abstinence from fluid as well as foods; observance is particularly hard when Ramadan falls in the summer, with a combination of heat and long hours of daylight. Nightly prayer services, the performance of 'good deeds', and the need to meet daily food and fluid needs during the hours of darkness disturb sleep patterns and lead to falling carbohydrate and fluid reserves as the day progresses. These factors seem likely to challenge maintenance of both training and optimal competitive performance, although the extent of this handicap has yet to be agreed.

Key Terms

Anorexia nervosa: A clinical disorder marked by a combination of obsessive exercise and a rigorous limitation of food intake that reduces the patient's body mass to a dangerously low level. Sometimes, the patient may further reduce food intake by deliberate vomiting (the condition of 'bulimia').

Body mass index (BMI): The ratio of body mass (M, kg) to height^2 (H, m), M/H^2. If the BMI exceeds 25 kg/m^2, a person is regarded as overweight, and if the BMI is over 30 kg/m^2, they are classed as obese.

Catechumen: A person receiving instruction in the principles of the Christian religion with a view to baptism.

Daniel fasting: A rigorous form of fasting approaching a vegan diet, practised as a spiritual discipline by some Christians for periods of 10–40 days.

Fatwā: For Muslims, a fatwa is a legal judgment made by a qualified expert on an issue pertaining to Islamic law. For the Sunni Muslims, it is non-binding, but for Shia Muslims, it is a binding ruling.

Female athletic triad: A disorder encountered in athletes who diet excessively in an attempt to improve physical appearance; it is characterized by an inadequate intake of food energy, amenorrhea (absence of the normal menses) and osteoporosis (a decrease in bone mass predisposing to fractures) or osteopenia (a lower than normal bone density, predisposing to osteoporosis).

Imam: Refers to the spiritual leader of a Muslim community. He leads congregations in prayer at the mosque. His role may be compared with that of the clergy in the Christian church.

Sabbatarianism: Restrictions upon Sunday engagement in secular activities by some Protestant Christians, as specified in the British 'Lord's Day Observance Act' and by 'blue laws' in other jurisdictions.

Key Points

1. Continuous fasting is defined as food restriction that could be partial or total, with or without water ingestion.
2. Food restriction should not exceed 40% of the normal total daily dietary energy intake. More drastic dieting is sometimes practised in attempts to

enhance appearance or to make a specific athletic weight category, but such efforts are dangerous to health and can have adverse effects upon performance.

3. Ramadan observance calls for abstinence from food and fluids during the hours of daylight. Because of nighttime feeding and mosque attendance, normal sleep patterns are disturbed, and during the daytime, carbohydrate and fluid reserves are progressively depleted.

4. Sedentary individuals who observe Ramadan can meet most of their daily food and fluid requirements during the hours of darkness. Such adjustments are more difficult for the athlete, as food and fluid needs are greater. However, the extent of the impact of Ramadan observance upon training and competitive performance for various categories of athlete has yet to be clarified.

5. Greek Orthodox fasting and Daniel fasting involve periods during the year when a vegan-type diet is adopted; the intake of energy, protein and fat is commonly reduced during the period of the fast.

Questions for Discussion

1. What precautions should be taken during a period of continuous fasting?
2. How onerous do you think the various requirements of Ramadan observance would be for an international athlete?
3. Which categories of athlete do you think would be affected most by Ramadan observance?
4. How far does religious belief impact upon athletic involvement in Western Society? Do you think the influence of religion should be increased or decreased?

References

1. Al Hadramy MS, Zawawi TH, Abdelwaham SM. Altered cortisol levels in relation to Ramadan. *Eur J Clin Nutr* 1988;42:359–362.
2. Bouhlel E, Salhi Z, Bouhlel H et al. Effect of Ramadan fasting on fuel oxidation during exercise in trained male rugby players. *Diabetes Metab* 2006;32:617–624.
3. Maughan RJ, Al-Kharusi W, Binnett, MS et al. Fasting and sports: A summary statement of the IOC workshop. *Br J Sports Med* 2012;46:457.
4. O'Malley TP. *Tertullian and the Athlete: Language, Imagery, Exegesis*. Dekker, Nijmegen, the Netherlands, 1967.
5. Roky R, Chapotot F, Benchekron MT et al. Daytime sleepiness during Ramadan intermittent fasting: Polysomnographic and quantitative waking EEG study. *J Sleep Res* 2003;12:95–101.
6. Sarri KO, Tzanakis NE, Linardakis MK et al. Effects of Greek Orthodox Christian Church fasting on serum lipids and obesity. *BMC Public Health* 2003;3:16.
7. Shephard RJ. The developing understanding of human health and fitness: 3. The classical era. *Health Fitness J Can* 2012;5(3):18–46.

8. Taylor J. London 2012: Islamic Olympians embrace Ramadan fasting despite UK's long summer days making it a grueling ordeal. *The Independent* (*newspaper*), 2012.
9. Trepanowski JF, Bloomer RJ. The impact of religious fasting on human health. *Nutr J* 2010;9:57.
10. Weeks P. *Make Yourself Better: A Practical Guide to Restoring Your Body's Wellbeing through Ancient Medicine*. Singing Dragon, London, U.K., 2012.
11. Williams R. *The Miracle Results of Fasting: Discover the Amazing Benefits in Your Spirit, Soul, and Body*. Harrison House, Tulsa, OK, 2004.

Further Reading

Guénard H. *Physiologie humaine*. Pradel Editions, Paris, France, 1996, pp. 520–548.
Keys A, Brožek J, Henschel A et al. *The Biology of Human Starvation*. University of Minnesota Press, Minneapolis, MN, 1950.
Robinson N. *Islam: A Concise Introduction*. Georgetown University Press, Washington, DC, 1999.

2

Changes of Body Mass and Energy Balance during Fasting and Dietary Restriction

Ezdine Bouhlel and Roy J Shephard

Learning Objectives

1. To identify the principles and main components of energy balance in humans
2. To understand different forms of partial, total, and selective restriction of food and fluid intake in relation to both sedentary individuals and athletes
3. To appreciate the impact of such restrictions upon energy balance, body mass, and body composition in sedentary subjects and athletes
4. To compare the effects of Ramadan observance on energy balance, body mass, and body composition in sedentary subjects and athletes
5. To formulate some dietary guidelines for those facing dietary restrictions, with particular reference to maximizing fat loss and conservation of lean tissue

Introduction

The energy balance of the body depends upon a close matching of energy intake to energy expenditure; even a small but repeated discrepancy can have major consequences over the course of several months. If energy expenditure is greater than energy intake, there will inevitably be a decrease of body mass; on the contrary, if energy intake is greater than energy expenditure, body mass will necessarily increase. However, it is important to underline that a calculation of energy balance does not indicate the nature of the associated change in body composition; there may be gains or losses of both fat and lean tissue, determined in part by the type of nutriments ingested. Increases of carbohydrate and proteins intake favour the stimulation of their oxidation, whereas a greater fat intake predisposes to both fat storage in adipose tissue and also an increase in the oxidation of fat [84].

After discussing the two sides of the energy balance equation in more detail, summarizing body reserves of energy, and examining the specific issue of ketosis, we will present data about the general effects of dietary restriction and/or high levels of energy expenditure upon energy balance and body mass in relation to various forms of fasting in both sedentary and well-trained subjects.

Energy Balance

Energy Intake

An appropriate energy intake, with a good balance of protein, fat, and carbohydrate is important, because it influences not only a person's body mass and thus the energy that must be expended during physical activity [25], but it also determines a person's body composition and athletic performance. Although the body can absorb small amounts of energy in the form of heat, its energy input depends almost entirely upon the food that is ingested. The energy yields of various foodstuffs were examined many years ago by Professor Max Rubner (Figure 2.1), who determined the amounts of heat produced when various food products were burned in laboratory calorimeters [154]. In these experiments, he established that each gram of carbohydrate, protein or alcohol yielded approximately 16.5 kJ of energy, but that a gram of fat yielded almost 37.5 kJ; notice, however, that if body fat is broken down because of dietary restrictions, the yield is closer to 28 kJ/g, since fat tissue comprises also protein and water. Rubner also confirmed that the general physical principle that energy could be neither created nor destroyed applied to determinations of energy balance within the human body [154,155].

Laboratory determinations of food intake are made in a metabolic ward, where all food that is provided is carefully identified and weighed, and all excreta are also collected and analysed. However, in most studies of athletes, reliance is placed upon dietary records. For high accuracy, participants are instructed by a dietician, who uses models to demonstrate portion sizes, but more commonly the athlete simply completes a daily checklist of the types and amounts of foods and fluids consumed over 3 or 7 days. Because it provides more data, and the routine of many people follows a 7-day cycle, the 1-week record is to be preferred. Computer programmes based upon the composition of locally available

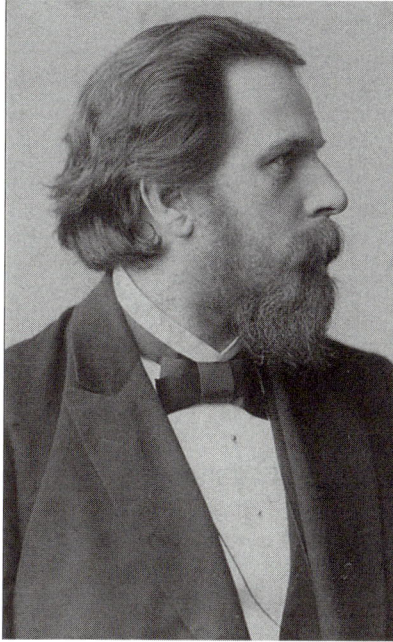

Figure 2.1 Max Rubner (1854–1932 CE) determined the energy yields of food-stuffs and gave the earliest known lecture on sports nutrition.

foods have now been developed to convert such information into estimates of total energy, nutrient and fluid intakes [113]. The values obtained often some-what underestimate intake, in part because people tend to forget snacks and soft drinks when completing their records; this is particularly a problem with athletes who may consume fluids with a high carbohydrate content [146]. Another issue in some western countries is that portion sizes have increased since the pro-grammes used for computer analysis were first developed. Based on the dietary records, a nutritionist can offer dietary recommendations enabling an athlete to improve his or her eating behaviour.

The amount of energy required to achieve energy balance varies widely, depending on daily activity patterns, from under 10 MJ/day in a sedentary person to as high of 32.7 MJ/day for participants in the Tour de France [161]. Athletes may encounter physical difficulties in ingesting large quantities of food repeatedly over the course of a day. This has been a particular problem for individuals attempting cross-Canada runs, which have taken 2–3 months to complete [169]. The World Health Organization (WHO), in collaboration with the Food and Agricultural Organization (FAO) and the United Nations University (UNU), has recommended that planners assure a daily provision of 185–200 kJ/kg of body mass in young adults [57], with the requirement decreasing slightly with aging.

Energy Expenditure

Basal Metabolic Rate

The main component of a sedentary individual's daily energy expenditure is the basal metabolic rate (BMR), the energy required to maintain the pumping actions of the heart and lungs, a minimum of muscle tone, digestion, and the various processes needed to sustain the integrity of the tissues. The BMR varies with sex, age, and body size, as shown in the original Harris/Benedict prediction equations [77], which estimated BMR in kcal/day, based on the individual's body mass (M, kg), standing height (H, cm), and age (A, years):

For men, $13.7516M + 5.0033H - 6.755A + 66.473$
For women, $9.5634M + 1.8496H - 4.6756A + 655.0955$

Thus, with a mass of 70 kg, a height of 1.7 m, and an age of 30 years, a man would have a daily BMR of 1676.5 kcal (6.97 MJ) and a woman a BMR of 1498.6 kcal (6.23 MJ) per day; the lower figure in the women reflects a higher fat mass for a given total body mass. A decade of aging would decrease the daily value by 68 kcal (281 kJ) in men and 47 kcal (194 kJ) in women (due to an increase in body fat and a slowing of the metabolic rate in most tissues with aging). Values at any given age are influenced by the relative proportions of muscle and fat in the individual concerned. Muscles have a high metabolic rate; thus, an athlete will have a high BMR for a given body mass, because the muscles are well developed, and a loss of muscle mass with food restriction will reduce the BMR for any given overall body mass. The BMR also has a genetic component; moreover, it tends to show a compensatory reduction with food restriction, perhaps in reduction to feedback signals from fat stores, thus frustrating the efforts of dieters [51]. Further, Bullough et al. [27] found an interactive effect of training upon the resting metabolic rate (RMR); the RMR was greater in trained than in untrained subjects, but only when the trained subjects were in a state of high energy flux (days when they undertook 90 minutes of exercise at 75% of their maximal oxygen consumption).

Physical Exercise

Even with the most efficient type of machine, such as a cycle ergometer, the mechanical efficiency of exercise does not exceed 25% [170]. Most of the energy that is not converted to external work appears as heat that must be dissipated from the body by sweating and other mechanisms, although additional energy is also consumed internally through the greater pumping activity of the heart and respiratory muscles and in maintaining the particular posture demanded by the activity that is being performed. During all-out effort, 10% of the observed oxygen consumption may be attributable to the activity of the heart and chest muscles [167], and this figure can rise further if the environment is cold and the individual is susceptible to an exercise-induced bronchospasm. As noted earlier, the energy cost of physical activity in an endurance athlete can add as much as 20–25 MJ/day to a person's total daily energy expenditure.

Physical activity also increases energy expenditures by creating an excess post-exercise oxygen consumption (EPOC), reflecting not only the need to dispose of accumulated metabolites such as lactate, but also the metabolic cost of replenishing food reserves such as glycogen, tissue repair, and hypertrophy, metabolic stimulation from a continuing increase of body temperature, and the continued circulation of hormones such as the catecholamines. The magnitude of EPOC depends on many factors, such as the intensity and duration of exercise [4,5], the physical fitness level of the subject [6,7], and the total dietary intake [27]. One study found metabolism was still increased by 13% at 3 hours post exercise and by 4% at 16 hours, with measurable effects persisting to 38 hours post exercise [165].

Other Sources of Energy Expenditure

In a very cold environment, energy must be expended to maintain body temperature, through a combination of shivering and non-shivering heat production, and there is some evidence that weight-loss programmes are more effective if conducted under arctic conditions [135]. Energy may also be expended in synthesizing muscle tissue, during a resistance training programme; the energy cost of such synthesis will be several times the energy equivalent of the new protein that is accumulated. In women, energy is similarly required for development of the foetus during pregnancy and for milk formation during the period of lactation.

Body Stores of Energy and Fluids

If the energy intake of energy and/or fluids does not match demands, due to either dietary restrictions or very high rates of energy expenditure, the body is obliged to draw upon its stores of carbohydrate, fat, protein, and fluids to cover the deficiency.

Carbohydrate

The carbohydrate reserves of the body are quite limited. In addition to small amounts of glucose in the plasma and tissues, glycogen is stored in the muscle (normally about 400 g) and in the liver (about 100 g), giving a total reserve equivalent to some 8 MJ of energy [170]. These reserves can be increased by at least 50% if the person concerned adopts a high-carbohydrate diet [79,185].

The rate of depletion of carbohydrate reserves depends not only on the daily energy expenditure, but also upon its nature. During moderate intensity rhythmic activity, much of the energy requirement can be met from the metabolism of fat; moreover, a higher proportion of energy is derived from fat in an endurance athlete than in a sedentary individual. At an intensity of effort demanding more than 70% of maximal oxygen intake (80%–90% in an endurance athlete), a large and growing fraction of the total energy requirement is met from the metabolism of carbohydrates [67]. The energy required for vigorous resisted muscular contractions, also, is derived almost exclusively from carbohydrate [170].

A physically active person is likely to deplete their carbohydrate stores within 24 hours or less of commencing a total fast. Any subsequent need for carbohydrate is met by the formation of glucose in the liver, the process known as hepatic gluconeogenesis. Such glucose formation depends mainly upon the breakdown of tissue protein and the metabolism of circulating amino acids, although the process is supplemented by the use of available glycerol and lactate [170].

Fat

Fat stores provide the body's main long-term reserve of energy. In sedentary North Americans, initial stores of fat can be quite large. An obese individual may store 20–30 kg of fat. If there is a major reduction in body fat stores during a period of fasting or dieting, there is a roughly corresponding decrease in body mass [171,174]; this reduces the energy cost of most tasks that require the displacement of body mass [25], although because of a loss of subcutaneous fat, a person may also need to spend more energy to compensate for heat loss in a very cold environment.

If the customary patterns of physical activity were to be maintained during fasting, then energy needs would amount to perhaps 6 MJ/day in a totally sedentary person, but 10–12 MJ/day in most athletes. Given that, the energy yield of stored body fat is about 28 kJ/g, if a person began a fast with 15 kg of surplus fat, this could provide a total reserve of some 435 MJ of energy, sufficient to sustain the energy needs even of a moderately active individual for a month or longer [170]. However, the tolerance of fasting would be much shorter in a typical athlete, who would begin any period of food deprivation with much smaller reserves of body fat and would face much higher daily energy demands.

Protein

The body has a labile reserve of some 300 g of protein [180], much of which is found in the liver. Over the first 5 days of starvation, this provides the main basis for the synthesis of glucose, at a rate of about 60 g/day. Thereafter, the main resource for continued hepatic gluconeogenesis is a progressive breakdown of muscle tissue. The American Heart Association has argued that unless dieters consume a minimum of 100 g of carbohydrate per day, a loss of tissue protein will be inevitable [176]. Unfortunately, about 1.6 g of protein is needed to provide the equivalent of 1 g of glucose [118], and the issue is further complicated in that not all amino acids can contribute to the synthesis of glucose.

The total muscle mass varies widely between a strength athlete, an endurance performer, and a sedentary adult. However, the typical muscle mass for a sedentary man would be about 35 kg [101,171]. A progressive breakdown of 100 g of lean tissue per day would provide a little over 1 MJ of energy per day, but would reduce lean mass by almost a third over 100 days of food shortage. The lack of circulating amino acids would also limit any local response to strength training [79,153,184] and would likely lead to a progressive decrease in muscular strength. Because of loss of plasma protein, tissue oedema might also develop, together with a natriuresis (excretion of sodium) and a secondary loss of potassium from the body [141,147].

Fluid

The body normally contains 45–50 L of water [170]. The maximal safe loss depends on circumstances, including the amount of exercise that must be performed, whether water has been liberated by the metabolism of intramuscular glycogen (a potential reserve of up to 2 L), and environmental conditions [168]. If a person is performing endurance exercise in a temperate climate, a loss of 5–6 L seems to be quite well tolerated [168].

Under resting conditions, normal fluid losses from the body amount to about 2.5 L/day (a urine flow of 1.2–1.5 L, water loss at the skin surface of 0.5 L/day, respiratory losses of 0.4 L/day, and the water content of the feces of about 0.15–0.2 L/day) [170]. However, if exercise is performed in the heat, an endurance athlete may lose an additional 2 L/hours or more by sweating, and there is a rapid deterioration of function if body fluid reserves cannot be replenished [170].

Issue of Metabolic Ketosis

Classical View of Metabolic Ketosis

The classic dictum of the biochemist was that 'fat burns in the flame of carbohydrate metabolism'. In the absence of sufficient carbohydrate metabolism, it was argued that body fats were partially broken down to ketone bodies and that these substances could not be metabolized in the liver because it lacked the necessary mitochondrial enzyme, succinyl CoA:3-ketoacid CoA transferase. It was thus suggested that ketone bodies would accumulate in the bloodstream, and by analogy with diabetic ketosis (where fat metabolism is increased because of a lack of insulin, and there is a massive and uncontrolled production of acidic ketone bodies), there was a fear that the end result of an inadequate carbohydrate intake in an active individual would also be a fatal ketotic coma.

Many nutritional scientists further argued that an adequate metabolism of carbohydrate was important to optimizing physical performance. Patients following low-carbohydrate diets commonly complained of weakness and early fatigue. Thus Christensen and Hansen [41] demonstrated that relative to a high-carbohydrate diet, a low-carbohydrate intake cut the time to exhaustion during submaximal cycle ergometer exercise from 206 to 81 minutes.

Impact of Circumpolar Research

Investigations conducted in the High Arctic led to a questioning of classical views on metabolic ketosis. Studies of the traditional Inuit demonstrated a very high level of daily physical activity, with daily energy expenditures of 13–16 MJ [172], but little or no access to dietary carbohydrate during their hunting expeditions [144]. Possibly, their adaptation to a protein/fat diet was helped by an increased intake of salt from the drinking of brackish water and the ingestion of caribou blood (which itself has a high salt content) [144].

Europeans living in the Arctic can also develop a remarkable tolerance to a fat and protein diet over the course of several weeks. The U.S. Schwatka Expedition, organized between 1878 and 1880 CE to seek evidence of the ill-fated Franklin expedition, provides a good example of this phenomenon. Lieutenant Frederick Schwatka and a party from the U.S. Army spent nearly a year searching the arctic tundra. They travelled by foot and by dog sled, covering a distance of 4360 km in just over 11 months. They had no sources of food other than the Inuit diet of fish and game after the first month of their journey. Schwatka commented [175]: 'When first thrown wholly upon a diet of reindeer meat, it seems inadequate to properly nourish the system, and there is an apparent weakness and inability to perform severe exertive fatiguing journeys. But this soon passes away in the course of two or three weeks'. At the end of the year, Schwatka and an Inuit companion remained in sufficiently good condition to cover the final 105 km of their trek in less than 2 days.

Laboratory Trials of a Ketotic Diet

The Schwatka observations were replicated in a nutrition laboratory in 1929, as a volunteer ate a diet comprising only meat and fat for an entire year. He remained in apparently good health [122,123]. In a more recent study, volunteers were given 1.2 g of protein per kg of body mass each day, essentially living off their fat reserves for 6 weeks [144]. No decline of maximal oxygen intake was seen.

A third experiment [142,143] provided well-trained cyclists with less than 20 g of carbohydrate per day for 4 weeks. Carbohydrate oxidation fell by 30%, but subjects maintained a normal blood glucose concentration throughout and showed no change in either maximal oxygen intake or endurance when cycling at 62%–64% of their maximal oxygen intake. Further tests in elite gymnasts have shown no deterioration in any of a series of gymnastic performance tests after 30 days of consuming a high-protein ketogenic diet [137].

Other reports have shown effects ranging from enhanced through unchanged to impaired physical performance. Brinkworth et al. [23] assigned 60 middle-aged obese individuals to a 30% energy deficit, an isoenergetic, or a hyperenergetic diet. The energy deficit diet had no effect on maximal or submaximal aerobic activity or muscle strength over 30 days of dieting. Walberg et al. [195] exposed obese women to a diet that met protein needs but was very low in carbohydrate for 4 weeks; their study participants showed a decrease in body mass of about 2 kg/week and a final 12% decrease of maximal oxygen intake, measured in L/min. Russell et al. [156] assessed muscle function by electrical stimulation of the adductor pollicis muscle. After 2 weeks of partial and 2 weeks of complete fasting, there was an increase of muscle force, but a slowing of relaxation and greater fatigue. White and associates [200] found that after 2 weeks on a low-carbohydrate diet, the perceived fatigue at any given intensity of exercise was increased, and they argued that this could have a negative impact upon the habitual physical activity of a person who was attempting to decrease his or her body mass. Bogardus et al. [15] examined the effects of a very-low-carbohydrate diet (<1%); in this study, there was a 50% decrease of endurance time on a cycle ergometer when exercising at 75% of maximal oxygen intake, but this could reflect either a physiological change such as the reduction in glycogen stores or a decrease in motivation of the subjects when their diet was restricted.

Conclusion

It seems that in general, healthy people have, or at least can acquire, a good tolerance of a prolonged ketotic diet, with no great change in performance capacity. An active person can maintain a normal blood pH and ketone bodies can provide a useful substrate for brain metabolism, thus sparing any glucose in the bloodstream [14]. Moreover, the muscles can metabolize at least seven amino acids directly. It thus may be more correct to claim that 'fat and carbohydrate burn in the flame of protein metabolism' [118]. Assuming that the energy intake of a dieter is 6 MJ/day less than the energy requirement, this deficit can be covered by metabolizing a combination of 150 g of stored fat and 100 g of tissue protein. Ketosis will develop if fats are metabolized in the absence of a substantial quantity of carbohydrate, and if this leads to an acidosis, it can impair athletic performance, but this will not invariably be the case [144].

There remain several important caveats. Firstly, protein intake must be augmented to permit adequate hepatic formation of glucose without a progressive breakdown of muscle protein. Athletes must also accept that because intramuscular glycogen reserves are depleted, their ability to perform sustained muscular efforts is likely to be compromised. Further, if a person's protein intake does not match the demands of augmented gluconeogenesis, there will be a greater loss of lean tissue than seen in dieting with a non-ketotic diet [193], and this will have adverse effects upon both aerobic and muscular activity, much as in the starvation experiments of Keys et al. [98]. Thus, moderately obese women with a daily food intake of 2.1 MJ, a carbohydrate intake <10 g/day, and a protein intake of 1.5 g/kg of body mass showed no significant decrease of maximal oxygen intake when their body mass had decreased by 17 kg, but a parallel group who ate what normally would have been regarded as an adequate protein intake (1.1 g/kg) showed a 15% decline of maximal aerobic power [47]. The group with the lower protein intake also showed a 13% decrease in the peak force of an isokinetic muscle contraction [47].

Severe Food Deprivation

Studies of severe food deprivation have mainly been conducted on experimental volunteers in order to assess human potential for wilderness survival, although there have also been a few observations on patients with clinical disorders limiting energy intake or availability. If food deprivation is prolonged, metabolic ketosis is likely.

Minnesota Starvation Study

Keys et al. [98] made a very thorough evaluation of the physiological effects of prolonged semistarvation (24 weeks) in experiments upon a panel of 36 moderately active and healthy conscientious objectors during and immediately following the Second World War.

The initial body fat stores of their subjects averaged 9.6 kg. During the 24-week trial, the subjects were given a very limited diet of the type that might be anticipated under famine conditions (mainly potatoes, rutabagas, turnips, bread, and macaroni), reducing their total intake of food energy from a normal figure of 14.5 to 6.5 MJ/day. In addition to any required laboratory exercise tests, the subjects continued to undertake about 15 hours of light housekeeping per week, as their physical condition allowed. Subjective complaints included hunger and an enhanced sensitivity to cold (probably related to a loss of subcutaneous fat). Clinical examination showed ankle oedema and an accumulation of fluid in the knee joints, suggestive of a decrease in plasma proteins.

The course of weight loss was carefully documented (Table 2.1). On average, the men lost 16.8 kg (24% of their body mass) over the 24 weeks. Specific gravity measurements suggested that 6.5 kg of the total loss was fat; some of the remainder was likely water, but 9–10 kg, or about a third of the subjects' initial lean tissue mass, was also metabolized. Decreases in limb circumference were consistent with such losses. However, the plasma volume showed only a small decrease. There was also a 56% increase in extracellular fluid volume, and since the abdominal circumference showed relatively little change, an intra-abdominal accumulation of ascitic fluid may be presumed, again probably a reflection of low plasma protein concentrations.

The changes of physical performance were much as would be predicted (Table 2.1). As the fast continued, the oxygen cost of submaximal treadmill walking at a speed of 5.6 km/h declined in almost direct proportion to the decrease of body mass. One measure of the decline in aerobic performance was the score obtained on a treadmill version of the Harvard Fitness Test (a score based on the rapidity of recovery of the heart rate following the exercise bout). The tolerated length of a treadmill run to exhaustion also decreased from an initial 242 to 106 seconds at 12 weeks and 50 seconds at 24 weeks of food restriction [28]. The maximal oxygen intake (measured in L/min) showed a substantial deterioration

TABLE 2.1 Main Changes of Physical Performance Seen in Minnesota Starvation Experiment (24% Loss of Body Mass over 24 Weeks)

Decline in oxygen cost of walking at 5.6 km/h, proportional to decrease in body mass
Harvard fitness test scores: control 64 units; 12 weeks 33 units; 24 weeks 18 units
Duration of run to exhaustion: control 242 seconds; 12 weeks 106 seconds; 24 weeks 50 seconds
Decrease of heart volume on PA radiograph
22% decrease of red cell count
Decrease of maximal oxygen intake and grip strength when 12%–16% loss of body mass

when the body mass had decreased by 12%–16% [182]. Furthermore, the heart size as seen in postero-anterior radiographs decreased over the experiment, and there was also a 22% decrease in the red cell count.

In terms of muscular performance, there were large decrements of hand-grip force and a marked deterioration in coordination as fasting continued [26]. Scores on a back-lift dynamometer had decreased by 16% at 12 weeks and 31% at 24 weeks; decreases of handgrip at 12 and 24 weeks were 22% and 40%, respectively. Clinical observations also suggested deterioration in the patellar reflex [98], and pattern tracing ability was impaired. Finally, there were increases of apathy and introversion as the experiment progressed, and these changes could have had a negative effect upon scores in tests requiring subject cooperation.

Other Studies of Severe Food Deprivation

Further studies of severe food deprivation have been conducted on military volunteers. In 1953, subjects were restricted to a diet of 2.41 MJ/day for 12 days and in 1955 to 4.2 MJ/day for 24 days [182]. In contrast to the earlier experiments on the conscientious objectors, the observers in this study considered that apprehension and loss of motivation contributed to a poor and variable performance, and many tests showed no consistent difference between controls and those undergoing semistarvation.

The reductions in maximal oxygen intake in absolute units (L/min) were for acute starvation (4.5 days) 7.5%, for severe food restriction (2.41 MJ/day for 12 days) 4.1%, and for prolonged but more moderate food restriction (4.2 MJ/day for 180 days) 37.3%. However, the maximal aerobic power per unit of body mass remained unchanged throughout. Some acidosis and dehydration developed, but the heart rate when walking at 5.6 km/h was actually less than in the control period [28].

Finally, studies in patients with chronic malnutrition due to gastrointestinal disorders or deliberate anorexic dieting have shown a slowing of muscular relaxation and a decrease of muscular endurance [115].

Prolonged Moderate Food Restriction

Dieting Alone

Sedentary subjects usually accept dietary restrictions that create an energy deficit in an attempt to reduce their body mass and lose surplus fat. The U.S. National Institutes of Health and the WHO have both recommended creating an energy deficit of 2–4 MJ/day in order to reduce body mass. In theory, this should reduce body mass by 0.5–1 kg/week, assuming that 0.5 kg fat mass yields approximately 14.5 MJ of energy. Unfortunately, the energy deficit needed to achieve this result is larger, because of adaptive changes. The RMR is reduced, because of decreases in the amount of metabolically active tissue in the body and possibly hormonal changes initiated from the depleted fat depots [51]. Moreover, the energy costs of most daily activities are decreased by the reduced body mass [25]. Nevertheless, some authors have demonstrated that dietary restriction can be an efficient method of inducing at least an initial loss of body mass and especially a loss of fat [9]. Diets that create a much larger energy deficit may lead to a greater initial decrease in body mass, but long-term benefits seem no greater than with more moderate regimens. Debate continues on the optimum composition of a low-energy diet; some authors maintain that a low-carbohydrate dietary intake is more efficient than a low-fat regime as a means of reducing body fat content [203].

Dieting Plus Exercise

The achievement of a negative energy balance by inclusion of an increase in physical activity is recommended, as this appears to concentrate the tissue loss in fat depots, with a sparing of lean tissue.

Physical activity is in itself a major factor in preventing and treating obesity. Trost [191] argued that the number of obesity cases could be reduced by 10% if youngsters undertook 1 h/day of moderate to intense exercise, and obesity increased by 12% for each hour that was spent watching TV. Kimm et al. [102] also pointed to an association between the reduction of daily physical activity and increases in BMI and in fat mass in girls who were followed for 10 years, beginning at an age of 9 years. Many studies have shown that the initiation of a physical exercise programme reduces body mass and body fat content in those who are overweight [22,111]. Public health agencies have recommended that adults take a minimum of 30 minutes of moderate physical activity on most days of the week [57]. In a supervised setting, the intensity of effort may be regulated as a percentage of the individual's anaerobic threshold, maximal oxygen intake, or maximal heart rate; moderate exercise is usually considered as activity between 50% and 70% of maximal oxygen intake [18]. Some investigators have suggested that the best results in terms of fat loss are obtained when exercise is set at the maximal fat oxidation point (LIPOXmax), as measured by indirect calorimetry in a metabolic laboratory [22,52]. Brandou et al. [22], for example, demonstrated that 2 months of training at an individually determined LIPOXmax increased the fat utilization of obese adolescents, enhancing their insulin sensitivity.

Many studies [178,183,202] have shown that exercise training programmes alone generally have a relatively small impact upon body mass and body fat content and that a combination of diet and exercise is more effective in producing long-term favourable changes of body composition (both a decrease of fat mass and an increase of fat-free mass). Benefits are particularly likely if behavioural techniques are used to increase the frequency of exercise and to modify eating patterns [19]. Weltman et al. [201] found that growth hormone (GH) supplementation enhanced the beneficial effects of combined dietary restriction and exercise, and it is worth noting that exercise is a powerful stimulus to GH release.

Dietary programmes intended to decrease body fat loss should include elements of both aerobic and resistance training to ensure that lean tissue is conserved as excess fat is metabolized. The value of training when decreasing body fat applies not only to obese individuals but also to athletes who wish to reduce their body fat stores. During diet programmes, CHO and proteins should be maintained to assure the continued effectiveness of aerobic and force training in athletes. Thus, Bouhlel et al. [19] found that in rugby players who maintained training during Ramadan observance, there was a decrease in body mass, but their lean mass was maintained.

Vegan-Type Dietary Restrictions

Commitment to a vegan-type diet is sometimes adopted by environmentalists on the basis that animal husbandry makes an excessive use of the earth's resources and contributes large quantities of methane to the atmosphere, with resultant global warming. Shorter periods of vegan-type dieting are associated with Greek Orthodox and Daniel fasting.

If carefully managed to ensure a balanced intake of essential amino acids, a vegan-type diet is quite compatible with an outstanding performance in some types of athletic competition [133], one striking example of this being the American track and field star Carl Lewis. One study found no difference in performance over a 1000 km race between those eating a vegan diet and their omnivorous peers [53]. A potential issue is that phytoestrogens may suppress testosterone levels and thus reduce the response to training in strength athletes [198]; a low intake of creatine may also have adverse effects on muscular performance [119]. In one study from Holland, vegetarian children had normal growth patterns and a normal level of aerobic fitness, but had below normal scores on strength and explosive power tests [81]. Others have found greater strength training responses in omnivores than in vegans [31,148].

There has been little study of the performance implications of shorter periods of previously motivated vegan-type dieting, either in sedentary individuals or in athletes. Often, there is some reduction of body mass, but this is not inevitable, and because of limitations in fat intake, there are often changes in blood lipid concentrations that are favourable from the viewpoint of arterial health [138,162,190].

Restrictions of Fluid Intake

The absence of fluid intake during the hours of daylight is a feature of Ramadan observance, but in general even athletes are able to replenish their fluid reserves at night, without developing a cumulative deficit. The biggest deficits of body fluids are incurred by those who undertake prolonged endurance events under hot conditions and those who deliberately restrict fluid intake in order to make a specific weight category in their final competition. In the latter case, the loss includes fat, lean tissue, and water, although water is the major component.

Fluid Needs

The fluid requirements of the body depend largely upon the individual's rate of sweating, as determined by the volume of activity that is being performed and environmental conditions of temperature, humidity, and wind speed. The impact of a given sweat loss upon athletic performance depends also on the extent to which intramuscular glycogen is depleted [173]; the release of bound water from glycogen can in some circumstances contribute as much as 2% to the overall pool of body fluids [170]. Thus, in an endurance event, a person can incur up to a 2 kg decrease of body mass without dehydration of the tissues.

The minimum fluid need has been estimated at about 250 mL/kJ of energy expended. However, most experimental studies of fluid deprivation have been of relatively short duration; possibly, the body may make some adaptations to longer periods of water deprivation. Empirical data show a consistent deterioration of aerobic performance as the body fluid reserves are depleted, and muscle force is also reduced as fluid loss becomes more extensive.

Aerobic Performance

The endurance of sustained, submaximal aerobic effort commonly deteriorates if any type of fluid deprivation or loss causes the body mass to decrease by >2%. Both running speeds and times to exhaustion are decreased [29,32,36,38,46,63, 106,196,199].

A 1.6%–2.1% diuretic-induced dehydration increased the times for performance of 5,000 and 10,000 m runs by 8% and 6%, respectively [5]; an increased cardiovascular strain, an impaired thermoregulation, and metabolic disturbances all contribute to a decrease of performance over such distances. Nadel et al. [132] noted that with 2.2% diuretic-induced dehydration, the cardiac stroke volume during exhausting exercise was decreased by an average of 17 mL/beat (about 15%).

Yoshida et al. [204] tested four differing levels of dehydration, induced by exercise in the heat; in their study, scores on a Harvard fitness test were decreased with 2.5% dehydration.

Caldwell and associates [30] tested a group of boxers, wrestlers, and judoka. After a diuretic-induced 3.1% loss of body mass, they observed a 2.9% decrease of maximal oxygen intake and the work rate during maximal exercise was also decreased; a weight loss achieved in 24 hours or less by use of a sauna or diuretics was more detrimental to performance than a loss that developed over 48 hours. Webster et al. [199] also found a 6.7% decrease of peak oxygen intake with a 4.9% weight loss.

Saltin [158] found no change of maximal aerobic power when 5% dehydration was induced by a period of sauna exposure, but subjects did show a substantial decrease of endurance during submaximal effort. During submaximal effort, heart rates were also higher with dehydration [159]. Two other studies found no adverse effects of 3.3% dehydration upon the outcome of a 2000 m rowing event [139], or scores on a Harvard fitness test [71].

Muscular Performance

There is general agreement that substantial dehydration can have adverse effects upon muscular performance [62,93], although there remains a need to clarify the critical amount of dehydration needed for a significant functional limitation (Table 2.2). One report concluded that hypohydration could decrease strength by 2%, muscular power by 3%, and high intensity endurance by as much as 10% [93]. The consensus of a recent review [108] was that maximal isometric strength and peak torque remained unchanged up to 4% dehydration, but that the torque during slower contractions was impaired with >2% dehydration. However, individual responses differ, depending on the method of dehydration, other possible associated stressors such as prolonged exercise, heat exposure or food restriction, and alleviating factors such as high initial fluid reserves (Table 2.2).

Individual studies confirm the impression that losses of performance are larger for power and endurance than for isometric strength. Serfass and associates [166] found no deterioration of handgrip force or ability to make 180 repeated contractions in wrestlers after dehydration equal to 5% of body mass.

Judelson et al. [94] also found no deterioration of back-mounted squat performance, even with 5% dehydration. However, there were substantial hormonal changes, including increased levels of cortisol and noradrenaline and a reduced testosterone response to exercise. Evetovich et al. [55] found no deterioration in maximal or submaximal isometric or isokinetic performance of the biceps with 2.9% dehydration. Even 4.2% dehydration had little effect on knee strength; in contrast, muscular endurance was reduced by 15%, although a part of this loss could reflect a loss of motivation and central drive [128]. Webster et al. [199] observed a decrease in upper limb but not lower limb torque with 4.9% dehydration. In one of the few studies of female subjects, Greenleaf et al. [71] tested young women following a 3.2% dehydration induced by a combination of exercise and heat; there were no changes in maximal isometric force of knee extension or elbow flexion, nor were there changes in scores for sit-ups, push-ups, and 100 and 400 yard runs.

Furosemide-induced dehydration (a 2.2% decrease of body mass) did not alter the performance of sprinters in 50, 200, and 400 m races, nor did it change their vertical jump heights [197], although in all of these and other jumping events, a smaller body mass was being propelled after dehydration. Others, also, have found no change of jump height with a rapid 1.8%–2% dehydration [73,86], and jump performance has even been improved with a 3%–6% decrease in body mass [193].

A few studies have found changes in isometric performance. Thus, Hickner et al. [84] observed a decreased power output on an isometric arm-cranking test with 4.5% dehydration. Hayes and Morse [80] produced dehydration by jogging in the heat; no deterioration was seen in vertical jump height or isokinetic leg extension at a rotation speed of 120 degrees/s, but isokinetic extension torque at 30 degrees/s was impaired by >2.6% dehydration, and isometric leg extension was impaired with as little as 1% dehydration. Bosco et al. [17] also saw a

TABLE 2.2 Some Reported Effects of Dehydration on Muscular Strength and Power

Author	Extent of Dehydration (% Body Mass)	Variable	Reported Change	Dehydration Method
Bigard et al. [11,12]	2.95	Knee extension strength and endurance	No change of strength, trend to faster fatigue	Sauna
Bijlani and Sharma [13]	2, 3	Forearm extension	Reduced endurance at 3%	Heat
Bosco et al. [17]	2.5	Maximal isometric strength	Strength/mass ratio decreased, 11% decrease in strength	Water deprivation
Caterisano et al. [33]	3	Cybex muscular endurance	Decrease in sedentary and anaerobically trained but not in aerobically trained	Sauna
Evetovich et al. [55]	2.9	Maximal and submaximal isometric, isokinetic biceps strength	No significant change	Water deprivation
Fogelholm et al. [61]	5–6	Sprint and 1 minute anaerobic test	Unchanged performance	Combination of dehydration techniques
Greenleaf et al. [71]	3.3	Maximal isometric strength	No significant change in elbow flexion or knee extension	Exercise/heat (female subjects)
Gutiérrez et al. [73]	1.8 (men) 1.4 (women)	Rowing and handgrip strength, squat and countermovement jumps	No effect in men; decrease of squat jump in women after rehydration	sauna
Hayes and Morse [80]	1.0, 2.6	Isometric, isotonic leg torque, vertical jump	Isometric force reduced at 1%, isokinetic torque reduced at 2.6%, no change of jump	Exercise/heat
Hickner et al. [84]	4	Isometric arm cranking	4.5% decreased power	Combination of dehydration techniques
Hoffman et al. [86]	1.9	Squat and countermovement jumps, 30 seconds anaerobic test	No significant changes	Exercise/water deprivation

(Continued)

TABLE 2.2 (*Continued*) Some Reported Effects of Dehydration on Muscular Strength and Power

Author	Extent of Dehydration (% Body Mass)	Variable	Reported Change	Dehydration Method
Houston et al. [87]	4.5	Isokinetic knee extension	10.5%–11.5% decrease at speeds of 30–300 degrees/s	Combination of dehydration techniques
Judelson et al. [94]	5	Squat performance	No change	Heat/water deprivation
Kraemer et al. [107]	6.0	Isometric and isokinetic strength	11.4% decrease of handgrip force, decrease of isokinetic force in extension and flexion of knee and elbow at various speeds	Combination of dehydration techniques
Montain et al. [128]	4.2	Knee extension	Strength unchanged, time to exhaustion—15%	Exercise/heat
Périard et al. [140]	3.2	Knee extensors	No change of isometric strength or fatiguability	Exercise/heat
Saltin [158,159]	3.8	Isometric strength elbow flexors, knee extensors	No significant change	Exercise/heat
Saltin [158,159]	3.8	Isometric strength elbow flexors, knee extensors	No significant change	Sauna
Schoffstall et al. [164]	1.5	Repetition maximum bench press	5.6% decrease	Sauna
Serfass et al. [166]	5	Isometric and isokinetic tests on biceps	No change in performance	Combination of dehydration techniques
Viitasalo et al. [194]	3.4, 3.8	Vertical jump	Improved performance	Sauna, diuretic
Watson et al. [197]	2	100, 200, 400 m sprints, vertical jump	No changes	Furosemide induced
Webster et al. [199]	4.9	Peak torque, average work per repetition	Decreased performance in upper limb, no change in lower limb	Exercise in sweat suit

decline of maximal isometric strength with dehydration, probably related to electrolytic disturbances within the muscle cytoplasm. Further, the time to muscular exhaustion and the tolerance of repeated muscular efforts was impaired with >2% dehydration [108].

Anaerobic Power and Capacity

Some authors have found no effect of fluid deprivation upon measures of anaerobic power and capacity, as seen in all-out sprints on a cycle ergometer. Others have seen some impact, but nevertheless, the fluid deficit needed to have an adverse effect upon anaerobic function has generally been larger than that needed for a decrease of aerobic power, commonly in the range of 3%–4% dehydration [108].

In one trial, a 2.7% decrease of body mass had no effect on anaerobic power, anaerobic capacity, or the fatigue index as measured by a Wingate all-out cycle ergometer test [37]. Other authors found that scores on a 30 seconds Wingate test were unchanged by thermal dehydration of as much as 5% [86,90]. However, Webster et al. [199] noted a 21% decrease of anaerobic power and a 10% decrease of anaerobic capacity when wrestlers reduced their body mass by 5% over 36 hours; in their study, the anaerobic sprint test continued for 40 rather than the customary 30 seconds. Likewise, Jones et al. [92] found that 3.1% dehydration reduced the peak anaerobic power by 14.5% when using the upper body muscle and by 19.2% when using the lower body. Yoshida et al. [204] tested four differing levels of dehydration, induced by a combination of exercise in the heat and partial fluid deprivation; they concluded that anaerobic power was decreased with 3.9%, but not with 2.5% dehydration.

Times for both 5 and 10 m dashes were also increased with 3% dehydration [116].

Thermoregulation

Quite small decreases in body fluids have adverse effects upon the body's capacity for thermoregulation [42,105], probably because they induce substantial reductions in cardiac stroke volume and skin blood flow. There was no evidence of any attenuation of sweating when subjects cycled for 2 h in the heat without fluid replacement [127].

Cerebral Function

The maintenance of blood flow to the brain depends on maintaining an adequate cardiac output, and cerebral function is thus adversely affected by the substantial decrease of cardiac stroke volume. A deterioration of many aspects of cognitive performance (particularly the motivation to maximal effort) is seen with a cumulative fluid loss that decreases body mass by >2% [131]. Greater dehydration impairs coordination and eventually leads to a loss of consciousness [170]. Degoutte et al. [48] examined the cerebral effects in judoka who reduced their body mass by 5% in the week preceding competition. Compared to competitors who maintained their body mass, food intake was reduced by some 4 MJ/day, there was a 5% decrease in handgrip force, and a standard sports psychology test (the Profile of Mood States questionnaire) suggested a loss of vigor, with increases of fatigue and tension.

Other Adverse Effects

Other adverse effects of exercising while dehydrated include an increase of oxidant stress (Chapter 8) that could potentially increase muscular soreness post exercise, seen with a 3% depletion of water [136] and a deterioration in some aspects of immune function, particularly a slowing of lymphocyte proliferation rates [139] that could increase an athlete's susceptibility to infection.

Time Needed for Rehydration

If an athlete has been 'making weight' in order to qualify for a particular weight category, performance is commonly restored over about 5 hours of rapid rehydration; however, attempts at rehydration may leave a persistent 2% deficit of body mass, and this can lead to a continuing impairment of physical working capacity [83]. A full recovery from rapid dehydration can take as long as 24–36 hours, thus potentially compromising the performance of athletes who attempt a rapid rehydration after completing their 'weigh-in'.

Intermittent (Ramadan) Fasting

Food intake and energy balance during the intermittent fasting of Ramadan differ between sedentary individuals and competitive athletes. The sedentary individuals often use Ramadan observance as an opportunity to reduce their body fat, with an energy intake of less than their anticipated energy expenditure [1,95], whereas most athletes attempt to maintain energy balance by eating large meals and drinking large volumes of fluid during the hours of darkness. Dietary records provide better evidence of changes in food intake than measurements of body mass, since the latter may be influenced largely by the accompanying dehydration [112].

Sedentary Subjects

Several studies of sedentary subjects have shown decreases of food intake during Ramadan observance, accompanied by reductions in body mass [4,12]. However, other reports have seen no change, and in a few reports there has even been an increase of food intake and body mass, perhaps associated with some of the ceremonial meals attended during Ramadan (Table 2.3).

TABLE 2.3 Changes in Energy Intake, Body Mass, and Body Composition during Ramadan Fasting in Sedentary Subjects

Authors	Subjects	Effects of Fasting
Adlouni et al. [1]	32 healthy adult men	2.4% decrease of body mass despite apparent increased intake of total energy, carbohydrate, and protein
Afrasiabi et al. [2]	58 hyperlipidemic men, 22 on hypocaloric diet	Energy intake shows n.s., trend to decrease of 1.2 MJ/day
Angel and Schwarz [4]	Adult men	Decreased energy intake
Al-Hourani and Atoum [3]	57 healthy females	Significant decrease of body mass, non-significant trend to decrease of energy intake
Bakhotmah [6]	173 female university students	Increase of body mass in 60% of subjects, activity decreased in 31%, food intake increased in 15%
Barkia et al. [8]	Healthy adults (19 M, 6 F)	Energy intake decreased 5.6%
Beltaifa et al. [9]	20 healthy adults	10% decrease of energy intake
Bigard et al. [12]	17 Air Force pilots	3 kg (2.7%) decrease of body mass
Born et al. [16]	12 healthy men	1.8 kg decrease of body mass
El Ati et al. [54]	16 healthy women	No change of total dietary intake or body mass. Increase of fat oxidation
Fakhrzadeh et al. [56]	Healthy adults (50 M, 41 F)	Decrease of BMI in men but not in women
Fedail et al. [59]	20 men and 4 women	Reduction of body mass by 1.8 kg, increases in uric acid, cholesterol, and thyroxin levels
Finch et al. [60]	Healthy adults (15 M, 26 F)	No significant change of body mass
Frost and Pirani [64]	15 young adults	Increase of energy intake and body mass
Gharbi et al. [65]	130 healthy adults	Increased energy intake
Grantham et al. [68]	42 young men	n.s. trend to 7% decrease of energy intake
Hallack et al. [76]	16 healthy men	Body mass decreased by 2.4 kg
Hajek et al. [75]	202 healthy adults (mostly men)	Body mass decreased by 1 kg
Hussain et al. [88]	Healthy adults (12 M, 9 F)	Body mass decreased 2.5% in men, 3.2% in women, associated with decreased energy intake
Ibrahim et al. [89]	Healthy adults (9 M, 5 F)	No significant decrease of total or lean mass
Kassab et al. [97]	6 lean and 18 obese women	Small decrease of body mass (0.4 kg) and fat mass (3.6 kg) in obese subjects
Khaled and Belbraouet [99]	276 women receiving oral antidiabetic drugs	3.1 kg decrease of body mass, 1.4 MJ/day decrease of energy intake
Khan and Kharzak [100]	10 healthy men	3.6 MJ/day decrease of energy intake
Lamine et al. [109]	Healthy adults (9 M, 21 F)	No change of body mass despite increased energy intake

(*Continued*)

TABLE 2.3 (*Continued*) Changes in Energy Intake, Body Mass, and Body Composition during Ramadan Fasting in Sedentary Subjects

Authors	Subjects	Effects of Fasting
Maislos et al. [117]	Healthy adults (14 M, 8 F)	No change of body mass
Morilla et al. [129]	Adolescents (24 M, 31 F)	No change of energy intake in males, increase in females
Muazzam and Khaleque [130]	13 adults (men and women)	1.4 kg decrease of body mass
Norouzy et al. [134]	Healthy adults (158 M, 82 F)	Reductions of body mass, greatest in men <35 year; decreases of both fat mass and fat-free mass
Poh et al. [145]	51 boys, 66 girls	Energy intake decreased 19% in boys, 23% in girls
Rahman et al. [150]	20 students	Reduction of dietary intake by 6% and body mass by 2 kg
Rakicioğlu et al. [151]	21 lactating women	Energy intake during Ramadan below recommended level, but no significant change in body mass index
Ramadan et al. [152]	6 active and 7 sedentary subjects	No change of body mass or body fat (0.4 kg)
Salehi and Neghab [157]	28 overweight men	Decrease of body mass (eating diet of 8.3 MJ/day during Ramadan)
Schmahl et al. [163]	27 men	3.6 kg decrease of body mass
Stannard and Thompson [177]	8 healthy subjects	Reduction of dietary intake and body mass (0.8%). Increase of fat oxidation
Sweileh et al. [179]	No indications	Reduction of body mass by 1.9 kg and fat mass by 2.8%, maintained values of fat-free mass, reduction of fluid intake during the first week, but correction at the end of Ramadan
Yucel et al. [206]	Healthy adults (21 M, 17 F)	No change of body mass or body fat
Zebidi et al. [207]	15 healthy men	2.6 kg decrease of body mass
Ziaee et al. [209]	Medical students (41 M, 39 F)	Significant decrease of body mass in both sexes, also decrease of blood glucose

Athletic Individuals

Most studies on athletes have shown relatively little change in body mass or body composition during Ramadan observance (Table 2.4). It seems that with appropriate encouragement from the coach, an athlete can often ingest sufficient food and fluid during the hours of darkness to compensate for the daytime fast [24]. However, there are some exceptions to this generalization, probably related to the volume of physical activity undertaken during Ramadan and the willingness to eat extra food at night. Bouhlel et al. [19–21] showed a decrease of body mass in

TABLE 2.4 Changes of Energy Intake, Body Mass, and Body Composition during Observance of Ramadan by Athletes

Authors	Subjects	Effects of Fasting
Bouhlel et al. [19]	9 rugby players	Reduction of body mass by 1.8 kg, fat mass by 1.3%; initial 1.1 kg of lean mass, but no change at the end of fourth week of fasting. Reduction of fluid intake and plasma volume, increase of fat oxidation
Briswalter et al. [24]	Nine 5000 m runners	No change of energy intake and no effect upon body composition
Chaouachi et al. [34]	15 judoku	No change of energy intake, but 1.3 kg decrease of body mass
Chennaoui et al. [35]	8 middle-distance runners	n.s. trends to 9% decrease of energy intake, 0.55 kg loss of body fat
Chiha et al. [39]	30 junior soccer players	Loss of 4.7 kg of lean mass, 0.4 kg fat
Chiha et al. [40]	12 junior soccer players	13.6% decrease of energy intake
Faye et al. [58]	10 middle-distance runners	Reduction of body mass and substantial decrease of blood glucose
Güvenç [74]	16 young male soccer players	No change of body mass, fat mass, or fat-free mass during Ramadan
Karli et al. [96]	10 elite male power athletes	No significant change of body mass or fat-free mass
Maughan et al. [121]	59 soccer players	No change of dietary intake, but small reduction of body mass (0.7 kg). Increase of haematocrit at the fourth week of fasting
Meckel et al. [124]	19 young soccer players	Small increase in dietary intake in final week of Ramadan, no change of body mass
Memari et al. [126]	12 female athletes	Decrease of body mass and energy intake during Ramadan
Racinais et al. [149]	11 moderately active men	No change of body mass or daily energy expenditure
Ramadan et al. [152]	6 active subjects	No change of body mass or body fat
Trabelsi et al. [188]	8 male bodybuilders	Body mass and body fat unchanged
Trabelsi et al. [187]	9 male body builders	Body mass unchanged (but increased in controls)
Trabelsi et al. [186]	12 male recreational sevens players	15.4% decrease of energy intake (increased proportion of protein and fat)
Trabelsi et al. [189]	10 physically active men	Decrease of body mass and 6.2% decrease in body fat relative to controls
Zerguini et al. [208]	64 soccer players	No change of dietary intake, reduction of body mass (0.7 kg)

rugby players, associated with reductions in body fat, although fat-free mass was unchanged by the end of Ramadan. The individuals studied were all members of the national team and did not relax their training schedule during Ramadan. Kordi et al. [104] also found that body mass and body mass index (BMI) decreased during Ramadan in 34 male volunteer athletes from different sports, training at the end of the day (just before or 3 hours after their evening meal). Memari et al. [126] reported decreases of body mass and BMI in 12 female athletes, although in their case the dietary intake was reduced during Ramadan. Faye et al. [58] also found a reduction of body mass and performance in sprinters (200 and 400 m), associated with severe hypoglycaemia. Meckel et al. [124] noted that in their subjects, Ramadan fasting resulted in a significant reduction in daily intense physical activity, but no change of daily energy intake or body mass.

Total Fasting

Studies of the impact of total fasting have been relatively few, although several papers have reported responses to short-term (12–36 hours) and longer (3–10 days) periods of total food deprivation (Table 2.4).

Some investigators have suggested that fasting might actually improve physical performance during endurance effort, in part because the resting plasma fatty acid concentration is increased [43], thus sparing the remaining glycogen reserves [45,85], and in part because a decrease of body fat reduces body mass and thus the energy cost of displacing both the limbs and the entire body [25]. If there is any such benefit, it seems more apparent in laboratory animals than in human subjects.

Short-Term Fasting (12–36 hours)

Over the first 12–36 hours of fasting, much of the energy needed by a person who is resting is found from a depletion of glycogen reserves, and there is a relatively limited usage of protein and fat stores. The early decrease of body mass is also relatively small, reflecting the metabolism of <1 kg of stored food and the loss of up to 2 kg of body water associated with stored molecules of glycogen [170]. At this stage, a decrease of blood glucose may impair cerebral function and have a negative effect upon motivation. Moreover, the depletion of glycogen reserves is likely to have an adverse effect upon sustained or repeated muscular contractions and the endurance of sustained submaximal aerobic activity.

Empirical observations during short-term fasting have looked mainly at changes in the endurance of submaximal aerobic exercise (Table 2.5). There is perhaps less likelihood of a decrease in motivation due to a decrease in blood glucose levels in animals than in humans.

Dohm et al. [49] observed a dramatic improvement in the treadmill endurance of rats after they had undergone a 24-hour fast. A 18% decrease in body mass in the fasted animals was associated with an increase of the time to exhaustion when running on a treadmill, 284 minutes, as compared with 158 minutes for the

TABLE 2.5 Influence of Short- and Medium-Term Total Fasting upon Physical Performance

Author	Subjects	Fast Duration	Exercise Intensity	Change with Fasting
Short-term fasting (12–36 hours)				
Dohm et al. [49]	Male Holtzman rats	24 hours	Treadmill, 28 m/ minutes 0% grade	80% increase in time to exhaustion with fast
Loy et al. [115]	10 young male competitive cyclists	24 hours	Cycle ergometry at 86% or 79% of maximal oxygen intake	73.5% decrease at 86%, 25.7% decrease at 79%
Dohm et al. [50]	9 healthy active young males	23 hours	Treadmill running at 70% of maximal oxygen intake	7.7% decrease when fasting; increased perception of exertion at 60 minutes
Gleeson et al. [66]	6 healthy young males	24 hours	Cycle ergometry at 100% of maximal oxygen intake	13% decrease when fasting
Maughan and Gleeson [120]	5 healthy males	36 hours	Cycle ergometry at 70% of maximal oxygen intake	35% decrease when fasting
Johnson and Leek [91]	22 healthy young women	12 hours	Reach and balance	Deterioration when fasting
Medium-term fasting (2.5–10 days)				
Uyeno and Graham [192]	Rats	3 days	Swimming time	Increased after fast
Young [205]	Dogs	5 days	Treadmill running	Time to exhaustion increased with fasting
Gutiérez et al. [72]	8 healthy young males	3 days	PWC_{170}, handgrip force, and perception reaction time	Decrease of PWC170 (23%–28%) but no change in other variables
Knapik et al. [103]	8 healthy young men	3.5 days	Cycle ergometry at 45% of maximal aerobic power	No change
Knapik et al. [103]	8 healthy young men	3.5 days	Isokinetic and isometric strength	No change of isometric strength or anaerobic capacity, but small decreases of isokinetic strength (8.6%–11% at 2 speeds of rotation)
Lategola [110]	6 healthy men	7 days	Treadmill maximal oxygen intake	31.6% decrease (less marked loss at 10 days of fasting)
Consolazio et al. [44]	6 healthy men	9 days	Handgrip force	9.3% decrease

control animals. The augmentation of endurance performance was judged too large to attribute simply to the decrease in body mass. Dohm et al. [49] suggested that glycogen sparing from an increased level of circulating fatty acids may also have been a contributing factor. The earlier data of Uyeno and Graham [192] support these findings; they showed an increased swimming time in fasted rats; gains were seen within 6 hours of food deprivation and surprisingly were still present after 3 days without food.

In contrast with these animal experiments, human data have consistently shown a negative effect of fasting upon endurance performance, possible contributing factors including a loss of motivation and a decrease in the plasma alkaline reserve. Loy et al. [115] tested competitive cyclists at 79% or 86% of their maximal oxygen intake. Initial muscle glycogen stores were unchanged by 24 hours of fasting, but plasma free fatty acid levels were increased, thus potentially sparing carbohydrate usage during the test exercise. Nevertheless, the time over which the required pedal cadence could be maintained was drastically shortened with fasting, from 115 to 42 minutes at 86% of maximal aerobic power and from 191 to 142 minutes at 79% of maximal aerobic power.

Dohm et al. [50] tested nine well-conditioned young men after 23 hours of total fasting. They noted that this period of food deprivation was associated with a small decrease (7.7%) in the duration of treadmill running at 70% of maximal oxygen intake, with an increased rating of perceived exertion after 60 minutes of running and increased plasma levels of free fatty acids and beta-hydroxybutyrate. Under fasting conditions, the respiratory gas exchange ratio indicated a substantial increase of fat usage during the first half of the submaximal exercise period.

Gleeson et al. [66] compared times to exhaustion in six young men pedaling a cycle ergometer at 100% of their personal maximal oxygen intake; times were significantly shorter after a 24-hour fast (212 seconds) than when they were eating a normal diet (243 seconds). During fasting, the pre-exercise buffering capacity (bicarbonate and base excess) were also reduced, and blood levels of glycerol, free fatty acids, and beta-hydroxybutyrate were increased. The deterioration of performance was thus thought due mainly to a worsening of the pre-exercise acid/base status during fasting [69,70], although there may also have been some effects from a decrease of motivation.

A 36-hour fast [120] reduced the cycle ergometer endurance time at 70% of maximal oxygen intake from 120 to 78 minutes, despite increased plasma levels of free fatty acids. None of the group became hypoglycaemic, despite the likely depletion of hepatic glycogen stores, and none reached high blood lactate levels. In this study, one controversial factor that was suggested as contributing to the impaired performance during fasting was a fall in the plasma concentration of branch-chained amino acids, leading to alterations in brain tryptophan levels and central fatigue.

There has been only limited examination of the impact of fasting upon the various components of cerebral function. However, Johnson and Leck [91] found that 12 hours of fasting was sufficient to cause a decline in functional reach and the ability to balance on a single limb (whether the eyes were opened or closed).

They linked these changes to other typical manifestations of a low blood glucose (loss of coordination, a staggering gait, fatigue, disorientation, dizziness, and vertigo), although they did not make any specific measurements of blood glucose concentrations.

Medium-Term Fasting (3–10 days)

As in short-term fasting, periods of 3–10 days without food have very different effects in animals and in humans. Loy et al. [115] found that the swimming time to exhaustion was increased in rats after 3 days of food deprivation. This confirmed earlier observations on rats that had been forced to exercise to exhaustion in activity cages during periods of starvation [160]. Likewise, Young [205] found that in dogs, the time to exhaustion during treadmill running was increased even after 5 days without food. One factor contributing to the increased performance of the experimental animals during these several studies of sustained fasting was a substantial decrease of body mass.

In contrast to the response seen in animals, fasting humans typically show a reduced absolute maximal oxygen intake or peak aerobic power (measured in L/minutes), a shortening of the endurance time during sustained submaximal aerobic effort, and in some instances a decreased isokinetic muscle strength. Factors differentiating these responses from those of animals may include a greater loss of motivation in humans and a lesser compensation of the fluid and mineral losses that are associated with the development of a metabolic ketosis [202].

Gutiérez et al. [72] fasted eight young men for 3 days. This led to a decrease of physical working capacity at a heart rate of 170 beats/minutes, irrespective of whether the subjects rested or exercised during their fast. However, handgrip force and perception reaction time were unchanged. The body mass decreased by 3.5 kg over the 3-day study, but muscle mass decreased by only 0.5% and body fat by 0.4%, so much of the 3.5 kg loss must have reflected a loss of fluid from the body.

Knapik et al. [103] studied the effects of a 3.5-day total fast in eight young men. There was no change of cycle ergometer endurance at 45% of maximal oxygen intake. Anaerobic power and the isometric strength of the torso and the hand also remained unchanged, but a small decrease of isokinetic elbow flexion strength was seen at two speeds of rotation (11% at 0.52 rad/seconds and 8.6% at 3.14 rad/seconds).

In a study where 12 subjects engaged in substantial physical work during 5 days of fasting (walking at 5.6 km/hours, 10% grade for 3 hours 15 minutes/day), Henschel et al. [82] noted a 7.7% decrease of absolute maximal oxygen intake (L/minutes). Scores for the Harvard fitness index also showed a substantial decrease by day 4. The authors attributed the decrease in performance to an acidosis, although the 5.5 kg decrease of body mass was also a likely factor.

Lategola [110] observed a 31.6% decrease of absolute maximal oxygen intake (L/minutes) over a 7-day fast, although this loss was slightly attenuated by the 10th day of fasting. In the same study, there was a small decrease of handgrip strength, statistically significant at 9.3% by the ninth day of fasting [44].

As in shorter periods of starvation, effects upon cerebral function have received only limited attention. Taylor et al. [181] noted a deterioration of motor speed and coordination in subjects who were required to exercise for 3 hours 15 min/day during a fast that lasted for 2.5 days.

There are numerous hormonal effects of total fasting that may influence the availability of metabolites, the rate of tissue breakdown, and tolerance of ketosis. In particular, the normal secretory bursts of growth hormone are augmented in both number and amplitude after 2 days of fasting [78], and secretions of insulin and insulin-like growth factor 1 are decreased [7]. These changes encourage the release of amino acids from muscle for gluconeogenesis [46] and decrease the anabolic response to any sort of muscle training.

Severe dietary restriction leads to a progressive loss of fat-free mass, particularly muscle mass. Meckling et al. [125] found that 10 weeks of dietary restriction (an energy deficit of 3.2 MJ/day) reduced fat-free mass by about 1.9 kg. An individual's level of daily energy expenditure depends in great measure upon the fat-free mass, so that in a medium- and long-term perspective if fat-free mass is reduced and energy intake is unchanged, there is likely to be an increase of body mass [183].

Dietary Guidelines

Whether a restricted diet is introduced to correct obesity or to allow an athlete in a sport such as karate, judo, or boxing to compete in a specific weight category, there is a risk that severe dieting will reduce physical performance and predispose to injuries. The aim should be to decrease body mass by no more than 0.5–1.0 kg/week, with an energy deficit no greater than 6–7 MJ/day for men and 5–6 MJ/day for women. An adequate intake of vitamins and micronutrients should be assured, and dieting should not be envisaged during periods of intensive training. During Ramadan observance, it is advantageous for athletes to increase the relative intake of carbohydrates and proteins to about 60%–70% and 20% (1.2–1.8 g of protein per kg of body mass) of total energy intake [2] in order to maintain carbohydrate reserves and minimize losses of lean tissue. It may also be helpful to reduce training volumes during Ramadan, replacing endurance training by technical exercises, agility, stretching, throwing, jumping, and sprinting.

Other Practical Implications

Although it is difficult to separate reduced motivation from the physiological effects of fasting and dehydration, any substantial reduction in the intake of food or fluid generally has negative implications for athletic performance. Where possible, athletes should thus maintain energy and fluid balance and correct any deficit that is incurred as rapidly as is practical. Although the decrease of body mass associated with fasting can increase the tolerance of running or swimming to exhaustion in laboratory animals because of reductions in total body mass, in humans, even brief periods of total fasting (24–36 hours) generally decrease times to exhaustion and impair sustained muscular contractions, often with a deterioration in motor coordination and balance. Longer periods of fasting (2.5– 10 days) reduce the maximal oxygen intake (as measured in absolute units of L/ min), the submaximal working capacity, and the endurance of aerobic activity. Some studies also show decreases in isokinetic and isometric strength. Further, the Minnesota starvation experiments demonstrate that over 24 weeks of grossly inadequate food intake, maximal oxygen intake, the Harvard fitness test score, the duration of treadmill running, and the handgrip force are all reduced, with a decrease in red cell count and radiographic estimates of heart volume. The only positive effect of a limited food intake is a decrease in the oxygen cost of walking, seemingly due to a decrease in body mass.

Athletic performance is also vulnerable to relatively small disturbances of fluid balance. A dehydration of 2% is often sufficient to impair aerobic function, thermoregulation, and cerebral function, although larger fluid losses (4%–5%) are usually needed to reduce anaerobic power, anaerobic capacity, and muscular performance. Athletes seeking to 'make weight' following deliberate dehydration may require at least 24 hours to achieve full rehydration and thus a recovery of performance.

Ketosis is associated with a lack of dietary carbohydrate, but this seems less detrimental to physical performance than was once believed. The traditional Inuit population can sustain high daily energy expenditures very well on a diet that is mainly protein and fat, and Europeans also seem capable of adapting to a very small dietary intake of carbohydrate. As adaptation develops, ketotic products can be metabolized by the brain, thus sparing body glucose reserves.

Although athletic performance is likely to be less than optimal, studies of athletes observing the intermittent fasting required by Ramadan have not to date demonstrated any dangers to health, and changes in physical performance have been small [173,174]. Potential issues include a reduced period for sleeping, disturbances of circadian rhythm, a decrease of plasma glucose and fluid reserves in the afternoon and evening, and a decrease in the levels of plasma amino acids needed for an optimal training response. However, most of these issues can be circumvented within the requirements of Islam, given a very careful regulation of food and fluid intake during the hours of darkness. The one caveat is that most of those studied have been engaged in team sports, and further information is needed on the possible risks of serious dehydration and glycogen depletion in longer events such as marathon and ultramarathon runs.

Conclusions

Athletic performance can be threatened by either short periods of total fasting or longer periods of severe dietary restriction. However, the functional losses are less than might be imagined, and (given the smaller effects that are seen in experimental animals) loss of motivation may well account for some of the observed negative effects in tests that require maximal effort from the subject. Two factors contribute to the limited effects of food deprivation: The decrease of body mass reduces the energy cost of performing tasks where the body mass is displaced, and the body has a surprising ability to adapt to the metabolism of stored fat and tissue protein. Fluid stores are fairly small in relation to the demands of vigorous exercise, and many aspects of physical performance are impaired with dehydration equivalent to 2%–5% of body mass.

Key Terms

Anaerobic capacity: The power that can be developed during a brief sprint, due mainly to an accumulation of lactate, and usually measured by a 30 seconds all-out ride on a cycle ergometer.

Anaerobic power: The power that can be developed during a very short sprint, mainly by the breakdown of phosphagen energy reserves in the muscle, measured by a 5 seconds all-out effort on a cycle ergometer.

Anaerobic threshold: The anaerobic threshold is an intensity of exercise where significant accumulation of lactate occurs, with an increase in ventilation that is disproportionate to the increase in effort.

Basal metabolic rate (BMR): The energy expenditure of the individual lying relaxed at least 12 hours after a meal.

Body mass index (BMI): The BMI is a simple epidemiological measure of obesity. It is calculated as the individual's body mass in kilograms (kg) divided by his or her height in meters squared.

Calorie: The calorie is the quantity of heat sufficient to increase the temperature of a kilogram of water by 1°C. Scientists have now replaced this unit by the joule. 1 calorie = 4.16 J.

Cardiac stroke volume: The volume of blood expelled from the left ventricle during a single heart beat.

Catecholamines: Hormones such as norepinephrine and epinephrine.

Diabetic ketosis: Diabetic ketosis is a condition where fat metabolism is increased because of a lack of insulin, and there is a massive and uncontrolled production of acidic ketone bodies that, if untreated, can lead to coma and death.

Excess post-exercise oxygen consumption (EPOC): The increase of oxygen consumption over initial resting values during recovery from exercise.

Exercise-induced bronchospasm: An increased resistance to airflow through the bronchi, commonly caused by the inhalation of cold dry air through the mouth during exercise.

Hepatic gluconeogenesis: The formation of glucose in the liver, using amino acids, glycerol, and lactate.

Isokinetic strength: A measurement of muscular force against a rotating resistance, so that the muscle is neither shortened nor lengthened by external forces as it contracts.

Isometric strength: A measurement of muscular force against a static resistance, with no substantial muscle shortening during contraction.

Natriuresis: An excessive loss of sodium in the urine.

Oedema: Formerly known as dropsy, oedema is an accumulation of fluid beneath the skin and in body cavities, usually caused by a reduction of protein and thus osmotic pressure in the plasma.

Resting metabolic rate (RMR): The energy expenditure of the individual under resting conditions.

Key Points

1. There is a relationship between energy intake and body mass. However, the association is somewhat complex because of variables influencing energy expenditures, including age, sex, physical activity level, training status, and environmental conditions.
2. Physical activity plays a major role in changing a person's overall energy balance and body composition.
3. Dietary restrictions should be both quantitative and qualitative when seeking to promote changes in body composition and body mass.
4. When seeking to reduce obesity, a combination of physical activity and dietary restriction is more effective than either an increase of physical activity or dietary restriction acting alone.
5. The intermittent fasting of Ramadan observance, when combined with physical exercise, can reduce body fat stores while conserving fat-free mass.

Questions for Discussion

1. How far does the concept of energy balance apply to human subjects?
2. What factors might influence an individual's metabolic rate?
3. What pattern of dietary restriction would you recommend to a person who is overweight?
4. Is dehydration an effective tactic for gaining a competitive advantage in weight-classified sports?
5. What recommendations would you suggest to conserve fat-free mass during dieting?

References

1. Adlouni A, Ghalim N, Benslimane A et al. Fasting during Ramadan induces a marked increase in high-density lipoprotein cholesterol and decrease in low-density lipoprotein cholesterol. *Ann Nutr Metab* 1997;41:242–249.
2. Afrasiabi A, Hassanzadeh S, Sattarivand R et al. Effects of Ramadan fasting on serum lipid profiles on 2 hyperlipidemic groups with or without diet pattern. *Saudi Med J* 2003;24:23–26.

3. Al-Hourani HM, Atoum MF. Body composition, nutrient intake and physical activity patterns in young women during Ramadan. *Singapore Med J* 2007;48(10):906–910.

4. Angel J, Schwarz N. Metabolic changes resulting from decreased meal frequency in adult male Muslims during Ramadan fast. *Nutr Rep Int* 1975;11:29–38.

5. Armstrong LE, Costill DL, Fink W. Influence of diuretic-induced dehydration on competitive running performance. *Med Sci Sports Exerc* 1985;17:456–461.

6. Bakhotmah BA. The puzzle of self-reported weight gain in a month of fasting (Ramadan) among a cohort of Saudi families in Jeddah, Western Saudi Arabia. *Nutr J* 2011;10:84.

7. Bang P, Brismar K, Rosenfeld RG et al. Fasting affects serum insulin-like growth factors (IGFs) and IGF-binding proteins differently in patients with noninsulin-dependent diabetes mellitus versus healthy nonobese and obese subjects. *J Clin Endocrinol Metab* 1994;78(4):960–967.

8. Barkia A, Mohammed K, Smaoui M et al. Change of diet, plasma lipids, lipoproteins and fatty acids during Ramadan: A controversial association of the considered Ramadan model with atherosclerosis risk. *J Health Popul Nutr* 2011;29:486–493.

9. Beltaifa L, Bouguerra R, Ben Slama C et al. La prise de nourriture, et les paramètres anthropométriques et biologiques dans Tunisiens adultes pendant le jeûne de Ramadan (Food intake, and anthropometrical and biological parameters in adult Tunisians during fasting at Ramadan). *East Mediterr Health J* 2002;8:603–611.

10. Beltaifa L, Chaouachi A, Zérifi R et al. Walk-run transition speed training as an efficient exercise adjunct to dietary restriction in the management of obesity: A prospective intervention pilot study. *Obes Facts* 2011;4(1):45–52.

11. Bigard AX, Boussif M, Chalabi H et al. Alterations in muscular performance and orthostatic tolerance during Ramadan. *Aviat Space Environ Med* 1998;69:341–346.

12. Bigard AX, Sanchez H, Claveyrolas G et al. Effects of dehydration and rehydration on EMG changes during fatiguing contractions. *Med Sci Sports Exerc* 2001;33(10):1694–1700.

13. Bijlani RL, Sharma KN. Effect of dehydration and a few regimes of rehydration on human performance. *Ind J Physiol Pharmacol* 1980;24(4):255–266.

14. Bistrian BR. Clinical use of protein-sparing modified fast. *JAMA* 1978;240(21): 2299–2302.

15. Bogardus C, LaGrange BM, Horton ES et al. Comparison of carbohydrate-containing and carbohydrate-restricted hypocaloric diets in the treatment of obesity. Endurance and metabolic fuel homeostasis during strenuous exercise. *J Clin Invest* 1981;68(2):399–404.

16. Born M, Elmadfa I, Schmahl FW. Auswirkungen eines periodischen Flüssigkeits- und Nahrungsentzuges. *Muench Med Wschr* 1979;121:1569–1572.

17. Bosco JS, Terjung RL, Greenleaf JE. Effects of progressive hypohydration on maximal isometric muscular strength. *J Sports Med Phys Fitness* 1968;8(2):81–86.

18. Bouchard C, Shephard RJ, Stephens T. *Physical Activity, Fitness and Health*. Human Kinetics, Champaign, IL, 1994.

19. Bouhlel E, Salhi Z, Bouhlel H et al. Effect of Ramadan fasting on fuel oxidation during exercise in trained male rugby players. *Diabetes Metab* 2006;32(6):617–624.

20. Bouhlel E, Zaouali M, Miled A et al. Ramadan fasting and the GH/IGF-1 axis of trained men during submaximal exercise. *Ann Nutr Metab* 2008;52(4):261–266.

21. Bouhlel E, Denguezli M, Zaouali M et al. Ramadan fastings effect on plasma leptin, adiponectin concentrations, and body composition in trained young men. *Int J Sport Nutr Exerc Metab* 2008;18(6):617–627.

22. Brandou F, Dumortier M, Garandeau P et al. Effects of a two-month rehabilitation program on substrate utilization during exercise in obese adolescents. *Diabetes Metab* 2003;29(1):20–27.

23. Brinkworth GD, Noakes M, Buckley JD et al. Long-term effects of a very-low-carbohydrate weight loss diet compared with an isocaloric low-fat diet after 12 mo. *Am J Clin Nutr* 2009;90(1):23–32.

24. Brisswalter J, Bouhlel E, Falola JM et al. Effects of Ramadan intermittent fasting on middle-distance running performance in well-trained runners. *Clin J Sport Med* 2011;21:422–427.
25. Brown JR. The metabolic cost of physical activity in relation to weight. *Med Serv J Can* 1966;22:262–272.
26. Brožek J, Guetzkow H, Mickelson O et al. Motor performance of young men maintained on restricted intakes of Vitamin-B complex. *Am J Psychol* 1946;30:359–379.
27. Bullough RC, Gillette CA, Harris MA et al. Interaction of acute changes in exercise energy expenditure and energy intake on resting metabolic rate. *Am J Clin Nutr* 1995;61(3):473–481.
28. Buskirk EL. Standard work tests in man: Some illustrative results. In: Spector H, Brožek J, Peterson MS (eds.), *Performance Capacity*. National Academy of Sciences, Washington, DC, 1957, pp. 115–131.
29. Buskirk EL, Iampietro PF, Bass DE. Work performance after dehydration: Effects of physical conditioning and heat acclimatisation. *J Appl Physiol* 1958;12(2):189–194.
30. Caldwell JE, Ahonen E, Nousianen U. Differential effects of sauna-, and diuretic-, and exercise-induced hypohydration. *J Appl Physiol* 1984;57(4):1018–1023.
31. Campbell WW, Barton ML Jr, Cyr-Campbell D et al. Effects of an omnivorous diet compared with a lactoovovegetarian diet on resistance-training-induced changes in body composition and skeletal muscle in older men. *Am J Clin Nutr* 1999;70:1032–1039.
32. Casa DJ, Clarkson PM, Roberts WO. American College of Sports Medicine round-table on hydration and physical activity; consensus statements. *Curr Sports Med Rep* 2005;4(3):115–127.
33. Caterisano A, Camaione DN, Murphy RT et al. The effect of differential training on isokinetic muscular endurance during acute thermally induced hypohydration. *Am J Sports Med* 1988;16(3):269–273.
34. Chaouachi A, Chamari K, Roky R et al. Lipid profiles of judo athletes during Ramadan. *Int J Sports Med* 2008;29:282–288.
35. Chennaoui M, Desgorces F, Drogou C et al. Effects of Ramadan fasting on physical performance and metabolic, hormonal, and inflammatory parameters in middle-distance runners. *Appl Physiol Nutr Metab* 2009;34:587–594.
36. Cheuvront SN, Carter R, Sawka MN. Fluid balance and endurance exercise performance. *Curr Sports Med Rep* 2003;2(4):202–208.
37. Cheuvront SN, Carter R, Haymes EM et al. No effect of moderate hypohydration or hyperthermia on anaerobic exercise performance. *Med Sci Sports Exerc* 2006;38(6):1083–1087.
38. Cheuvront SN, Montain SJ, Sawka MN. Fluid replacement and performance during the marathon. *Sports Med* 2007;37(4–5):353–357.
39. Chiha F. Effets du jeûne de Ramadan sur l'aptitude aérobie et les paramètres anthropométriques et biochimiques chez des footballeurs (15–17 ans) (Effects of Ramadan fasting on aerobic performance and anthropometric and biochemical parameters in footballers). *Sci Hum* 2008;30:25–41.
40. Chiha F. Variations du métabolisme énergétique à l'effort des footballeurs lors du jeûne de Ramadan (Changes in metabolism and the energetics of exercise in footballers during Ramadan fasting). PhD thesis, University of Algiers, Algiers, Algeria, 2008/09.
41. Christensen EH, Hansen O. Zur Methodik der respiratorischen Quotient-Bestimmungen in Ruhe und bei Arbeit (Methodology for the respiratory quotient determinations at rest and at work). *Skand Arch Physiol* 1939;81(1):137–171.
42. Claremont AD, Nagle F, Reddan WD et al. Comparison of metabolic, temperature, heart rate and ventilation responses to exercise at extreme ambient temperatures (0°C and 35°C). *Med Sci Sports Exerc* 1975;7(2):150–154.
43. Conlee RK, Rennie MJ, Winder WW. Skeletal muscle glycogen content: Diurnal variation and effects of fasting. *Am J Physiol* 1976;231(2):614–618.

44. Consolazio CF, Nelson RA, Johnson HL et al. Metabolic aspects of acute starvation in normal humans: Performance and cardiovascular evaluation. *Am J Clin Nutr* 1967;20(7):684–693.
45. Costill DL, Coyle E, Dalsky G et al. Effects of elevated plasma FFA and insulin on muscle glycogen usage during exercise. *J Appl Physiol* 1977;43(4):695–699.
46. Craig FN, Cummings EG. Dehydration and muscular work. *J Appl Physiol* 1966;21(2):679–684.
47. Davis PG, Phinney SD. Differential effects of two very low calorie diets on aerobic and anaerobic performance. *Int J Obesity* 1990;14(9):779–787.
48. Degoutte F, Jouanel P, Bègue RJ et al. Food restriction, performance, biochemical, psychological, and endocrine changes in judo athletes. *Int J Sports Med* 2006;27(1):9–18.
49. Dohm GL, Tapscott EB, Barakat HA et al. Influence of fasting on glycogen depletion in rats during exercise. *J Appl Physiol* 1983;55(3):830–833.
50. Dohm GL, Beeker RT, Israel RG et al. Metabolic response to exercise after fasting. *J Appl Physiol* 1986;61(4):1363–1368.
51. Dulloo AG, Jacquet J. Adaptive reduction in basal metabolic rate in response to food deprivation in humans: A role for feedback signals from fat stores. *Am J Clin Nutr* 1998;68:599–606.
52. Dumortier M, Brandou F, Perez-Martin A et al. Low intensity endurance exercise targeted for lipid oxidation improves body composition and insulin sensitivity in patients with the metabolic syndrome. *Diabetes Metab* 2003;29(5):509–518.
53. Eisinger M, Plath M, Jung K et al. Nutrient intake of endurance runners with ovo-lacto-vegetarian diet and regular western diet. *Z Ernahrungswiss* 1994;33:217–229.
54. El Ati J, Beji C, Danguir J. Increased fat oxidation during Ramadan fasting in healthy women. An adaptative mechanism for body weight maintenance. *Am J Clin Nutr* 1995;62:302–307.
55. Evetovich TK, Boyd JC, Drake SM et al. Effect of moderate dehydration on torque, electromyography, and mechanography. *Muscle Nerve* 2002;26(2):225–231.
56. Fakhrzadeh H, Larijani B, Sanjari M et al. Effect of Ramadan fasting on clinical and biochemical parameters in healthy adults. *Ann Saudi Med* 2003;23:223–226.
57. FAO/WHO/UNU. Human energy requirements. Report of a joint FAO/WHO/UNU consultation, Rome, Italy, October 17–24, 2001. FAO, Geneva, Switzerland, 2004.
58. Faye J, Fall A, Badji L et al. Effects of Ramadan fast on weight, performance and glycemia during training for resistance. *Dakar Med* 2005;50(3):146–151.
59. Fedail SS, Murphy D, Salih SY et al. Changes in certain blood constituents during Ramadan. *Am J Clin Nutr* 1982;36(2):350–353.
60. Finch GM, Day JE, Razak et al. Appetite changes under free living conditions during Ramadan fasting. *Appetite* 1998;31(2):159–170.
61. Fogelholm GM, Koskinen R, Laasko J et al. Gradual and rapid weight loss: Effects on nutrition and performance in male athletes. *Med Sci Sports Exerc* 1993;25(3):371–377.
62. Fogelholm GM. Effects of body weight reduction on sports performance. *Sports Med* 1994;18(4):249–267.
63. Fritzsche RG, Switzer TW, Hodgkinson BJ et al. Water and carbohydrate ingestion during prolonged exercise increase maximal neuromuscular power. *J Appl Physiol* 2000;88(2):730–737.
64. Frost G, Pirani S. Meal frequency and nutritional intake during Ramadan: A pilot study. *Hum Nutr Appl Nutr* 1987;41(1):47–50.
65. Gharbi M, Akrout M, Zouari B. Food intake during and outside Ramadan (article in French). *East Mediterr Health J* 2003;9(1–2):131–140.
66. Gleeson M, Greenhaff PL, Maughan RJ. Influence of a 24 h fast on high intensity cycle exercise performance in man. *Eur J Appl Physiol* 1988;57(6):653–659.
67. Gmada N, Marzouki H, Haboubi M et al. The cross-over point and maximal fat oxidation in sedentary healthy subjects: Methodological issues. *Diabetes Metab* 2012;38(1):40–45.

68. Grantham JR, Belhaj J, Balasekaran J. The effect of four weeks' fasting during Ramadan on body composition in Muslim Arab males. *Med Sci Sports Exerc* 2007;37(Suppl. 5):293.
69. Greenhaff PL, Gleeson M, Maughan RJ. The effects of dietary manipulation on blood acid–base status and the performance of high intensity exercise. *Eur J Appl Physiol* 1987;56(3):331–337.
70. Greenhaff PL, Gleeson M, Maughan RJ. Dietary composition and acid-base status: Limiting factors in the performance of maximal exercise in man? *Eur J Appl Physiol* 1987;56(4):444–450.
71. Greenleaf JE, Prang RM, Averkin JE. Physical performance of women following heat-exercise dehydration. *J Appl Physiol* 1967;22(1):55–60.
72. Gutiérez A, González-Geross M, Delgado M et al. Three days fast in sportsmen decreases physical work capacity but not strength or perception-reaction time. *Int J Sport Nutr Exerc Metab* 2001;11(4):420–429.
73. Gutiérrez A, Mesa JL, Rutz JR et al. Sauna-induced rapid weight loss decreases explosive strength in women but not in men. *Int J Sports Med* 2003;24(7):518–522.
74. Güvenç A. Effects of Ramadan fasting on body composition, aerobic performance and lactate, heart rate and perceptual responses in young soccer players. *J Hum Kinet* 2011;29:79–91.
75. Hajek P, Myers K, Dhanji AR et al. Weight change during and after Ramadan fasting. *J Public Health (Oxf)* 2012;34(3):377–381.
76. Hallack MH, Nomani MZ. Body weight loss and changes in blood lipid levels in normal men on hypocaloric diets during Ramadan fasting. *Am J Clin Nutr* 1988;48:1197–1210.
77. Harris J, Benedict F. Abiometric study of human basal metabolism. *Proc Natl Acad Sci USA* 1918;4(12):370–373.
78. Hartman ML, Veldhuis JD, Johnson ML et al. Augmented growth hormone (GH) secretory burst frequency and amplitude mediate enhanced GH secretion during a two-day fast in normal men. *J Clin Endocrinol Metab* 1992;74(4):757–765.
79. Hawley JA, Schabort EJ, Noakes TD et al. Carbohydrate-loading and exercise performance. *Sports Med* 1997;24(2):73–81.
80. Hayes LD, Morse CI. The effects of progressive dehydration on strength and power: Is there a dose response? *Eur J Appl Physiol* 2010;108(4):701–707.
81. Hebbelinck M, Clarys P, de Malsche A. Growth, development, and physical fitness of Flemish vegetarian children, adolescents, and young adults. *Am J Clin Nutr* 1999;70:579S–585S.
82. Henschel A, Taylor HL, Keys A. Performance capacity in acute starvation with hard work. *J Appl Physiol* 1954;6:624–633.
83. Herbert W, Ribisl PM. Effects of dehydration upon physical working capacity of wrestlers under competitive conditions. *Res Q* 1972;43(4):416–422.
84. Hickner RC, Horswill CA, Welker JM et al. Test development for the study of physical performance in wrestlers following weight loss. *Int J Sports Med* 1991;12(6):557–562.
85. Hickson RC, Rennie MJ, Conlee RK et al. Effects of increased plasma free fatty acids on glycogen utilization and endurance. *J Appl Physiol* 1977;43(5):829–833.
86. Hoffmann JR, Stavsky H, Falk B. The effect of water restriction on anaerobic power and vertical jumping height in basketball players. *Int J Sports Med* 1995;16(4):214–218.
87. Houston ME, Marrin DA, Green HJ et al. The effect of rapid weight loss on physiological function in wrestlers. *Phys Sportsmed* 1981;9:73–78.
88. Hussain SA. Medication during Ramadan. *Lancet* 1989;1(8650):1331.
89. Ibrahim WH, Habib HM, Jarrar AH et al. Effect of Ramadan fasting on markers of oxidative stress and serum biochemical markers of cellular damage in healthy subjects. *Ann Nutr Metab* 2008;53:175–181.
90. Jacobs I. The effects of thermal dehydration on performance of the Wingate anaerobic test. *Int J Sports Med* 1980;1(1):21–24.
91. Johnson S, Leck K. The effects of dietary fasting on physical balance among healthy young women. *Nutr J* 2010;9:18.

92. Jones LC, Cleary MA, Lopez RM et al. Active dehydration impairs upper and lower body anaerobic muscular power. *J Strength Cond Res* 2008;22:455–463.
93. Judelson DA, Maresh CM, Anderson JM et al. Hydration and muscular performance. Does fluid balance affect strength, power and high-intensity endurance? *Sports Med* 2007;37(10):907–921.
94. Judelson DA, Maresh CM, Yamamoto LM et al. Effect of hydration state on resistance exercise-induced endocrine markers of anabolism, catabolism, and metabolism. *J Appl Physiol* 2008;105(3):816–824.
95. Karaağaoğlu N, Yücecan S. Some behavioural changes observed among fasting subjects, their nutritional habits and energy expenditure in Ramadan. *Int J Food Sci Nutr* 2000;51(2):125–134.
96. Karli U, Güvenç A, Aslan A et al. Influence of Ramadan fasting on anaerobic performance and recovery following short time high intensity exercise. *J Sports Sci Med* 2007;6:490–497.
97. Kassab SE, Abdul-Ghaffar T, Nagalla DS et al. Serum leptin and insulin levels during chronic diurnal fasting. *Asia Pac J Clin Nutr* 2003;12:483–487.
98. Keys A, Brožek J, Henschel A et al. *The Biology of Human Starvation*. University of Minnesota Press, Minneapolis, MN, 1950.
99. Khaled BM, Belbraouet S. Effect of Ramadan fasting on anthropometric parameters and food consumption in 276 type 2 diabetic obese women. *Int J Diabetes Dev Ctries* 2009;29:62–68.
100. Khan A, Kharzak AMAK. Islamic fasting: An effective strategy for prevention of obesity. *Pak J Nutr* 2002;1:185–187.
101. Kim J, Wang Z, Heymsfield SB et al. Total-body skeletal muscle mass: Estimation by a new dual-energy X-ray absorptiometry method. *Am J Clin Nutr* 2002;76:378–383.
102. Kimm SY, Glynn NW, Obarzanek E et al. Relation between the changes in physical activity and body-mass index during adolescence: A multicentre longitudinal study. *Lancet* 2005;366(9482):301–307.
103. Knapik JJ, Jones BH, Meredith C et al. Influence of a 3.5 day fast on physical performance. *Eur J Appl Physiol* 1987;56(4):428–432.
104. Kordi R, Abdollahi M, Memari AH et al. Investigating two different training time frames during Ramadan fasting. *Asian J Sports Med* 2011;2(3):205–210.
105. Kovacs MS. A review of fluid and hydration in competitive tennis. *Int J Sports Physiol Perf* 2008;3(4):413–423.
106. Kozlowski S. Physical performance and maximum oxygen uptake in exercise dehydration. *Bull Acad Pol Sci Biol* 1966;14(7):513–519.
107. Kraemer WJ, Fry AC, Rubin MR et al. Physiological and performance responses to tournament wrestling. *Med Sci Sports Exerc* 2001;33(8):1367–1378.
108. Kraft JA, Green JM, Bishop PA et al. The influence of hydration on anaerobic performance: A review. *Res Q Exerc Sport* 2012;83(2):282–292.
109. Lamine F, Bouguerra R, Jabrane J et al. Food intake and high density lipoprotein cholesterol levels changes during Ramadan fasting in healthy young subjects. *Tunis Med* 2006;84:647–650.
110. Lategola AMT. Effects of 5-day complete starvation on cardiopulmonary functions of aerobic work capacity and orthostatic tolerance. *Fed Proc* 1965;24:560.
111. Lazzer S, Boirie Y, Montaurier C et al. A weight reduction program preserves fat-free mass but not metabolic rate in obese adolescents. *Obes Res* 2004;12(2):233–240.
112. Leiper JB, Molla AM, Molla AM. Effects on health of fluid restriction during fasting in Ramadan. *Eur J Clin Nutr* 2003;57(Suppl. 2):S30–S38.
113. Lennernäs M. Dietary assessment and validity: To measure what is meant to measure. *Scand J Nutr* 1998;42:63–65.
114. Lopes J, Russell DM, Whitwell J, Jeejeebhoy KN. Skeletal muscle function in malnutrition. *Am J Clin Nutr* 1982;36(4):802–810.
115. Loy SF, Conlee RK, Winder WW et al. Effects of a 24 h fast on cycling endurance time at two different intensities. *J Appl Physiol* 1986;61(2):654–659.

116. Magal M, Webster J, Sistrunk LE et al. Comparison of glycerol and water hydration regimens on tennis-related performance. *Med Sci Sports Exerc* 2004;35(1):150–156.
117. Maislos M, Abou-Rabiah Y, Zuili I et al. Gorging and plasma HDL-cholesterol—The Ramadan model. *Eur J Clin Nutr* 1998;52(2):127–130.
118. Manninen AH. Metabolic effects of the very low carbohydrate diets: Misunderstood "villains" of human metabolism. *J Int Soc Sports Nutr* 2004;1(2):7–11.
119. Maughan R. Nutritional ergogenic aids and exercise performance. *Nutr Res Rev* 1999;12(2):255–280.
120. Maughan RJ, Gleeson M. Influence of a 36 h fast followed by refeeding with glucose, glycerol or placebo on metabolism and performance during prolonged exercise in man. *Eur J Appl Physiol* 1988;57(5):570–576.
121. Maughan RJ, Bartagi Z, Dvorak J et al. Dietary intake and body composition of football players during the holy month of Ramadan. *J Sports Sci* 2008;26(Suppl. 3):S29–S38.
122. McClellan WS, DuBois EF. Clinical calorimetry. Prolonged meat diets with a study of kidney function and ketosis. *J Biol Chem* 1930;87:651–668.
123. McClellan WS, Rupp VR, Toscani V. Clinical calorimetry. Prolonged meat diets with a study of the metabolism of nitrogen, calcium, and phosphorus. *J Biol Chem* 1930;87:669–680.
124. Meckel Y, Ismaeel A, Eliakim A. The effect of the Ramadan fast on physical performance and dietary habits in adolescent soccer players. *Eur J Appl Physiol* 2008;102(6):651–657.
125. Meckling KA, O'Sullivan C, Saari D. Comparison of a low-fat diet to a low-carbohydrate diet on weight loss, body composition, and risk factors for diabetes and cardiovascular disease in free-living, overweight men and women. *J Clin Endocrinol Metab* 2004;89(6): 2717–2723.
126. Memari AH, Kordi R, Panahi N et al. Effect of Ramadan fasting on body composition and physical performance in female athletes. *Asian J Sports Med* 2011;2(3):161–166.
127. Montain SJ, Coyle EF. Influence of graded dehydration on hyperthermia and cardiovascular drift during exercise. *J Appl Physiol* 1992;73(4):1340–1450.
128. Montain SJ, Smith SA, Mattot RP et al. Hypohydration effects on skeletal muscle performance and metabolism: A 31P-MRS study. *J Appl Physiol* 1998;84:1889–1894.
129. Morilla RG, Rodrigo JR, Caravaca AS et al. Modificaciones dietéticas, en jóvenes musulmanes que practican el ayuno del Ramadán (Dietary modifications in young Muslims who practice Ramadan fasting). *Nutr Hospitalaria* 2009;24:738–743.
130. Muazzam MG, Khaleque KA. Effect of fasting in Ramadhan. *J Trop Med Hyg* 1959;62: 292–294.
131. Murray B. Hydration and physical performance. *J Am Coll Nutr* 2007;26(5 Suppl.): 542S–548S.
132. Nadel ER, Fortney SM, Wenger CB. Effect of hydration status on circulatory and thermal regulations. *J Appl Physiol* 1980;49(4):715–721.
133. Nieman DC. Physical fitness and vegetarian diets: Is there a relation? *Am J Clin Nutr* 1999;70:570S–575S.
134. Norouzy A, Salehi M, Philippou E et al. Effect of fasting in Ramadan on body composition and nutritional intake: A prospective study. *J Hum Nutr Diet* 2013;26(Suppl. 1):97–104.
135. O'Hara WJ, Allen G, Shephard RJ. Loss of body weight and fat during exercise in a cold chamber. *J Appl Physiol* 1977;37:205–218.
136. Paik IY, Jeong MH, Jin HE et al. Fluid replacement following dehydration reduces oxidative stress during recovery. *Biochem Biophys Res Commun* 2009;383(1):103–107.
137. Paoli A, Grimaldi K, D'Agostino D et al. Ketogenic diet does not affect strength performance in elite artistic gymnasts. *J Soc Sports Nutr* 2012;9(1):34.
138. Papadaki A, Vardavas C, Hatzis C et al. Calcium, nutrient and food intake of Greek Orthodox Christian monks during a fasting and nonfasting week. *Public Health Nutr* 2008;11:1022–1029.
139. Penkman MA, Field CJ, Sellar CM et al. Effect of hydration status on high intensity rowing performance and immune function. *Int J Sports Med* 2008;3(4):531–546.

140. Périard JD, Tammam AH, Thompson WM. Skeletal muscle strength and endurance are maintained during moderate dehydration. *Int J Sports Med* 2012;33(6):607–612.
141. Phinney SD, Horton ES, Sims EAH et al. Capacity for moderate exercise in obese subjects after adaptation to a hypocaloric ketogenic diet. *J Clin Invest* 1980;66(5):1152–1161.
142. Phinney SD, Bistrian BR, Wolfe RR et al. The human metabolic response to chronic ketosis without caloric restriction: Physical and biochemical adaptation. *Metabolism* 1983;32(8):757–768.
143. Phinney SD, Bistrian BR, Evans WJ et al. The human metabolic response to chronic ketosis without caloric restriction: Preservation of submaximal exercise capability with reduced carbohydrate oxidation. *Metabolism* 1983;32(8):768–778.
144. Phinney SD. Ketogenic diets and physical performance. *Nutr Metabol* 2004;1:2 (on-line publication).
145. Poh B, Zawiah H, Ismail M et al. Changes in body weight, dietary intake and activity pattern of adolescents during Ramadan. *Malays J Nutr* 1996;2:1–10.
146. Poslusna K, Ruprich J, de Vries JH et al. Misreporting of energy and micronutrient intake estimated by food records and 24 hour recalls, control and adjustment methods in practice. *Br J Nutr* 2009;101(Suppl. 2):S73–S85.
147. Pozefsky T, Tancredi RG, Moxley RT et al. Effect of brief starvation on muscle amino acid metabolism in nonobese man. *J Clin Invest* 1976;57(2):444–449.
148. Raben A, Kiens B, Richter EA et al. Serum sex hormones and endurance performance after a lacto-ovovegetarian and a mixed diet. *Med Sci Sports Exerc* 1994;24:1290–1297.
149. Racinais S, Périard JD, Li CK et al. Activity patterns, body composition and muscle function during Ramadan in a Middle-East Muslim country. *Int J Sports Med* 2012;33:641–646.
150. Rahman M, Rashid M, Basher S et al. Improved serum HDL cholesterol profile among Bangladeshi male students during Ramadan fasting. *East Mediterr Health J* 2004;10(1–2):131–137.
151. Rakicioğlu N, Samur G, Topcu A et al. The effect of Ramadan on maternal nutrition and composition of breast milk. *Pediatr Int* 2006;48:278–283.
152. Ramadan J, Telahoun G, Al-Zaid NS et al. Responses to exercise, fluid, and energy balances during Ramadan in sedentary and active males. *Nutrition* 1999;15(10):735–739.
153. Rasmussen BB, Tipton KD, Miller SL et al. An oral essential amino acid-carbohydrate supplement enhances muscle protein anabolism after resistance exercise. *J Appl Physiol* 2000;88(2):386–392.
154. Rubner M. Kalorimetrische Untersuchungen (Calorimetric Investigations). *Z Biol (Munich)* 1885;3:337–410.
155. Rubner M. Ernährung bei Leibesübungen (Nutrition in physical exercise). In: Kohlrausch W (ed.), *Sportärztzetagung 1925 des Deutschen Ärztebundes zur Förderung der Leibunsübungen*. Gustav Fischer, Jena, Germany, 1925, pp. 36–62.
156. Russell DM, Leiter LA, Whitwell J et al. Skeletal muscle function during hypocaloric diets and fasting: A comparison with standard nutritional assessment parameters. *Am J Clin Nutr* 1983;37(1):137–138.
157. Salehi M, Neghab M. Effects of fasting on a medium calorie balanced diet during the holy month of Ramadan on weight, BMI and some blood parameters of overweight males. *Pak J Biol Sci* 2007;10(6):968–971.
158. Saltin B. Circulatory response to submaximal and maximal exercise after thermal dehydration. *J Appl Physiol* 1964;19(6):1125–1132.
159. Saltin B. Aerobic and anaerobic work capacity after dehydration. *J Appl Physiol* 1964;19(6):1114–1118.
160. Samuels LT, Gilmore RC, Reinecke RM. The effect of previous diet on the ability of animals to do work during subsequent fasting. *J Nutr* 1948;36(5):639–651.
161. Saris WH, van Erp-Baart MA, Brouns F et al. Study on food intake and energy expenditure during extreme sustained exercise: The Tour de France. *Int J Sports Med* 1989;10 (Suppl. 1):S26–S31.

162. Sarri KO, Tzanakis NE, Linardakis MK et al. Effects of Greek Orthodox Christian Church fasting on serum lipids and obesity. *BMC Public Health* 2003;3:16.

163. Schmahl FW, Metzler B, Born M et al. Ramadan, Gesundheitsgefährdung während des Fastenmonats. *Dtsch Ärztebl* 1988;85:B-842–B-844.

164. Schoffstall JE, Branch JD, Leutholz BC et al. Effects of dehydration and rehydration on the one-repetition maximum bench press of weight-trained males. *J Strength Cond Res* 2001;15(1):102–108.

165. Schuenke MD, Mikat RP, McBride JM. Effect of an acute period of resistance exercise on excess post-exercise oxygen consumption: Implications for body mass management. *Eur J Appl Physiol* 2002;86(5):411–417.

166. Serfass RC, Stull GA, Alexander JF et al. The effects of rapid weight loss and attempted rehydration on strength and endurance of the handgripping muscles in college wrestlers. *Res Q Exerc Sport* 1984;55(1):46–52.

167. Shephard RJ. Oxygen cost of breathing during vigorous exercise. *Q J Exp Physiol* 1966;51:336–350.

168. Shephard RJ, Kavanagh T. Biochemical changes with marathon running. Observations on post-coronary patients. In: Howald H, Poortmans JR (eds.), *Metabolic Adaptations to Prolonged Physical Exercise*. Birkhauser Verlag, Basel, Switzerland, 1975, pp. 245–252.

169. Shephard RJ, Kavanagh T, Conway S et al. Nutritional demands of sub-maximum work: Marathon and trans-Canadian events. In: *Proceedings of the Third International Symposium on Sportsmen Nutrition*, Warsaw, Poland, October 22–24, 1975. Polish Sports Federation, Warsaw, Poland.

170. Shephard RJ. *Physiology and Biochemistry of Exercise*. Praeger Publications, New York, 1982.

171. Shephard RJ. *Body Composition in Biological Anthropology*. Cambridge University Press, Cambridge, U.K., 1991.

172. Shephard RJ, Rode A. *The Health Consequences of 'Modernization'*. Cambridge University Press, Cambridge, U.K., 1996.

173. Shephard RJ. The impact of Ramadan performance upon athletic performance. *Nutrients* 2012;4:491–505.

174. Shephard RJ. Ramadan and sport: Minimizing effects upon the observant athlete. *Sports Med* 2013;43:1217–1241.

175. Stackpole EA. *The Long Arctic Search: The Narrative of Lieutenant Frederick Schwatka*. Marine Historical Society, Mystic, CT, 1965.

176. St Jeor ST, Howard BV, Prewitt E et al. Dietary protein and weight reduction: A statement for health care professionals from the Nutrition Committee of the Council on Nutrition, Physical Activity and Metabolism of the American Heart Association. *Circulation* 2001;104:1869–1874.

177. Stannard SR, Thompson MW. The effect of participation in Ramadan on substrate selection during submaximal cycling exercise. *J Sci Med Sport* 2008;11(5):510–517.

178. Stiegler P, Cunliffe A. The role of diet and exercise for the maintenance of fat-free mass and resting metabolic rate during weight loss. *Sports Med* 2006;36(3):239–262.

179. Sweileh N, Schnitzler A, Hunter GR et al. Body composition and energy metabolism in resting and exercising Muslims during Ramadan fast. *J Sports Med Phys Fitness* 1992;32(2):156–163.

180. Swick RW, Benevenga NJ. Labile protein reserves and protein turnover. *J Dairy Sci* 1977;60(4):505–515.

181. Taylor HL, Brozek J, Henschel A et al. The effect of successive fasts on the ability of men to withstand fasting during hard work. *Am J Physiol* 1945;143:148–155.

182. Taylor HJ, Buskirk ER, Brismar K et al. Performance capacity and effects of caloric restriction with hard physical work on young men. *J Appl Physiol* 1957;10(3):421–429.

183. Thompson JL, Manore MM, Thomas JR. Effects of diet and diet-plus-exercise programs on resting metabolic rate: A meta-analysis. *Int J Sport Nutr* 1996;6:41–46.

184. Tipton KD, Elliot TA, Cree MG et al. Timing of amino-acid carbohydrate ingestion alters anabolic response of muscle to resistance exercise. *Am J Physiol* 2001;281(2): E197–E206.

185. Thomas CD, Peters JC, Reed GW et al. Nutrient balance and energy expenditure during ad libitum feeding of high-fat and high-carbohydrate diets in humans. *Am J Clin Nutr* 1992;55(5):934–942.

186. Trabelsi K, el Abed K, Stannard R et al. Effects of fed- versus fasted-state aerobic training during Ramadan on body composition and some metabolic parameters in physically active men. *Int J Sports Nutr Exerc Metab* 2012;22(1):11–18.

187. Trabelsi K, Stannard SR, Maughan RJ et al. Effect of resistance training during Ramadan on body composition and markers of renal function, metabolism, inflammation, and immunity in recreational bodybuilders. *Int J Sports Nutr Exerc Metab* 2012;22(4):267–275.

188. Trabelsi K, Rebai H, el Abed K et al. Effect of Ramadan fasting on renal function markers and serum electrolytes after a rugby sevens match. *IOSR. J Pharm* 2013;2:42–50.

189. Trabelsi K, Stannard SR, Ghlissi Z et al. Effect of fed- versus fasted state resistance training during Ramadan on body composition and selected metabolic parameters in bodybuilders. *J Int Soc Sports Nutr* 2013;10(1):23.

190. Trepanowski JF, Bloomer RJ. The impact of religious fasting on human health. *Nutr J* 2010;9:57.

191. Trost SG. Objective measurement of physical activity in youth: Current issues, future directions. *Exerc Sport Sci Rev* 2001;29(1):32–36.

192. Uyeno ET, Graham RA. The effect of food deprivation of rats on swimming to exhaustion. *Behaviour* 1965;26(3):351–356.

193. Vasquez JA, Adibi SA. Protein sparing during treatment of obesity: Ketogenic versus nonketogenic very low calorie diet. *Metabolism* 1992;41:406–414.

194. Viitasalo JT, Kyrolainen H, Bosco C et al. Effects of rapid weight reduction on force production and vertical jumping height. *Int J Sports Med* 1987;8(4):281–285.

195. Walberg JL, Ruiz VK, Tarlton SL et al. Exercise capacity and nitrogen loss during a high or low carbohydrate diet. *Med Sci Sports Exerc* 1988;20(1):34–43.

196. Walsh RM, Noakes TD, Hawley JA et al. Impaired high-intensity cycling performance time at low levels of dehydration. *Int J Sports Med* 1994;19(7):392–398.

197. Watson G, Judelson DA, Armstrong LE et al. Influence of diuretic-induced dehydration on competitive sprint and power performance. *Med Sci Sports Exerc* 2005;37(7): 1168–1174.

198. Weber KS, Setchell KD, Stocco DM et al. Dietary soy-phytoestrogens decrease testosterone levels and prostate weight without altering LH, prostate 5 alpha-reductase or testicular steroidogenic acute regulatory peptide levels in adult male Sprague-Dawley rats. *J Endocrinol* 2001;170:591–599.

199. Webster S, Rutt R, Weltman A. Physiological effects of a weight-loss regimen practiced by college wrestlers. *Med Sci Sports Exerc* 1990;22(2):229–234.

200. White AM, Johnston CS, Swan PD et al. Blood ketones are directly related to fatigue and perceived effort during exercise in overweight adults adhering to low-carbohydrate diets for weight loss: A pilot study. *J Am Diet Assoc* 2007;107(10):1792–1796.

201. Weltman A, Weltman JY, Veldhuis JD et al. Body composition, physical exercise, growth hormone and obesity. *Eat Weight Disord* 2001;6(3 Suppl.):28–37.

202. Wilmore JH. Increasing physical activity: Alterations in body mass and composition. *Am J Clin Nutr* 1996;63(3 Suppl.):456S–460S.

203. Yancy WS Jr, Olsen MK, Guyton JR et al. A low-carbohydrate, ketogenic diet versus a low-fat diet to treat obesity and hyperlipidemia: A randomized, controlled trial. *Ann Intern Med* 2004;140(10):769–777.

204. Yoshida T, Takanishi T, Nakai S et al. The critical level of water deficit causing a decrease in exercise performance: A practical field study. *Eur J Appl Physiol* 2002;87(6):529–534.

205. Young DR. Effect of food deprivation on treadmill running in dogs. *J Appl Physiol* 1959;14(6):1018–1022.

206. Yucel A, Degirmenci B, Acar M et al. The effect of fasting month of Ramadan on the abdominal fat distribution: Assessment by computed tomography. *Tohoku J Exp Med* 2004;204:179–187.
207. Zebidi A, Rached S, Dhidah M et al. The effect of Ramadan fasting on some plasmatic and urinary parameters. *Tunisie Med* 1990;68:367–372.
208. Zerguini Y, Dvorak J, Maughan RJ et al. Influence of Ramadan fasting on physiological and performance variables in football players: Summary of the F-MARC 2006 Ramadan fasting study. *J Sports Sci* 2008;26(Suppl. 3):S3–S6.
209. Ziaee V, Razaei M, Ahmadinejad Z et al. The changes of metabolic profile and weight during Ramadan fasting. *Singapore Med J* 2006;47:409–414.

Further Reading

Maughan RJ. *Nutrition in Sport*, 2nd edn. Blackwell Publishing, Oxford, U.K., 2004.
Shephard RJ. *Physiology and Biochemistry of Exercise*. Praeger Publications, New York, 1982.

Carbohydrate Metabolism and Fasting

Ezdine Bouhlel and Roy J Shephard

Learning Objectives

1. To review the nature of carbohydrates and the normal daily carbohydrate needs of the body
2. To understand the hormonal mechanisms regulating anabolic and catabolic activities
3. To examine the effects of exercise intensity and duration upon the need for carbohydrates
4. To explore the effects of carbohydrate supplements
5. To learn the impact of various types of fasting and/or dietary restriction upon carbohydrate intake
6. To discover the specific effects of Ramadan observance upon carbohydrate intake and blood glucose levels
7. To determine practical implications for athletes, coaches, and trainers

Nature of Carbohydrates and Normal Daily Requirements

Classification of Carbohydrates

Carbohydrates are classified according to the number and length of their carbon chains. The fundamental unit of carbohydrate is a single molecule, built from five atoms of carbon (*pentoses*) or six atoms of carbon (*hexoses*). We distinguish three types of carbohydrate: monosaccharides, disaccharides, and polysaccharides.

Monosaccharides

Monosaccharides comprise a single pentose or hexose molecule. *Hexoses* play an important metabolic role. Their biochemical formula is $C_6H_{12}O_6$. Monosaccharides such as glucose, fructose, and galactose are absorbed rapidly from the gastrointestinal tract and are also used quickly by the body. Glucose is transported across membranes by a facilitated transport mechanism involving five transporter substances, coded from 1 to 5, and called *GLUT 1–5*. It is because of the action of these transporters that monosaccharides are absorbed rapidly and appear in the circulating blood soon after their ingestion.

Disaccharides

Disaccharides are built from two monosaccharide molecules, for example, sucrose (glucose and fructose) and maltose (glucose and glucose). Disaccharides must be hydrolysed to their constituent monosaccharides by salivary and/or pancreatic enzymes in order for them to be absorbed into the body. The absorption of disaccharides thus occurs substantially less rapidly than that of monosaccharides.

Polysaccharides

Polysaccharides are built from many monosaccharide molecules, but they can be broken down to their constituents by a process of hydrolysis. Glycogen is the form of polysaccharide that is stored in the muscle and the liver. The body typically contains about 300–500 g of muscular glycogen and 50–150 g of hepatic glycogen [52]. However, glycogen stores vary, depending on the dietary regimen and physical activity patterns. One gram of carbohydrate is equivalent to about 17 kJ of energy. According to standard dietetic recommendations, carbohydrate intake should account for 50%–55% of the total dietary intake in a normal moderately active individual. The body stores 3 g of water with each gram of glycogen, and this water is liberated as glycogen is broken into its constituent glucose molecules; it is important to allow for this increase in the *free* water component of the body when calculating fluid balances.

Carbohydrate Stores and Physical Performance

Many studies have shown the importance of carbohydrates to physical performance [26,29]. Carbohydrates are the main carburant for brief and intense periods of exercise [39,40], for sustained aerobic activity [10,29,55,56], for the performance of repeated heats during sprinting contests, and for sustained isometric activity (for example, in dinghy sailing [49]). During prolonged bouts of exercise, energy is initially derived mainly from carbohydrate, but the contribution of fats becomes progressively more important as the glycogen stores are depleted; in an endurance event such as a marathon run, glycogen depletion is relatively complete after 90 minutes of activity, accounting for the 'wall' that many marathon runners report encountering at this stage in their event. If dietary means are taken to boost the initial store of glycogen, this helps to avert premature fatigue and the resulting deterioration in physical performance. Carbohydrate supplementation is thus important to athletes, both before and after exercise. If a prolonged competitive event is contemplated, it may be advantageous to increase carbohydrate intake to 65%–70% of the total dietary energy per day in order to maximize glycogen reserves and thus prolong aerobic performance.

A low blood sugar also deprives the brain of its principal fuel and thus impairs various aspects of cognitive performance [46], with a loss of athletic skills, and a negative impact upon competitive performance [5,26,32,61].

In emergency situations in a cold environment, much energy is spent in shivering. Glycogen reserves can be depleted by shivering within a few hours, although survival can be prolonged by shifting shivering from slow-twitch muscle fibres that consume mainly glycogen to the fast-twitch fibres that have a greater ability to metabolize fat [42].

Hormonal Mechanisms Regulating Anabolic and Catabolic Activities

Anabolism is important for tissue repair, growth, and the training response. However, during fasting, the balance swings in favour of catabolism, as the breakdown of stored metabolites becomes necessary to provide the energy needed for physical activity and the maintenance of body function. Both anabolic and catabolic processes are regulated primarily by the hormones insulin and glucagon, but catecholamines, cortisol, growth hormone (GH), and thyroid hormone are also involved to a lesser degree. Together, the interaction of these hormones plays a major role in regulating blood glucose levels.

Insulin contributes to the penetration of both glucose and amino acids into the cells. It also facilitates biochemical reactions involving glucose and amino acids, particularly the oxidation of fats and the synthesis of glycogen. Insulin secretion is stimulated by an increase of blood glucose; this hormone is secreted after the absorption of food and is involved in storing energy. An absence or deficit of insulin secretion leads to excessive increases in blood glucose (hyperglycaemia); hyperglycaemia is one of the main manifestations of diabetic mellitus, which is caused essentially by a deficient pancreatic secretion of insulin.

Antagonist hormones stimulate a release of glucose as blood glucose falls, as in both fasting and prolonged periods of exercise. Glucagon, epinephrine, GH, and cortisol all contribute to the increase in blood glucose levels [60]. Glucagon and epinephrine stimulate the breakdown of glycogen stores (glycogenolysis) in both muscle and the liver. GH stimulates the synthesis of glucose from amino acids, glycerol, and lactate in the liver (hepatic gluconeogenesis). Epinephrine and GH also stimulate triglyceride oxidation. Furthermore, GH inhibits the cellular metabolism of glucose. A cortisol-induced increase of blood amino acid concentrations stimulates the action of glucagon and GH.

Effects of Exercise Intensity and Duration on Carbohydrate Oxidation

The relative contribution of carbohydrate to metabolism depends on the intensity and duration of exercise. The 'crossover' concept describes this impact of intensity upon the relative usage of carbohydrate and fat (Chapter 4). An augmentation of carbohydrate metabolism depends on an increased secretion of catecholamine and glucagon and a reduced output of insulin. During moderate exercise, fatty acids are the preferred substrates, but as the intensity of effort is increased, fat metabolism plateaus and then declines, and during intensive exercise, energy is derived largely from carbohydrate [8].

Muscle glycogenolysis develops as the intensity of exercise is increased. Muscle glycogen stores are typically depleted after about 90 minutes of exercise at 75% of maximal oxygen intake ($\dot{V}O_{2max}$), although endurance athletes (by developing their ability to metabolize fat) can often exercise for 90 minutes at 85%–90% of $\dot{V}O_{2max}$ before glycogen stores are depleted [11,12]. Muscle glycogen depletion leads to an inability to perform anaerobic activity and thus a reduction of most types of physical performance; the initial size of muscle glycogen stores is a major determinant of an individual's ability to sustain exercise at a high percentage of $\dot{V}O_{2max}$, when some of the active muscles are becoming underperfused relative to their oxygen needs [8,26].

Hepatic glucose release increases progressively during intensive exercise. There are two contributing mechanisms, glycogenolysis and gluconeogenesis; their relative importance depends upon the intensity and duration of exercise [60]. At the onset of exercise, glycogenolysis (the breakdown of hepatic glycogen stores) predominates, but gluconeogenesis (the hepatic synthesis of glycogen) becomes more important during prolonged exercise, as initial liver stores of glycogen become depleted. Lactate, alanine, and glycerol are the main precursors used in gluconeogenesis.

Since cerebral metabolism is normally almost entirely glucose dependent, central nervous system activity is impaired by reductions in blood glucose, whether due to prolonged exercise or dietary restrictions. A reduction of blood glucose contributes to perceptions of fatigue, and glycogen depletion thus becomes an important psychological factor limiting prolonged aerobic performance and impairing judgment and cooperation between players in team sports.

Impact of Carbohydrate Supplements upon Physical Performance

Many studies have shown that athletic performance can be enhanced by ingesting moderate quantities of carbohydrate during an event [53,54], this being particularly true for prolonged activities such as a marathon run or a 90-minute team game; however, the benefits of administering carbohydrates before an event are less clearly established.

Prior to Exercise

Various studies have shown no change, an increase or even a reduction in muscular performance when carbohydrate supplements were administered prior to exercise. These discrepancies are probably explained by differences in the time of ingestion before exercise, the quantity and the nature of the CHO ingested, the duration of the event, and the extent to which an athlete had engaged in preparation by long-term boosting of muscle glycogen reserves. Koivisto et al. [33] found that glucose ingestion 45 minutes before exercise led to hyperglycaemia, stimulation of insulin secretion, and in consequence hypoglycaemia during the activity. Horowitz et al. [28] also noted that carbohydrate ingestion 60 minutes before exercise stimulated insulin secretion, thus limiting fat oxidation during the effort and contributing to a reduction of aerobic capacity. Koivisto et al. [33] recommended the ingestion of fructose rather than glucose before exercise; because fructose had a low *glycaemic index*, the smaller increase of blood sugar induced only a modest rise of insulin, and in consequence hypoglycaemia did not develop during exercise. Fructose may be an interesting dietary option for athletes performing prolonged exercise, although in some competitors, it seems to cause more gastric distress than glucose [15].

In contrast to these negative reports, some studies have suggested that in terms of maintaining blood glucose availability and carbohydrate oxidation throughout an event, taking carbohydrate 30 minutes before exercise is as effective as ingesting it throughout a prolonged bout of exercise [10,63].

Considering the composition of the most recent meal, Rowlands and Hopkins [56,57] showed a reduction of fat oxidation rate in competitive cyclists who had eaten a high-carbohydrate meal. Fat oxidation following a high-protein meal was similar to that following a high-fat meal. However, they concluded that meal composition had no clear effect on either sprint or 50 km performance. Hargreaves [25] also argued that interventions increasing the availability of fat before exercise reduced carbohydrate utilization during exercise, but did not appear to have any ergogenic benefit.

In the context of the intermittent fasting of Ramadan, there may be an advantage in ingesting a substantial amount of carbohydrate at the evening meal in order to maximize glycogen stores, but a fat-containing meal that empties slowly from the stomach is probably a better breakfast-time choice.

During Exercise

Most studies have shown some ergogenic benefits from the ingestion of small amounts of carbohydrate during prolonged exercise [13,14,22]; in general, effects are greater with repeated administration of small quantities than when a larger amount is given as a single dose. The ingestion of a 6%–7% solution of carbohydrate increased times to exhaustion during a simulated soccer match [14,22]. Providing 30–60 g of carbohydrate in water throughout a physical test reduced fatigue and increased performance during a 30 km run [62]. Reliance upon carbohydrate is important during prolonged events and competitive team sports that require intermittent bursts of high intensity activity [14,22]. Rollo and Williams [54] also found that ingesting 2 mL/kg of a 6.4% carbohydrate–electrolyte drink every 15 minutes improved performance relative to a placebo fluid during a one-hour maximal treadmill run.

However, the benefits of pre-event carbohydrate ingestion are reduced by the boosting of initial glycogen stores. The consumption of a high dietary CHO intake (400–600 g/day) for several days can increase muscle hepatic glycogen stores by as much as 200%, with associated increases in aerobic endurance [29]. Hargreaves [25] noted the importance of boosting pre-exercise carbohydrate stores in order to minimize the risk of glycogen depletion during exercise. Hawley et al. [26] also pointed out that initial glycogen boosting could in itself improve endurance performance by 2%–3%. Rauch et al. [55] found that carbohydrate loading improved mean power output during a one-hour time trial and permitted the athletes to use more their muscle glycogen stores than during a trial when they had been following their normal diet; all seven of their subjects finished the event with a similar final glycogen reserve, and they thus speculated that there may have been a feedback signal from the leg muscles regulating running pace as glycogen became depleted. Noakes et al. [50] found that in endurance runners who had previously followed a 6-day programme of glycogen loading, glucose, glucose polymer, or fructose supplements during a race had no effect on the rate of glycogen depletion and performance over distances of up to 56 km.

High dietary carbohydrate intake enhances muscle and hepatic glycogen stores. This contributes to an increase in aerobic performance, particularly in prolonged exercise or if repeated sprints are performed. A low carbohydrate intake could compromise the capacity of athletes even for high-intensity exercise. Foods with a low glycaemic index should be eaten shortly before exercise in order to avoid an immediate hyperglycaemia, hyperinsulinaemia, and a subsequent hypoglycaemia. The ingestion of carbohydrates immediately before prolonged exercise only improves a competitor's aerobic performance if the carbohydrate ingestion is maintained throughout exercise. The ingestion of CHO (about 2 g/kg of body mass) during prolonged exercise generally improves a competitor's aerobic performance.

Effect of Fasting and/or Dietary Restrictions on Carbohydrate Metabolism

Given initial glycogen reserves of some 500 g in muscle and liver, this equates to a reserve of about 8 MJ of energy, and a resting subject is unlikely to develop hypoglycaemia with a fast that lasts for less than 24 hours; liver glycogen is broken down at a rate of about 4 g/h, and muscle glycogen may be used at about four times this rate. Nevertheless, shorter periods of fasting, as in Ramadan observance, have the consequence that an athlete will start an event with a reduced store of glycogen, particularly if competition is scheduled in the afternoon or early evening.

Mikulski et al. [47] noted that the metabolic and hormonal changes seen after carbohydrate restriction and depletion of glycogen stores are essentially similar to those seen during total fasting. Some authors have reported decreases in plasma glucose with a total fast of 23–24 hours [17,51], but other investigators have found unchanged blood glucose concentrations with 24 or 27 hours of fasting, either at rest or after exercise [21,48]. These differences are probably related to the subjects' diet, physical fitness, training load, and the resulting extent of initial glycogen stores. Despite the small decrease of resting blood glucose following 23 hours of fasting, Dohm et al. [16] found that a normal blood glucose concentration was maintained during exercise. Homeostasis was apparently achieved by increased gluconeogenesis and a decreased utilization of glucose in the muscle as a result of lowered pyruvate dehydrogenase activity.

As might be expected with a longer (36 hours) fast, Zinker et al. [65] found a significant decrease of blood glucose concentration and an altered pattern of substrate utilization in trained subjects both at rest and throughout exercise to exhaustion at 50% of $\dot{V}O_{2max}$. Despite CHO sparing, endurance performance was decreased. Maughan and Gleeson [43] also fasted their subjects for 36 hours. None of their group became clinically hypoglycaemic (blood glucose <4 mol/L), but nevertheless relative to control subjects, endurance of a cycle ergometer test was reduced, and during the exercise bout, there was an increased metabolism of fat and a decreased metabolism of carbohydrate.

The depletion of glycogen stores by repeated sprinting in normally fed subject is exacerbated by fasting or food restriction [9,36]. In lean rats, 48 hours of fasting reduced hepatic glycogen stores 45-fold [34], although the change was much smaller in obese rats. Lima-Silva et al. [39,40] had human volunteers follow a 25% carbohydrate diet for 48 hours. This restriction was sufficient to induce a 19% reduction in the endurance time when cycling at a loading equivalent to 115% of maximal oxygen intake; aerobic energy release was also reduced by 39%. Casey et al. [9] had subjects follow a low-carbohydrate diet (7.8% of total energy intake) or a diet rich in carbohydrate (81.5 [0.4]%) for 3 days. The resultant decline of muscle glycogen in the first group reduced their performance during the first three of four maximal cycle ergometer sprints. Langfort et al. [37] also observed that following a low-carbohydrate diet (5% CHO, 50% fat, 45% protein) for 3 days decreased the average power output achieved during a 30 seconds Wingate test. However, the lactate threshold and the maximal oxygen intake remained unchanged. Langfort et al. [37] suggested that aerobic power was conserved by a combination of increased sympathoadrenal activity, cortisol secretion, and a decrease of plasma insulin.

In addition, the low carbohydrate diet enhanced the activity of the sympathoadrenal system at rest and after exercise. Greenhaff et al. [23] provided their subjects with a very low carbohydrate intake (3%) for 4 days; the maximum rate of muscle glycogenolysis was reduced by low levels of muscle glycogen, and a further factor reducing the capacity for high-intensity exercise was metabolic acidosis. Maughan et al. [44] conducted a somewhat similar experiment where muscle glycogen was initially reduced by 60–90 minutes of exhausting cycle ergometer exercise, and a diet providing only 5% carbohydrate was then given for 3–4 days; a 10%–30% reduction of exercise capacity during a 5 minute all-out cycle ergometer test was associated with an increased accumulation of strong organic acids, particularly fatty acids and 3-hydroxybutyrate [44]. Jansson et al. [31] further found a greater oxygen uptake and heart rate and a lower respiratory quotient during submaximal exercise (25 minutes at 65% of $\dot{V}O_{2max}$) after 5 days of following a low-carbohydrate diet (5% CHO, 72% fat, and 23% protein). During exercise, plasma concentrations of free fatty acid, glycerol, and beta-hydroxybutyrate were higher than in control data, whereas concentrations of insulin and lactate were lower. Again, the low-carbohydrate diet increased the relative contribution of fat to metabolism and increased the sympathoadrenal response to exercise [31,36].

Mikulski et al. [47] found a decreased respiratory quotient even after a fast of 12–16 hours, indicating an increase of fat oxidation during 90 minutes of exercise at 70% of maximal heart rate. As expected, blood glucose was unchanged during this short fast.

Fasting or dietary restriction affecting glycogen reserves modifies the activity of a number of hormones regulating glucose homeostasis. Pérusse et al. [52] found no effect of brief exercise (a maximal oxygen intake test) upon plasma leptin concentrations. However, in the study of Hilton and Loucks [27], leptin levels were decreased by diet-induced glycogen depletion. They compared responses in subjects ingesting 18.7 kJ/kg of food energy versus those receiving only 4.2 kJ/kg of lean tissue mass for 4 days; the restricted diet reduced both the mean leptin concentration (−72%) and the amplitude of the diurnal fluctuation (−85%). Mikulski et al. [47] also observed decreased leptin levels when subjects depleted their glycogen reserves by 90 minutes of exercise at 70% of maximal heart rate and then undertook a 12–15-hour fast. GH levels also increased with glycogen depletion, especially during the period of fasting [47].

Some glucostatic mechanisms seem to be more efficient in endurance-trained athletes than in sedentary individuals. Thus, the reduction of insulin secretion during fasting was greater in trained athletes than in sedentary subjects [47]. Tissue sensitivity to insulin was also greater in endurance-trained athletes, and a decreased activity of the sympathetic nervous system reduced norepinephrine concentrations after glycogen depletion [47]. Pérusse et al. [52] further noted a decrease of plasma leptin levels after 20 weeks of training in male, but not in female subjects; in their studies, these changes were associated with decreases in fat mass.

Impact of Ramadan Observance on Carbohydrate Intake and Blood Glucose

During Ramadan observance, there are two dietary phases after the last meal of the night (Shur, taken shortly before sunrise):

1. *Phase one*: The digestion and absorption of food. The duration of this phase depends upon the size and composition of the meal; it would normally range from 3 to 4 hours.
2. *Phase two*: The remainder of the fast of 12–15 hours until the evening meal. During this phase, blood glucose levels are normally maintained through muscle and/or liver glycogenolysis.

Glucose homeostasis might be thought to present a challenge to athletes observing Ramadan, particularly if they are involved in endurance events. A commonly adopted tactic is to eat a high-carbohydrate diet at night in order to maximize their glycogen reserves [7,45,59]. However, it is not advisable to consume a high-carbohydrate meal pre-dawn. This would stimulate insulin secretion, inhibiting the mobilization and thus the oxidation of fatty acids during any exercise that is taken during the period of fasting.

There is no inherent reason why 12–15 hours of fasting should cause a decrease in blood glucose in a sedentary person. However, 7 of 11 empirical studies of sedentary subjects have shown a decrease of blood glucose during Ramadan (Table 3.1). In particular, Larijani et al. [38] found that blood glucose decreased

TABLE 3.1 Effects of Ramadan Observance on Fasting on Blood Glucose

Authors	Subjects	Effect on Blood Glucose
Sedentary Subjects		
Adlouni et al. [1]	32 healthy men	Reduction of blood glucose (5.1–4.4 mmol/L), decrease of cholesterol and triglycerides
Aybak et al. [2]	20 healthy men	Progressive decrease of glucose from 5.2 to 3.8 mmol/L
Ba et al. [4]	15 sedentary subjects	No significant change
Bigard et al. [6]	11 pilots	Maintenance of blood glucose at the beginning of Ramadan, reduction to 4.0 mmol/L at the end of Ramadan
El Ati et al. [18]	16 healthy women	Maintenance of blood glucose
Fakhrzadeh et al. [19]	50 men, 41 women	Significant decrease, but no symptoms of hypoglycaemia
Ibrahim et al. [30]	14 healthy men	Reduction of blood glucose at the end of Ramadan
Krifi et al. [35]	32 sedentary subjects	Hyperglycaemia and fall of insulin
Larijani et al. [38]	115 healthy men	Reduction of blood glucose from 4.9 to 3.5 mmol/L
Maislos et al. [41]	24 healthy men	Maintenance of blood glucose
Ziaee et al. [64]	41 men, 40 women	Decrease from 4.3 to 3.8 mmol/L
Athletes		
Ba et al. [4]	15 endurance athletes	Non-significant trend, 4.6–4.5 mmol/L
Bouhlel et al. [7]	9 trained rugby players	Maintenance of blood glucose both at rest and during exercise despite decreased carbohydrate intake
Gueye et al. [24]	12 male sports students	Decrease from 5.2 to 4.1 mmol/L at rest, but no change in post-exercise values
Krifi et al. [35]	26 athletes	Hyperglycaemia and decrease of insulin levels
Maughan et al. [45]	59 soccer players	Maintenance of blood glucose (but not all samples collected in the afternoon); carbohydrate intake increased during Ramadan

from 4.9 to 3.5 mmol/L, although this change was associated with a substantial decrease in energy intake. In some of the other groups where blood glucose decreased, it seems likely that those studied were not only observing Ramadan, but were also using this period of intermittent fasting as a means of decreasing body fat stores. In none of the studies cited did the blood glucose drop to the level associated with clinical hypoglycaemia (3 mmol/L).

A progressive reduction of blood glucose could develop in trained athletes over the course of the day [20], particularly if physical activity was required during the period of fasting, and it is unfortunate that not all investigators have collected blood samples during the late afternoon. Nevertheless, four of five studies of athletes have shown little change of either resting blood glucose or values post-exercise during Ramadan. Presumably, the athletes maintain glucose homeostasis through a combination of food absorbed from meals taken immediately before dawn, the breakdown of liver glycogen stores [3], and gluconeogenesis.

To our knowledge, there have been no studies examining the effect of Ramadan fasting on glycogen stores in athletes. This is an important gap in current knowledge. Such a study might show a cumulative glycogen depletion not revealed by measurements of plasma glucose measurements, developing either during an individual day or over the course of Ramadan, especially in endurance-trained subjects. More information is also needed on the possible effects of glycogen-depleting fasts upon the mental aspects of competitive performance.

Implications for Athletic Performance

Carbohydrate stores make a major contribution to endurance performance in athletes. The potential for a progressive reduction of glycogen stores and hypoglycaemia that could develop even with the brief intermittent fasting of Ramadan can be countered in part by ingesting high-carbohydrate meals in the evening. Other helpful tactics are to consume a high-fat diet and to maximize aerobic training in the period leading up to Ramadan; this will increase the ability of the body to metabolize fat rather than glucose during prolonged physical activity. Finally, stores of glycogen should be conserved by taking the minimum possible amount of daytime physical activity between events.

Conclusions

Fasting or a restricted diet, particularly if low in carbohydrates, can potentially lead to a progressive depletion of glycogen stores, with adverse effects upon both mental and physical performance. Those particularly affected are endurance athletes, those involved in cooperative team sports, and those where tactics make a substantial contribution to victory. These issues can be countered by maximal aerobic training and a high-fat diet in the weeks before fasting and, in the case of Ramadan observance, a high carbohydrate intake at the evening meal in order to replenish glycogen stores. Much of the available empirical data suggest that with careful dietary management, athletes face little change of blood glucose during Ramadan. However, existing observations relate mostly to participants in short- and medium-term events. Further study is needed, both to observe possible effects in long- and ultralong distance events and to determine possible pre-event deple- tion of muscle glycogen reserves. More research is needed to study the impact of Ramadan fasting on muscle glycogen levels and to assess the energetic balance at rest and during prolonged exercises in sedentary and trained athletes.

Key Terms

Catecholamines: The catecholamines are a family of neurotransmitters produced at nerve terminals, including epinephrine, norepinephrine, and dopamine.

Glucose transporters (GLUT): Glucose transporters are a family of membrane proteins that facilitate the transport of glucose across tissue membranes (GLUT1–GLUT4).

Glucostatic mechanisms: Glucostatic mechanisms regulate blood glucose lev- els within a narrow range, thus facilitating use of glucose by the cells. Regulation depends on receptors that are sensitive to blood glucose and insulin concentrations.

Glycogen: Glycogen is a polysaccharide formed by the complexing of a large number of glucose molecules. It provides the main store of carbohydrate in muscle and liver.

Glycaemic index: The glycaemic index provides a measure of the rise of blood glucose seen after the ingestion of a given carbohydrate foodstuff.

Hexose: A hexose is a monosaccharide carbohydrate formed from six atoms of carbon.

Insulin: Insulin is a hormone secreted by the beta cells of the pancreas. Insulin is concerned primarily with the regulation of blood glucose levels, but its actions also include a stimulation of glycogen and lipid synthesis, an inhibition of protein breakdown, and a stimulation of amino acid uptake by muscle cells.

Pentose: A pentose is a monosaccharide containing a 5-atom carbon ring.

Sympathoadrenal system: The sympathoadrenal system is that component of the nervous sympathetic system based upon the secretions of the adrenal medulla. It releases epinephrine and norepinephrine in stressful situa- tions such as vigorous exercise, fasting, and emotional disturbances.

Key Points

1. Carbohydrates are the main source of fuel for brief and intensive exer- cise and also for sustained aerobic activity.
2. Maintaining at least a limited store of carbohydrate is important in avoiding premature fatigue and a reduction of endurance performance.

3. There is a close relationship between the availability of carbohydrate and aerobic performance, particularly during sustained exercise (>90 minutes).
4. The contribution of fat stores to overall metabolism increases progressively as glycogen stores are depleted.
5. Further studies are needed to examine the effects of fasting in ultraendurance athletes, with particular reference to pre-event glycogen reserves.
6. The challenges of glucose homeostasis for fasting endurance athletes can be reduced by a high-fat diet and maximal aerobic training in the weeks preceding a fast, and during Ramadan observance by taking a high-carbohydrate meal during the evenings.

Questions for Discussion

1. How would you set about assessing the carbohydrate needs of an athlete?
2. What changes of hormonal profile would you expect to observe in an athlete during fasting or carbohydrate restriction?
3. What changes of carbohydrate metabolism would you anticipate with a reduction of glycogen stores?
4. What practical recommendations would you make to an athlete to minimize any adverse impact of fasting upon performance?

References

1. Adlouni A, Ghalim N, Benslimane A et al. Fasting during Ramadan induces a marked increase in high-density lipoprotein cholesterol and decrease in low-density lipoprotein cholesterol. *Ann Nutr Metab* 1997;41(4):242–249.
2. Aybak M, Türkoĝlu A, Sermet A et al. Effect of Ramadan fasting on platelet aggregation in healthy male subjects. *Eur J Appl Physiol* 1996;73:552–556.
3. Azizi F. Islamic fasting and health. *Ann Nutr Metab* 2010;56(4):273–282.
4. Ba A, Samb A, Seck D et al. Comparative study of the effect of fasting during Ramadan on the glycaemia at rest in sportsmen and sedentary individuals (in French). *Dakar Méd* 2005;50:22–25.
5. Bentley DJ, Cox GR, Green D et al. Maximizing performance in triathlon: Applied physiological and nutritional aspects of elite and non-elite competitions. *J Sci Med Sport* 2008;11:407–415.
6. Bigard AX, Boussif M, Chalabi H et al. Alterations in muscular performance and orthostatic tolerance during Ramadan. *Aviat Space Environ Med* 1998;69:341–346.
7. Bouhlel E, Salhi Z, Bouhlel H et al. Effect of Ramadan fasting on fuel oxidation during exercise in trained male rugby players. *Diabetes Metab* 2006;32:617–624.
8. Brooks GA, Mercier J. Balance of carbohydrate and lipid utilization during exercise: The "crossover" concept. *J Appl Physiol (1985)*. 1994 Jun;76(6):2253–2261.
9. Casey A, Short AH, Curtis S et al. The effect of glycogen availability on power output and the metabolic response to repeated bouts of maximal, isokinetic exercise in man. *Eur J Appl Physiol Occup Physiol* 1996;72:249–255.
10. Coggan AR, Coyle EF. Carbohydrate ingestion during prolonged exercise: Effects on metabolism and performance. *Exerc Sport Sci Rev* 1991;19:1–40.

11. Costill DL, Sparks K, Gregor R et al. Muscle glycogen utilization during exhausting running. *J Appl Physiol* 1971;31:353–356.
12. Costill DL, Fink WJ, Pollock ML. Muscle fiber composition and enzyme activities of elite distance runners. *Med Sci Sport* 1976;8:96–100.
13. Coyle EF, Coggan AR, Hemmert MK et al. Substrate usage during prolonged exercise following a preexercise meal. *J Appl Physiol* 1985 Aug;59(2):429–433.
14. Currell K, Conway S, Jeukendrup AE. Carbohydrate ingestion improves performance of a new reliable test of soccer performance. *Int J Sport Nutr Exerc Metab* 2009 Feb;19(1):34–46.
15. de Oliveira EP, Burini RC. Food-dependent, exercise-induced gastrointestinal distress. *J Int Soc Sports Nutr* 2011 Sep 28;8:12.
16. Dohm GL, Kasperek GJ, Tapscott EB et al. Protein metabolism during endurance exercise. *Fed Proc* 1985 Feb;44(2):348–352.
17. Dohm GL, Beeker RT, Israel RG et al. Metabolic responses to exercise after fasting. *J Appl Physiol* 1986;61:1363–1368.
18. El Ati J, Beji C, Danguir J. Increased fat oxidation during Ramadan fasting in healthy women: An adaptative mechanism for body-weight maintenance. *Am J Clin Nutr* 1995;62:302–307.
19. Fakhrzadeh H, Larihani B, Sanjari M et al. Effect of Ramadan fasting on clinical and biochemical parameters in healthy adults. *Ann Saudi Med* 2003;23:223–226.
20. Faye J, Fall A, Badji L et al. Effects of Ramadan fast on weight, performance and glycemia during training for resistance (Article in French). *Dakar Med* 2005;50(3):146–151.
21. Gleeson M, Greenhaff PL, Maughan RJ. Influence of a 24 h fast on high intensity cycle exercise performance in man. *Eur J Appl Physiol Occup Physiol* 1988;57(6):653–659.
22. Goedecke JH, White NJ, Chicktay W et al. The effect of carbohydrate ingestion on performance during a simulated soccer match. *Nutrients* 2013 Dec 16;5(12):5193–5204.
23. Greenhaff PL, Gleeson M, Maughan RJ. Diet-induced metabolic acidosis and the performance of high intensity exercise in man. *Eur J Appl Physiol Occup Physiol* 1988;57:583–590.
24. Gueye L, Samb A, Seck D et al. Influence of a 12-hour fast on maximal exercise. *Scripta Med (Brno)* 2005;(77):271–276.
25. Hargreaves M. Muscle glycogen and metabolic regulation. *Proc Nutr Soc* 2004 May;63(2):217–220.
26. Hawley JA, Schabort EJ, Noakes TD et al. Carbohydrate-loading and exercise performance. An update. *Sports Med* 1997 Aug;24(2):73–81.
27. Hilton LK, Loucks AB. Low energy availability, not exercise stress, suppresses the diurnal rhythm of leptin in healthy young women. *Am J Physiol Endocrinol Metab* 2000 Jan;278(1):E43–E49.
28. Horowitz JF, Mora-Rodriguez R, Byerley LO et al. Lipolytic suppression following carbohydrate ingestion limits fat oxidation during exercise. *Am J Physiol* 1997 Oct;273(4 Pt 1):E768–E775.
29. Hultman E. Liver as a glucose supplying source during rest and exercise with special reference to diet. In: Parizkova J, Rogozkin VA (eds.), *Nutrition, Physical Fitness and Health*. University Park Press, Baltimore, MD, 1978, pp. 9–30.
30. Ibrahim WH, Habib HM, Jarrar AH et al. Effect of Ramadan fasting on markers of oxidative stress and serum biochemical markers of cellular damage in healthy subjects. *Ann Nutr Metab* 2008;53(3–4):175–181.
31. Jansson E, Hjemdahl P, Kaijser L. Diet induced changes in sympatho-adrenal activity during submaximal exercise in relation to substrate utilization in man. *Acta Physiol Scand* 1982 Feb;114(2):171–178.
32. Kelly D, Hamilton JK, Riddell MC. Blood glucose levels and performance in a sports camp for adolescents with type 1 diabetes mellitus: A field study. *Int J Pediatr* 2010;2010:216167.

33. Koivisto VA, Karonen SL, Nikkilä EA. Carbohydrate ingestion before exercise: Comparison of glucose, fructose, and sweet placebo. *J Appl Physiol Respir Environ Exerc Physiol* 1981 Oct;51(4):783–787.
34. Koubi H, Duchamp C, Géloën A et al. Resistance of hepatic glycogen to depletion in obese Zucker rats. *Can J Physiol Pharmacol* 1991;69:841–845.
35. Krifi M, Ben Salem M, Ben Rayana MC et al. Food intake, and anthropometrical and biological parameters in adult Tunisians in Ramadan (in French). *J Méd Nutr* 1989;25:223–228.
36. Langfort J, Pilis W, Zarzeczny R et al. Effect of low-carbohydrate-ketogenic diet on metabolic and hormonal responses to graded exercise in men. *J Physiol Pharmacol* 1996 Jun;47(2):361–371.
37. Langfort J, Zarzeczny R, Pilis W et al. The effect of a low-carbohydrate diet on performance, hormonal and metabolic responses to a 30-s bout of supramaximal exercise. *Eur J Appl Physiol Occup Physiol* 1997;76(2):128–133.
38. Larijani B, Zahedi F, Sanjari M et al. The effect of Ramadan fasting on fasting serum glucose in healthy adults. *Med J Malaysia* 2003 Dec;58(5):678–680.
39. Lima-Silva AE, De-Oliveira FR, Nakamura FY et al. Effect of carbohydrate availability on time to exhaustion in exercise performed at two different intensities. *Braz J Med Biol Res* 2009 May;42(5):404–412.
40. Lima-Silva AE, Pires FO, Bertuzzi R et al. Effects of a low- or a high-carbohydrate diet on performance, energy system contribution, and metabolic responses during supramaximal exercise. *Appl Physiol Nutr Metab* 2013 Sep;38(9):928–934.
41. Maislos M, Khamaysi N, Assali A et al. Marked increase in plasma high-density-lipoprotein cholesterol after prolonged fasting during Ramadan. *Am J Clin Nutr* 1993 May;57(5):640–642.
42. Martineau L, Jacobs I. Muscle glycogen usage during shivering thermogenesis in humans. *J Appl Physiol* 1988;65(5):2036–2050.
43. Maughan RJ, Gleeson M. Influence of a 36 h fast followed by refeeding with glucose, glycerol or placebo on metabolism and performance during prolonged exercise in man. *Eur J Appl Physiol Occup Physiol* 1988;57(5):570–576.
44. Maughan RJ, Greenhaff PL, Leiper JB et al. Diet composition and the performance of high-intensity exercise. *J Sports Sci* 1997 Jun;15(3):265–275.
45. Maughan RJ, Bartagi Z, Dvorak J et al. Dietary intake and body composition of football players during the holy month of Ramadan. *J Sports Sci* 2008 Dec;26(Suppl. 3):S29–S38.
46. McNay EC, Cotero VE. Mini-review: Impact of recurrent hypoglycemia on cognitive and brain function. *Physiol Behav* 2010;100:234–238.
47. Mikulski T, Ziemba A, Nazar K. Metabolic and hormonal responses to body carbohydrate store depletion followed by high or low carbohydrate meal in sedentary and physically active subjects. *J Physiol Pharmacol* 2010 Apr;61(2):193–200.
48. Nieman DC, Carlson KA, Brandstater ME et al. Running endurance in 27-h-fasted humans. *J Appl Physiol (1985)* 1987 Dec;63(6):2502–2509.
49. Niinimaa V, Wright GR, Shephard RJ et al. Characteristics of the successful dinghy sailor. *J Sports Med Phys Fitness* 1977;17:83–96.
50. Noakes TD, Lambert EV, Lambert MI et al. Carbohydrate ingestion and muscle glycogen depletion during marathon and ultramarathon racing. *Eur J Appl Physiol* 1988;57(4):482–489.
51. Oliver SJ, Laing SJ, Wilson S et al. Endurance running performance after 48 h of restricted fluid and/or energy intake. *Med Sci Sports Exerc* 2007 Feb;39(2):316–322.
52. Pérusse L, Collier G, Gagnon J et al. Acute and chronic effects of exercise on leptin levels in humans. *J Appl Physiol (1985)* 1997 Jul;83(1):5–10.
53. Phillips SM, Sproule J, Turner AP. Carbohydrate ingestion during team games exercise: Current knowledge and areas for future investigation. *Sports Med* 2011 1; 41(7):559–585.
54. Rollo I, Williams C. Influence of ingesting a carbohydrate-electrolyte solution before and during a 1-hr running performance test. *Int J Sport Nutr Exerc Metab* 2009;19:645–658.

55. Rauch HG, St Clair Gibson A, Lambert EV et al. A signaling role for muscle glycogen in the regulation of pace during prolonged exercise. *Br J Sports Med* 2005;39(1):34–38.
56. Rowlands DS, Hopkins WG. Effect of high-fat, high-carbohydrate, and high-protein meals on metabolism and performance during endurance cycling. *Int J Sport Nutr Exerc Metab* 2002 Sep;12(3):318–335.
57. Rowlands DS, Hopkins WG. Effects of high-fat and high-carbohydrate diets on metabolism and performance in cycling. *Metabolism* 2002 Jun;51(6):678–690.
58. Shephard RJ. *Physiology and Biochemistry of Exercise*. Praeger, New York, 1982.
59. Shephard RJ. The impact of Ramadan observance upon athletic performance. *Nutrients* 2012 Jun;4(6):491–505.
60. Shephard RJ, Johnson N. Physical activity and the liver. *Eur J Appl Physiol* 2015;115(1):1–46.
61. Wax B, Brown SP, Webb HE et al. Effects of carbohydrate supplementation on force output and time to exhaustion during static leg contraction superimposed with electromyostimulation. *J Strength Cond Res* 2012;26:1717–1723.
62. Williams C, Serratosa L. Nutrition on match day. *J Sports Sci* 2006;24:687–697.
63. Wu CL, Williams C. A low glycemic index meal before exercise improves endurance running capacity in men. *Int J Sport Nutr Exerc Metab* 2006 Oct;16(5):510–527.
64. Ziaee V, Razaei M, Ahmadinejad Z et al. The changes of metabolic profile and weight during Ramadan fasting. *Singapore Med J* 2006;47:409–414.
65. Zinker BA, Britz K, Brooks GA. Effects of a 36-hour fast on human endurance and substrate utilization. *J Appl Physiol (1985)* 1990 Nov;69(5):1849–1855.

Further Reading

Henriksson J. Cellular metabolism and endurance. In: Shephard RJ, Åstrand P-O (eds.), *Endurance in Sport*. Blackwell Scientific, Oxford, U.K., 2000, pp. 118–135.
Maughan RJ. *Nutrition in Sport*. Blackwell Publishing, Cambridge, MA, 2005.
Poortmans JR, Boisseau N. *Biochimie des activités chimiques*. De Boeck Université, Paris, France, 2002.
Shephard RJ. *Biochemistry of Exercise*. C.C. Thomas, Springfield, IL, 1983.

4

Mobilization and Utilization of Lipids during Dietary Restriction Conditions

Ezdine Bouhlel and Roy J Shephard

Learning Objectives

1. To understand the mechanisms regulating fat metabolism under non-fasting conditions, both at rest and during exercise, with particular reference to the role of hormones and enzymes
2. To learn the influence of the intensity of exercise upon the oxidation of fat relative to carbohydrates
3. To discover the impact of endurance training and of aerobic fitness upon rates of lipolysis
4. To understand the use of indirect calorimetry in assessing the relative usage of fat and carbohydrate
5. To grasp the notions of maximal lipid oxidation and the crossover point
6. To understand the changes that may occur in fat metabolism during Ramadan and other forms of dieting, both at rest and during exercise
7. To explore relationships between glycogen breakdown, hepatic glucose synthesis and lipolysis during Ramadan and longer periods of fasting
8. To understand the potential impact of a high-fat diet upon lipolysis and athletic performance

Fat Metabolism under Non-Fasting Conditions

Characteristics and Functions of Adipose Tissue

Adipose tissue accounts for 10–15 kg of body mass in a healthy, non-obese subject, about 15%–20% and 20%–25% of body mass in men and women, respectively. The body fat content is substantially higher for many people in developed societies, due to a combination of overeating and a sedentary lifestyle [27]. Moreover, the proportion of the population who are overweight or obese has increased in recent years, to the point that health agencies speak of an obesity epidemic [27]. The body fat content is lower for most categories of competitor, but with substantial differences between athletic disciplines: values as low as 6%–8% are seen in long-distance runners [8] and among athletes such as gymnasts and figure skaters where performance is scored in part on physical appearance [81], but percentages are quite high in pursuits where body mass confers an advantage, such as North American football [57,64], and 26% in top Sumo wrestlers [26].

In adult humans, most of the body fat is white adipose tissue, which is made up of adipocytes, although there may be very small quantities of brown adipose tissue, which can generate heat during exposure to a cold environment [20]. Superficial body fat is important to the thermal insulation of the body [28] and protects against external trauma, but the main function of white adipose tissue is to provide a store of triacylglycerol metabolites. Triacylglycerols are formed from circulating fatty acids (the process of lipogenesis); these reserves can later be broken down to meet the energy needs of the body (the process of lipolysis). Fat is a highly concentrated form of energy storage, yielding some 37 kJ/g, compared with around 16 kJ/g for protein or carbohydrate; one author estimated that if energy was stored as glycogen rather than fat, the body mass of a typical man would increase by 55 kg [10].

Lipolysis is activated during physical exercise, when a person is exposed to a cold environment, and on other occasions when an individual develops a negative energy balance (as during prolonged fasting). Each adipocyte stores a large amount of triacylglycerol, individual droplets coalescing to form a large globule that fills most of the fat cell. White adipose tissue as a whole accounts for some 95% of the body's triacylglycerols, although small quantities are also found in muscle tissue [49] and fat can accumulate in the liver of sedentary individuals [74].

Other metabolic functions of the adipocyte include the synthesis of several peptide and non-peptide hormones. Leptin is the best known of these endocrine factors. It is the hormone of satiety, and it plays an important role in regulating an individual's dietary intake and body mass [48].

International recommendations are that lipids should account for between 20% and 35% of a person's total energy intake, with saturated fats accounting for less than 10% of this total [31]. However, athletes may sometimes opt to take a substantially larger fraction of their diet as lipid, for reasons discussed later in this chapter. Health authorities also advise limiting the proportion of trans fat; although trans fat lowers LDL cholesterol (LDL-C), it also reduces levels of high-density lipoprotein (HDL) cholesterol and appears to increase the risk of heart attacks [33].

Regulation of Lipolysis

The key enzyme controlling fatty acid mobilization is the intracellular *hormone-sensitive lipase*, found within the adipocytes. Activation of this enzyme promotes lipolysis, with hydrolysis of the stored triacylglycerols and the release of fatty acids and glycerol from the adipocytes into the blood stream. The fatty acids are bound to albumin during their transport in the blood.

Activation of the *hormone-sensitive lipase* can be brought about by two inter-related processes. One involves perilipin A, which normally protects the fat cells from the hormone-sensitive lipase [37]. However, the perilipin is phosphory-lated by beta-adrenergic activity; the shape of the molecule is changed, and this exposes the fat to lipase, with resultant lysis. The second mechanism also involves phosphorylation, but it depends upon a more complex chain of events. The enzyme *protein kinase A* is activated by a 'second messenger', *cyclic adenosine monophosphate* (cAMP). The cAMP is formed from adenosine triphosphate (ATP) through the action of *adenyl cyclase*, an enzyme activated by epinephrine (in muscle), glucagon (in the liver) and both epinephrine and glucagon (in the fat cells). In contrast, insulin reduces cAMP levels and thus inhibits the lipase and resulting lipolysis [24]. The increased catecholamine concentrations that initiate lipolysis are triggered by physical exercise, stressful situations and fasting, pro-viding metabolic fuel for a 'fight or flight' reaction.

Epinephrine plays a major metabolic role in the regulation of metabolism. It not only initiates the process of lipolysis in adipose tissue and muscle but also inhibits lipogenesis in both the liver and adipose tissues. It also stimulates gly-cogen breakdown in both muscle and liver, inhibits the synthesis and storage of glycogen in these same tissues and activates glucose synthesis (gluconeogenesis) in the liver (the last reaction being opposed by insulin).

Many other factors influence the rate of lipolysis. One consideration is the avail-ability of substrates such as fatty acids, phosphates, oxygen and adenosine diphos-phate (ADP). A second influence is the availability of membrane transporting molecules (transporters), and membrane-bound allosteric enzymes (enzymes that change their configuration upon binding with an effector); they also influence the rate of lipolysis. Among this last group of substances, we may note in the respiratory chain, *ATP/ADP translocase*; in the Krebs cycle, *isocitrate dehydrogenase*; and in the β-oxidation of fatty acid molecules, *carnitine palmityl transferase I* (CPT I).

Factors Limiting Lipolysis

The availability of body fat does not normally limit lipolysis except during pro-longed fasting, because triacylglycerol reserves are large. Many people have large enough fat stores to survive for 4 or 5 weeks. Nor do protons and phosphate nor-mally play a limiting role; their mitochondrial concentrations are usually suffi-cient to sustain the process. However, if the oxygen supply to a muscle is restricted (as when performing resisted exercise), the usage of fatty acids is slowed, because fatty acids cannot be metabolized anaerobically. The most important limiting factor is the concentration of ADP, the substrate of ATPase, which enters the mitochondria through the action of the enzyme *translocase*. When the ATP/ADP ratio is high, the amount of ADP that enters the mitochondria is quite small, and lipolysis is correspondingly reduced. However, the ATP/ADP ratio diminishes rapidly during exercise, allowing an increased flux of ADP and a reactivation of lipolysis, thus providing the fuel needed to sustain the activity.

Transport of Long-Chained Fatty Acids into the Mitochondria

Long-chained fatty acids are oxidized within the mitochondria, but they do not diffuse easily into the interior of mitochondria. Their penetration is under the control of a transport system facilitated by the enzymes CPT I and CPT II. Acyl-CoA is produced by lipolysis of circulating fat and a combination of the resulting carboxylic acids with coenzyme A. The acyl-Co-A is transformed to acyl-carnitine by combination with L-carnitine within the external membrane of the mitochondria, through the catalysing action of CPT I. CPT I is the slower enzyme involved in the β-oxidation of fats and thus sets a limiting rate upon fat metabolism. Subsequently, the acyl-carnitine is reconverted to acyl-CoA as it is liberated into the mitochondrial matrix by CPT II, making L-carnitine available for metabolism (Figure 4.1 [44]).

The CPT I is inhibited by malonyl-CoA, formed from acetyl-CoA as the latter leaves the mitochondria. The enzyme involved in this process (*acetyl-coA*

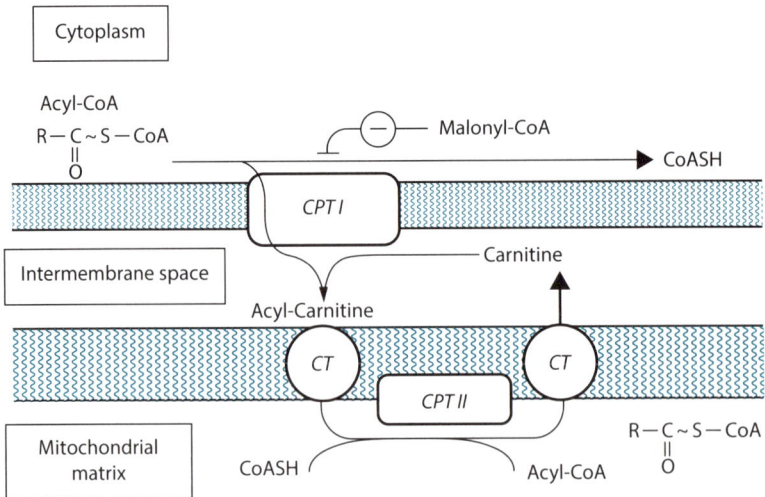

Figure 4.1 Role of *carnitine palmityltransferases* I and II in regulating the passage of fatty acids into the mitochondria. *Carnitine palmityltransferases*, CPT I and CPT II. CT, *carnitine translocase*. (Adapted from Jeukendrup, AE et al., *Int J Sports Med*, 19, 293, 1998.)

carboxylase, ACC) is inactivated by *5' adenosine monophosphate protein–activated kinase A* (AMPK). When the ATP/ADP ratio is high, the activity of the respiratory chain and the Krebs cycle is reduced, causing citrate to leave the mitochondria. Citrate is the substrate for the synthesis of fatty acids, with malonyl-CoA as an intermediary stage in this process.

The penetration of long-chained fatty acids into the mitochondria is controlled in great part by malonyl-CoA, which inhibits CPT I. There is thus an inverse relationship between the concentration of malonyl-CoA and the rate of lipolysis. During exercise, AMPK activity increases, inhibiting the activity of ACC activity, thus reducing concentrations of malonyl-CoA and increasing the penetration of fatty acids into the mitochondria.

Others metabolic factors also influence the penetration of fatty acid penetration into the mitochondria. Glucose stimulates ACC activity, increasing the synthesis of malonyl-CoA, inhibiting *carnitine palmityltransferase* activity, and thus diminishing lipid oxidation [26]. In addition, citrate and oxaloacetate, intermediary compounds in the Krebs cycle, stimulate ACC activity and thus inhibit lipid oxidation. The availability of fatty acids is also a major determinant of the type of substrate oxidized by muscle [67]. An increased concentration of fatty acids directly or indirectly inhibits the activity of glycolytic enzymes via citrate and acetyl-CoA (Figure 4.2). Other studies have confirmed that the availability of fatty acids can influence the rate of lipid oxidation [42,71], although lipid oxidation can also vary independently of any change in the availability of fatty acids [70].

A person's overall energy balance is regulated in part by the relative activity of the hormones leptin and adiponectin. Leptin is a protein hormone synthesized by the adipocytes; it inhibits food intake by its action upon satiety receptors in the hypothalamus and other receptors in the liver, spleen, pancreas, kidney and testes [79]. Adiponectin, also secreted by the adipocytes, has an opposing action; it increases feelings of hunger, has insulin-sensitizing properties and may modify substrate utilization [10]. High concentrations of adiponectin are correlated with adverse features of body composition, particularly an intra-abdominal accumulation of fat [25]. A third hormone involved in regulating food intake is ghrelin; this hormone is produced in the gastrointestinal tract when the stomach is empty. It acts on the same hypothalamic receptors as leptin, stimulating appetite [59].

Metabolism of Fat at Rest

Depending on the fitness and nutritional status of the subject, the breakdown of lipids accounts for 60%–90% of metabolism at rest. The percentage is typically higher in endurance athletes [70]. Fatty acids derived from adipose tissue were long considered as the main source of lipids for cellular metabolism, but it is now known that muscle can also use triacylglycerols directly. Some 300 g of fatty acid is stored as small droplets within muscle, quantities being relatively greater in slow twitch than in fast twitch muscle fibres. Both at rest and during exercise, triacylglycerols in plasma and muscle account for some 5%–10% of the lipids that are oxidized [68]. The main source of fatty acids is the plasma pool;

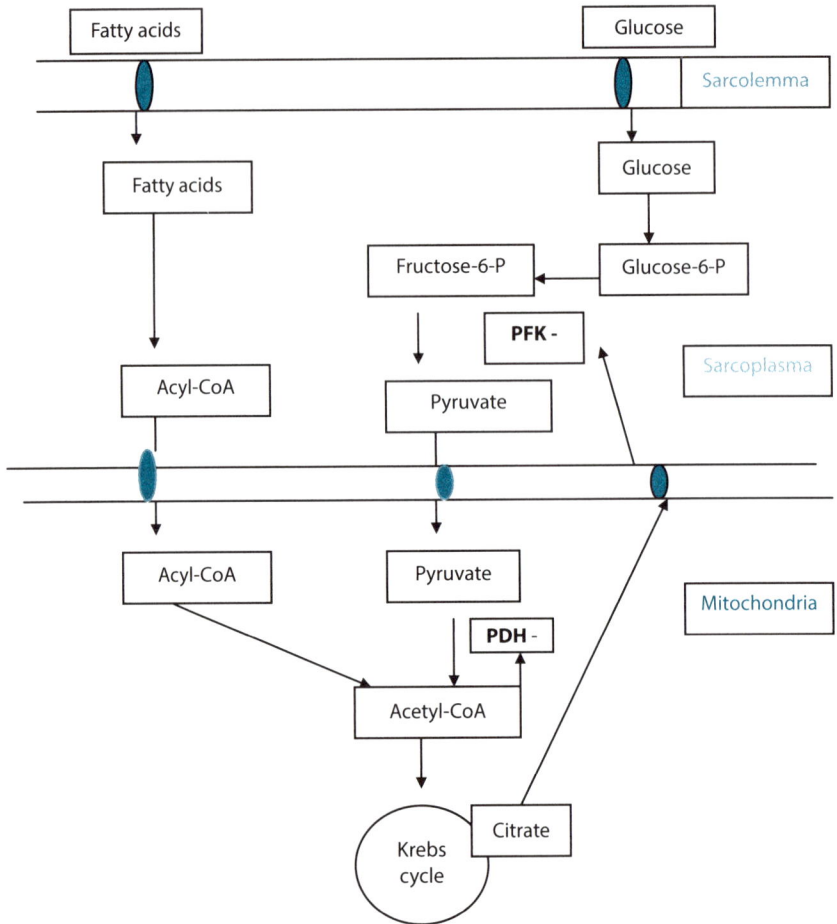

Figure 4.2 Illustrating the competition between glucose and fatty acids as potential fuels that release energy by entering the Krebs metabolic cycle. Note the enzymatic control of fat metabolism by *pyruvate dehydrogenase* and *phosphofructo-kinase*. (Adapted from Randle, PJ et al., *Lancet*, 1(7285), 785, 1963.)

here, the fatty acids are bound to albumin. On entering a muscle cell, the fatty acids are converted to acyl-CoA and in the mitochondria they undergo β-oxidation via the Krebs cycle (Figure 4.2), producing electrons that are carried by nicotin-amide adenine dinucleotide (NADH) to the mitochondrial respiratory chain in the process of releasing energy.

Metabolism of Fat during Exercise

During exercise, both intramuscular triglycerides and fatty acids transported from the adipose tissue depots are used as substrates for muscular contraction, provided that the local oxygen supply is adequate. Other factors influencing the relative use of lipids include the intensity and duration of exercise and the physical fitness and nutritional status of the individual. The intensity of exercise is perhaps the most important consideration. At rest, the percentage utilization of lipids is high, but the total quantity of lipids metabolized is quite small. During exercise, the percentage utilization of lipids decreases, but if the energy expenditure is high, the quantity of lipids metabolized can also be quite high. As the exercise intensity rises, a point is reached when the quantity of lipids oxidized is maximal; this intensity is called maximal fat oxidation (LIPOX$_{max}$ or Fat$_{max}$). It varies from one subject to another (20%–65% of $\dot{V}O_{2max}$). This metabolic parameter is largely used by clinicians to individualize training processes in the obese, in patients suffering from metabolic syndrome, and even in healthy subjects to enhance fat oxidation. The 'crossover' point is reached at a respiratory quotient (RQ) of about 0.90, corresponding to a higher carbohydrate contribution compared to lipids [19].

Determination of the Crossover Point

Assessments of the relative usage of fat and carbohydrate are based on the technique of indirect calorimetry, measuring respiratory gas volumes and the gaseous composition of expired air. The key calculation is the individual's RQ (the steady-state ratio of carbon dioxide output ($\dot{V}CO_2$) to oxygen consumption ($\dot{V}O_2$) [61]). The necessary calculations assume that protein breakdown makes a negligible contribution to overall metabolism, a postulate that is normally acceptable, but becomes open to question if the duration of fasting is sufficient to cause a progressive loss of lean tissue. The RQ is 0.71 if metabolism is attributable entirely to the breakdown of fat, but it rises to 1.0 if the energy source is entirely carbohydrate. Thus, if $\dot{V}O_2$ and $\dot{V}CO_2$ are expressed in L/min, the usage of carbohydrate and fat can be estimated from the following simple equations:

$$\text{\% of } \dot{V}O_2 \text{ attributable to carbohydrates} = [(RQ - 0.71)/0.29] \times 100$$

$$\text{\% of } \dot{V}O_2 \text{ attributable to lipids} = 100 - \text{\% of } \dot{V}O_2 \text{ attributable to carbohydrates}$$

$$\text{Rate of CHO usage (g/min)} = 4.585\dot{V}CO_2 - 3.2255\dot{V}O_2$$

$$\text{Rate of fat usage (g/min)} = 1.6946\dot{V}O_2 - 1.7012\dot{V}CO_2$$

This approach has been applied to determine the relative contributions of carbohydrate and fat to metabolism during both low- [13] and high-intensity exercises [50–52,60].

Effect of Exercise Intensity

The 'crossover' point is reached as the intensity of exercise is increased [19]; beyond this point, there is an increasing reliance upon carbohydrates as the energy

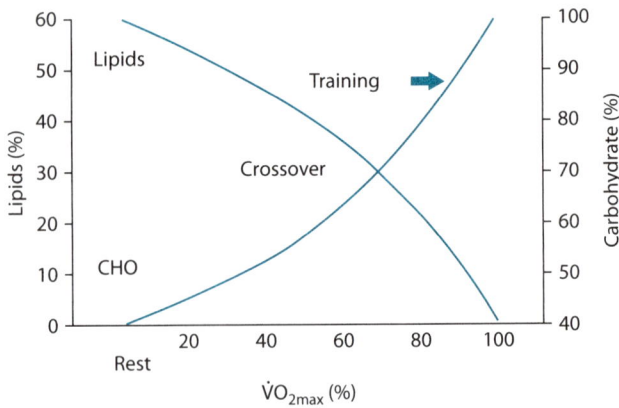

Figure 4.3 Illustration of crossover point where the oxidation of carbohydrate exceeds that of fat. (Adapted from Brooks, GA and Mercier, J, *J Appl Physiol*, 76, 2253, 1994.)

source (Figure 4.3). The oxidation of fat diminishes in part not only because of a decreased delivery of fatty acids to the exercising muscles, but also because a decreasing fraction of the active muscle fibers. The crossover is thus reached earlier if the activity involves only small muscles or if substantial resisted exercise is required.

Low-Intensity Exercise

During exercise demanding 20%–35% of a person's $\dot{V}O_{2max}$, substrates are essentially drawn from the plasma (fatty acids and glucose), and there are large interindividual variations in the relative usage of fat and carbohydrate [2].

Moderate-Intensity Exercise

In activities demanding 35%–60% of the individual's $\dot{V}O_{2max}$, intramuscular glycogen and triglycerides make an increasing contribution to energy supply, with an associated reduction in the reliance upon plasma substrates. Friedlander et al. [35] observed an increased oxidation of fatty acids in women at exercise intensities demanding 45% and 65% of $\dot{V}O_{2max}$, and Achten and Jeukendrup [3] reported that fat oxidation peaked at an exercise intensity between 45% and 65% of $\dot{V}O_{2max}$.

High-Intensity Exercise

At oxygen consumptions demanding more than 80% of $\dot{V}O_{2max}$, the utilization of carbohydrate is markedly increased, and a person derives much of the required energy from intramuscular reserves of glycogen. Romijn et al. [71] found that when exercising at 85% of $\dot{V}O_{2max}$, even the intravenous infusion of lipids could not restore the rate of lipid oxidation observed at lower intensities of effort. Plainly, other factors than availability reduce lipid usage during intensive exercise, including oxygen supply, and possibly a reduced transport of fatty acids into the mitochondria, due to a lesser availability of carnitine and/or a decrease of intracellular pH.

Effect of Exercise Duration

The respiratory exchange ratio (RER) at any given intensity of effort decreases progressively as the duration of exercise is extended. This reflects an increased contribution of lipids to the total energy needs of the body as carbohydrate reserves are depleted over 60–90 minutes of activity.

Effects of Endurance Training and Fitness Level

Endurance training increases the relative oxidation of fat during submaximal exercise, reducing the individual's dependence on carbohydrate as a source of energy [3,11,62]. The relative use of adipose and intramuscular triacylglycerols during exercise also depends on the aerobic fitness of the person. At any given absolute intensity of effort, endurance-trained subjects oxidize more fat, without necessarily any increase in lipolysis. This reflects both increases in the activity of aerobic enzymes within the muscle fibres, allowing a greater oxidation of intramuscular triacylglycerol stores [40], and also an increase of myocardial function, allowing a more effective perfusion of the contracting muscles.

Catecholamine concentrations increase with the intensity of exercise, and insulin levels diminish. However, the catecholamine secretion is smaller at any given intensity of exercise, either absolute or relative, and the decreased secretion of catecholamines is particularly marked during prolonged bouts of exercise. However, other factors must compensate for this, since lipolysis is greater in endurance athletes than in sedentary individuals.

General Effects of Fasting upon Fat Metabolism

Total Fasting

With total fasting, reserves of carbohydrate in the muscles and liver are depleted within a few hours. Thereafter, the body is totally dependent upon reserves of fat and protein; fat depots range from about 4 kg in an athletic male, through 14 kg in a healthy but sedentary adult, to as much as 30 kg in an obese individual, equivalent to reserves of about 120, 400 and 870 MJ of energy, respectively. If energy expenditure is held to a minimum, perhaps 8 MJ/day for an adult male, and 10% of this requirement is met from protein stores, there will be a potential for survival of up to 17, 55 and 121 days, respectively. In emergency situations, survival may be shorter, because of energy expended in attempts to escape and in a cold environment there is an ever-increasing energy cost of maintaining body temperature as subcutaneous fat is lost.

During short-term fasting, the reliance upon fat metabolism creates a ketosis, as acidic ketone bodies accumulate in the tissue (Chapter 2), with sensations of weakness and fatigue, and a substantial reduction of endurance times during submaximal cycle ergometer exercise [23]. Gleeson et al. [36] had subjects engage in an experimental fast for 24 hours. Following this fast, fat oxidation was increased when exercising, and the time to exhaustion was also reduced during intensive exercise (>80% of $\dot{V}O_{2max}$).

With periods of fasting of 24 hours or less, *glycogenolysis and gluconeogenesis* are likely the predominant sources of the glucose required by the brain and anaerobic muscular activity, but after prolonged and uninterrupted fasting (40 days), *ketones* account for an important fraction of the energy used by the skeletal muscle and even the brain [34]. Changes in other factors such as physical fitness [52], moderate aerobic training [13,62] and muscle blood flow (the last associated with dehydration) may play a secondary role in modifying fat usage during brief periods of fasting, even if the plasma glucose concentration remains unchanged.

van Loon et al. [78] found that after an overnight fast, the rate of free fatty acid oxidation increased during exercise, correlating well with increased plasma free fatty acid concentrations. They concluded that intramuscular triglyceride stores were an important source of substrate for endurance-trained male athletes when they undertook moderate-intensity exercise following an overnight fast; however, the usage of intramuscular and lipoprotein-derived triglycerides decreased as the duration of exercise was extended.

Experimental studies in both animals and humans have demonstrated increases of lipolysis during fasting. In this context, fasting has been proposed as a tool to enhance a person's lipid utilization and thus spare glycogen reserves during subsequent exercise. Dohm et al. [29] found increased fat oxidation and a sparing of intramuscular glycogen in rats that had been fasted for 24 hours. A 24-hour fast had similar effects in humans, both at rest and during moderate exercise [36]; fat oxidation was increased, intramuscular glycogen was conserved and endurance performance was enhanced. However, during high-intensity exercise (>80% of $\dot{V}O_{2max}$), physical performance was reduced, presumably because glycogen reserves were low [36]. One report saw a 200% increase of lipolysis after a 3-day fast. Lipolysis is increased by as much as 200% after 3 days of fasting. Possible mechanisms for this could be an increased secretion of epinephrine in response to the low blood glucose concentration and/or an increase in the sensitivity of adipose tissue to catecholamine.

Severe Dietary Restriction

Severe dietary restriction also increases the body's reliance upon depot fat as a source of energy, particularly if much of the energy that is allowed is in the form of fat, as in the Atkins diet. However, if a minimum of glucose or protein is made available, there seems adaptation to a high rate of fat metabolism in a longer-term perspective (Chapter 2), with little evidence of ketosis or a deterioration in physical performance [14,63], and ketone bodies may even serve as a substrate to sustain the metabolism of the brain [12].

Moderate Dietary Restriction

For a person who is overweight or who has moderate obesity, a typical recommendation is to create a moderate energy deficit of about 4 MJ/day, preferably by a combination of dietary restriction, increased physical activity and an adequate intake of protein in order to conserve lean tissue mass (Chapter 5). The loss of fat and muscle tissue and compensatory hormonal reactions may reduce the resting metabolism by as much as 15%, to less than 7 MJ/day, so that at most 3 MJ/day is derived from fat stores, equivalent to about 100 g of fat. Even with faithful adherence to the prescribed exercise and diet, it would thus take around 160 days to metabolize a 16 kg excess of fat. This is a hard lesson for both patients and those running obesity clinics. Fat was accumulated over many years by a very small excess of food intake relative to requirements, and it will also take quite a long time to metabolize this fat, particularly if damage to lean tissue is to be avoided.

Animal research is currently underway to explore the possibility of facilitating dieting by suppressing blood flow to parts of the stomach that synthesize ghrelin [7], and others are looking at the possibility of developing adiponectin receptor antagonists [58]. Because it increases catecholamine secretion, exercise in a cold environment may also favour fat loss relative to activity in a warmer environment [56]. A further useful tactic may be to plan exercise sessions so that the intensity of effort coincides approximately with the crossover point, when fat oxidation is maximal.

Ramadan Observance

Most studies of changes in fat metabolism during Ramadan fasting have been in sedentary individuals rather than athletes. Many sedentary individuals see the Ramadan month as an opportunity to reduce their body fat content, and thus they deliberately develop a negative energy balance, with a substantial loss of body fat. However, some enjoy the communal meals, particularly the feasting during the final 3 days of Ramadan, and may thus show an increase of body mass and body fat. Even in athletes, the pattern of weight and fat loss is very variable; in some cases, determined efforts to eat large amounts of food at night may help to maintain a balance between food intake and energy expenditures, but other athletes show a substantial reduction of fat stores, particularly in disciplines with high daily energy expenditures. Lipolysis is activated, particularly if prolonged bouts of exercise at low to moderate intensities must be undertaken in daylight hours, when food intake is prohibited. Once glycogen stores are depleted, triacylglycerol becomes the body's main energy source during the hours of fasting,

The observance of Ramadan fasting has indeed been proposed as a tool to increase fat oxidation and optimize the blood lipid profile in healthy sedentary subjects. For example, El Ati et al. [30] found an increase of lipolysis and a decreased utilization of carbohydrates in sedentary resting women during Ramadan. They noted a concomitant decrease of plasma insulin concentrations. Ramadan et al. [66] also found an increased utilization of fat during steady-state exercise at 70% of $\dot{V}O_{2max}$ in seven sedentary and six active subjects who were observing Ramadan. However, attribution of these various changes to intermittent fasting is uncertain, since the overall diet is frequently modified during Ramadan. Thus, in a study of serum lipids of 20 healthy male students, Rahman et al. [65] found a 6% decrease of energy intake and a 2 kg decrease of body mass; however, probably because there was a greater intake of fat during Ramadan, they observed an increase of HDL cholesterol. In contrast, the sedentary student volunteers of Ziaee et al. [80], who also lost weight during Ramadan, found reductions in blood glucose and HDL cholesterol, but no significant changes in total cholesterol (TC), triacylglycerols or very-low-density lipoprotein (VLDL).

Changes in substrate availability could have an impact on substrate utilization during Ramadan observance [15]. Bouhlel et al. [15] found an increase of fat oxidation in trained subjects both at rest and during submaximal exercise. They suggested that one likely cause was an increased fat intake during Ramadan. A second factor is probably the reduced availability of glucose and glycogen, particularly during the afternoon hours [4,43,45,70]. Sidossis and Wolfe [76] argued that it was the availability of glucose rather than fatty acids that was the primary determinant of the substrate that was oxidized. Horowitz et al. [41] pointed out that an energy deficit, increased fatty acid availability and an increased expression of *pyruvate dehydrogenase kinase* (PDK)-4 mRNA would all work to suppress carbohydrate oxidation, even if the dietary intake of carbohydrate was not curtailed.

The adoption of high-fat meals has been recommended as a way to increase fat oxidation [3]. Achten et al. [1] had seven runners trained daily while consuming a diet containing 45% CHO, 40% fat and 15% protein; this regimen brought about an increase in fat oxidation and a decrease in muscle glycogenolysis. Horowitz and Klein [40] also reported a 22% increase of fat oxidation as the plasma fatty acid concentration was increased from 0.15 to 0.48 mmol/L. Given the dietary changes that are seen in some groups observing Ramadan (a greater fat intake, with increased concentrations of plasma triglycerides and HDL cholesterol [16]), this could certainly contribute to the increased fat oxidation that is seen during submaximal exercise. Modifications in the type of fat consumed may also contribute to the change of blood lipid profile that is seen during Ramadan observance. Tunisian people often increase their intake of saturated fat during Ramadan [9,30], and a high intake of saturated fat is known to increase levels of TC and HDL cholesterol ([HDL-C] [5,53]).

Effects of Ramadan Observance upon Fat Metabolism in Athletes

During the observance of Ramadan, some athletes contrive to maintain their energy balance, with no change of body fat, but in others, body mass decreases by up to 3 kg, mainly due to the metabolism of body fat (Chapter 2). We will focus here upon the associated changes of metabolism and regulatory hormones.

Resting Conditions

There has been little discussion of the effects of Ramadan fasting on the metabolism of fat in trained subjects [15–17,22]. Chennaoui et al. [22] found metabolic, hormonal and inflammatory changes, but no disturbance of total energy intake, body mass or body fat content in eight middle-distance runners. Bouhlel et al. [15] noted an increased fat oxidation at rest. In their subjects, this was associated with a progressive decrease of body mass and body fat content. Dietary records showed a significant increase of fat intake during Ramadan.

Increases in HDL-C concentration in trained subjects at the beginning of Ramadan offer some evidence of greater fat metabolism [16]. The increase in HDL-C was of a similar order to that seen in sedentary subjects [6,69] and confirms other findings in endurance athletes such as runners, swimmers, rowers, boxers and soccer [21]. The change in lipid profile, if maintained subsequent to Ramadan, could offer some protection against the development of atherosclerosis. Reports on possible changes in LDL-C concentrations have been conflicting. Some studies have seen significant increases of LDL-C in healthy subjects during Ramadan fasting [9,38], but Bouhlel et al. [15] found no changes in a group of nine Rugby players. Filaire et al. [32] also saw no change in LDL-C concentrations over a longer (7 days continuous) period of food restriction [32].

Lipolysis is activated particularly during prolonged low- to moderate-intensity exercises and periods of food restriction.

During Exercise

Ramadan observance combined with prolonged low-intensity bouts of exercise is a good tactic to enhance fat oxidation [15]. The extent of fat mobilization is related also to the time of day when exercise is taken and to the cumulative duration of the fast [54]. Metabolic responses during a combination of exercise and fasting reflect two constraints: the need to maintain blood glucose and to provide sufficient energy for exercise. Neural and hormonal systems of regulation generate pivotal metabolic responses:

- Hepatic glucose production is stimulated by increases of both glycogenolysis (favoured by reduced insulin levels plus secretion of glucagon and catecholamine) and gluconeogenesis (favoured by reduced insulin levels, plus the secretion of glucagon, cortisol and growth hormone) [75].
- Muscular glycogenolysis is stimulated by reduced insulin levels plus the secretion of catecholamines.
- Lipolysis is stimulated by reduced insulin levels, plus the secretion of glucagon, catecholamines, cortisol and growth hormone.

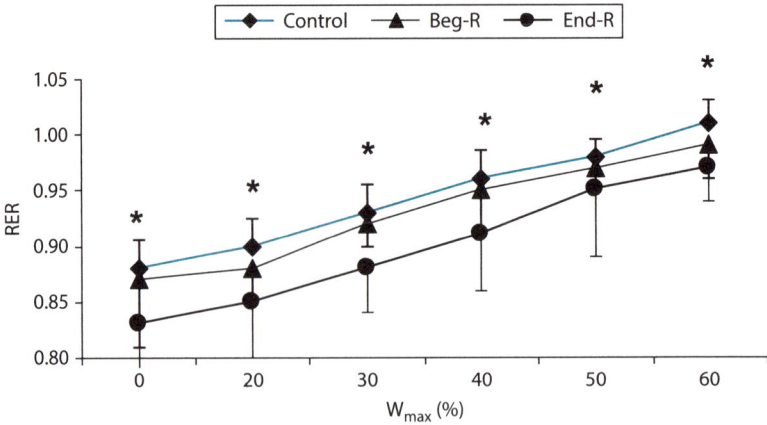

Figure 4.4 Comparison of respiratory exchange ratio in a group of rugby players at selected exercise intensities during a control period (C), at the end of the first week (Beg-R), and during the last week of Ramadan observance (End-R). * Significantly different from before Ramadan (control compared with End-R), $p < 0.001$. (Based on data of Bouhlel, E et al., *Diabetes Metab*, 32(6), 617, 2006.)

An overall trend to metabolism of fat is promoted by a combination of prolonged low-intensity exercise and fasting. Training further enhances these metabolic adaptations and attenuates neurohormonal responses. Empirical evidence of such a response is seen in a group of rugby players both at rest and during submaximal exercise (Figure 4.4 [15]); a reduced RER confirms a greater dependence upon lipid metabolism during Ramadan.

Determinations of the crossover point show a similar tendency, with a shift of the maximal lipid oxidation point to the right (i.e., it occurs at a larger fraction of maximal effort), particularly in trained athletes (Figure 4.5).

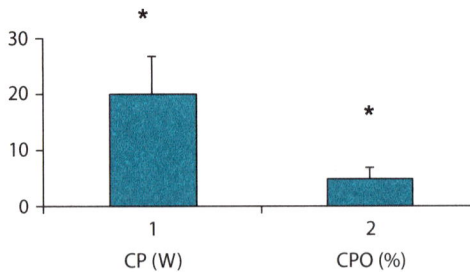

Figure 4.5 Changes of crossover point in a group of nine rugby players during Ramadan observance, expressed in absolute units (CP, W) and as a percentage of maximal power output (CPO, %). * Significantly different from before Ramadan, $p < 0.001$. (Based on data of Bouhlel, E et al., *Diabetes Metab*, 32(6), 617, 2006.)

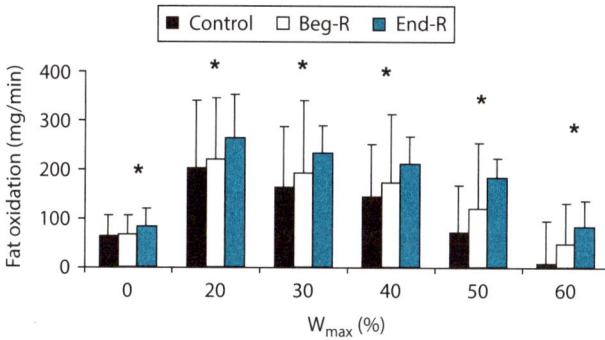

Figure 4.6 Lipid oxidation rates in a group of rugby players during submaximal exercise before (control), at the beginning (Beg-R) and at the end (End-R) of Ramadan observance. * Significantly different from before Ramadan (control compared with End-R), $p < 0.001$. (Based on data of Bouhlel, E et al., *Diabetes Metab*, 32(6), 617, 2006.)

During submaximal exercise, the rate of fat oxidation peaked at 20% of maximal working capacity and was significantly lower at 60% than at 20%–50% of maximal power output (Figure 4.6).

The increase in fat oxidation during Ramadan was accompanied by reductions in both body mass and fat mass. Insulin secretion was reduced [15], but there was no change in the GH/IGF-1 axis or leptin or adiponectin concentrations [15,16]. This group of athletes had continued to train regularly during Ramadan, and this may have played a major role in increasing their oxidation of fat. Aerobic training also induces muscular adaptations such as increased capillarization, a greater mitochondrial volume, an enhanced activity of oxidative enzymes [72] and an increase of fatty acid–binding protein in the sarcolemma [46].

Stannard and Thompson [77] studied healthy active men. They observed a significant increase in the average rate of lipid oxidation from 0.18 to 0.31 g/min during the first week of Ramadan observance, but by the end of the fast, any effect was much smaller (0.23 g/min). They concluded that a net energy deficit led to a reduction in body mass and that this probably mediated the increase of lipid oxidation seen during submaximal exercise; it seems likely that greater success in eating an optimal amount of food accounted for the decrease of lipid oxidation as Ramadan progressed.

Practical Applications

Moderate exercise will help to conserve lean tissue during fasting, and the rate of fat loss may be further increased by choosing an intensity of effort corresponding to the maximal oxidation of fat and by exercising in a cold environment. The relative metabolism of fat is greater at rest and during low to moderate effort than during intensive exercise [36].

However, evidence on the relationship between fat oxidation and aerobic performance is conflicting. One might anticipate that an increased metabolism of fat would spare glycogen and thus prolong performance. Some authors have indeed found that an increased dietary intake of fat increases fat oxidation and that this leads to an enhanced endurance performance. Thus, in one study, the maximal oxygen intake was increased and the running time to exhaustion with 30 minutes of exercise at 85% of maximal oxygen intake followed by sustained exercise at 75%–80% of maximum was longer after 7 days of a high-fat diet (about 38% of the total energy intake) than after a normal, mixed or carbo-hydrate-rich diet [55]. However, other authors have found no direct relation-ship between the percentage of energy derived from fat oxidation and aerobic performance. Satabin et al. [73] found that in nine trained individuals, fat oxi-dation was increased 1 hour following a high-fat meal, but there was no sig-nificant difference in the average endurance time at 60% of maximal oxygen intake with any of four dietary patterns (fasting, medium-chain triacylglycer-ols, long-chained fatty acids or glucose). The absence of effect upon endur-ance in their investigation probably reflects mainly the short-term nature of the dietary change, but it could also be that the uptake of fatty acids plateaus or that an increased oxidation of fatty acid is not an important factor for endurance [47], except during prolonged exercise at near-maximal power output. Helge et al. [39] investigated the effect of ingesting a very high-fat diet (62% of total energy) in initially sedentary individuals over 7 weeks of endurance training. The time to exhaustion at 81% of the initial maximal oxygen intake increased with training, but the gain in performance was much smaller on the high-fat diet than with a high-carbohydrate diet (65% of total energy).

The performance of aerobic activities lasting less than 10 minutes seems unaf-fected by Ramadan observance [74], and laboratory measures of maximal oxygen intake also remain unchanged [18].

Areas Requiring Further Research

The mechanisms underlying changes in fat oxidation, body composition and/or endurance performance during Ramadan remain poorly understood, particularly in trained subjects. It is still unclear whether short- or long-term increases in fat intake enhance endurance performance, and if so, how. There is thus a need for further investigation of adaptations to combinations of a fat-rich diet with training and intermittent or total fasting, assessing effects on sustained aerobic perfor-mance. There is a specific need to study participants from a wider range of ath-letic disciplines, looking particularly at those engaged in very prolonged events, where body stores of glycogen are likely to become depleted during competition. Finally, there have been almost no observations on the metabolic responses of female athletes during Ramadan and other types of fasting, although there are important sex-related differences in both the magnitude of initial fat reserves and hormonal control mechanisms.

Conclusions

The intermittent fasting of Ramadan can serve as a tactic to increase fat oxidation, and reduce body fat content while maintaining lean tissue mass. The intensity of exercise has a major influence upon changes in fat oxidation during fasting. At low intensities, fat oxidation is increased and endurance performance is enhanced. However, at higher intensities of effort, the metabolic dependence on fat diminishes. Initial fat oxidation is greater in aerobically trained individuals, due to enzymatic adaptations in skeletal muscle. In the categories of athlete studied to date, any changes of lipid metabolism induced by fasting have had little effect upon competitive performance. However, there remains a need for data on the performance of endurance and ultraendurance athletes, where a greater ability to metabolize fatty acids is likely to offset the depletion of glycogen reserves and thus to sustain their performance during periods of fasting.

Key Terms

Acyl-carnitine: A compound formed during the transport of fatty acids across membranes.

Acyl-CoA: A compound formed from carboxylic acids and coenzyme A that serves as an important intermediary stage in the oxidation of fatty acids; energy is liberated as it is converted to acetyl-CoA, and the latter substance can enter the Krebs cycle to yield further energy.

5′ Adenosine monophosphate protein–activated kinase A (AMPK): This enzyme plays a key role in stimulating the oxidation of fatty acids in muscle and liver and in inhibiting lipogenesis.

Adipocyte: Adipocytes are the cells forming white adipose tissue; each cell stores large quantities of triacylglycerol.

Allosteric enzymes: Enzymes that change their configuration after binding with an effector substance.

Beta-oxidation: Beta-oxidation is an aerobic process whereby fatty acids are broken down to acetyl-CoA and can enter the Krebs cycle for the liberation of energy.

Body mass index (BMI): The BMI is an individual's body mass in kilograms (kg) divided by his height in meters squared. It is commonly used as an epidemiological measure of obesity.

cAMP: Cyclic adenosine monophosphate (cAMP) is a second messenger that can transmit a signal arising from stimulation of an epinephrine receptor to the interior of the adipocyte.

Carboxylic acids: Carboxylic acids are long-chained fatty acids that can combine with glycerol to form fats.

Carnitine palmityl transferase: Carnitine palmityl transferase is a protein on the external membrane of mitochondria that catalyses the penetration of fatty acids into their interior.

Coenzyme A: Coenzyme A is a sulphur-containing compound that, among other functions, assists in the transfer of fatty acids across membranes.

Crossover point: The crossover point is the power output at which the energy derived from carbohydrate (CHO) predominates over the energy derived from lipids. Further increases in power output increase CHO utilization but decrease lipid oxidation (Brooks and Mercier [19]).

Dual-photon absorptiometry: This technique uses two x-ray beams of differing energy levels to assess tissue composition.

Enzymes: Enzymes are large biological molecules that speed specific chemical reactions, both inside and outside the body.

Epinephrine: Epinephrine is a neurotransmitter released by the adrenal medulla and by some nerve endings. In terms of metabolism, it stimulates the processes of glycolysis, gluconeogenesis and the mobilization of fat.

Gluconeogenesis: Gluconeogenesis is the synthesis of glucose from molecules such as amino acids, lactate and glycerol; it occurs mainly in the liver.

Glycogen: Glycogen is a complex carbohydrate that provides an energy reserve through stores in muscle and the liver.

Glycogenesis: Glycogenesis is the process of glycogen synthesis from glucose molecules.

Glycogenolysis: Glycogenolysis is the process of breaking down glycogen to provide energy for muscles and the liver; it serves to maintain the blood glucose level.

HDL cholesterol: HDL cholesterol is that component of plasma cholesterol that is associated with good cardiovascular health (the 'good' cholesterol).

Hormone-sensitive lipase: Hormone-sensitive lipase is a key enzyme promoting lipolysis within adipocytes.

Indirect calorimetry: Indirect calorimetry is a technique that estimates the rate of metabolism of fat and carbohydrate from an individual's oxygen consumption and carbon dioxide output.

Insulin: Insulin is a hormone produced by the beta cells of the pancreas. Insulin is concerned primarily with the regulation of blood glucose levels, but its actions also include a stimulation of glycogen and lipid synthesis, an inhibition of protein breakdown and a stimulation of amino acid uptake by muscle cells.

Krebs cycle: The Krebs or citric acid cycle is a sequence of aerobic reactions used by the body to generate energy that is transferred to ATP molecules.

Lipogenesis: Lipogenesis is the process by which acetyl-CoA is converted to fatty acids for storage in the adipocytes and liver.

Lipolysis: Lipolysis is the degradation of triacylglycerols to fatty acids and glycerol; lipolysis is linked to three metabolic processes allowing the phosphorylation of ADP to ATP: β-oxidation, the Krebs cycle and the respiratory chain.

Malonyl-CoA: Malonyl-CoA assists in the transfer of metabolites into the mitochondria; it is also a key compound in the synthesis of long-chained fatty acids.

Maximal fat oxidation (Fat$_{max}$) or lipid maximal oxidation (LIPOX$_{max}$): The intensity of exercise that elicits a maximal oxidation of lipids.

Maximal oxygen intake (V̇O$_{2max}$): The plateau of oxygen consumption reached in a laboratory exercise test where the work rate is increased progressively; it reflects the maximal ability of the circulation to deliver oxygen to the tissues.

Nicotinamide adenine dinucleotide (NADH): During metabolism, NADH serves to carry electrons from one reaction to another.

Perilipin: A molecule that normally protects fat cells from the action of lipases. Perilipin is phosphorylated by catecholamines, as during exercise, this alters the molecular shape, exposing stored fats to the action of lipases.

Protein kinase A: A family of enzymes activated by cAMP that can phosphorylate and thus activate hormone-sensitive lipase.

Protons: Protons are subatomic particles that carry a positive charge.

Respiratory exchange ratio: The respiratory gas exchange ratio is the ratio of carbon dioxide produced to oxygen consumed; it decreases from a value of 1.00 during the metabolism of carbohydrates to 0.7 during the metabolism of fat.

Respiratory quotient: The same as the RER, but measured under steady-state conditions.

Second messenger: Second messengers are molecules that can relay a signal from a surface receptor to target molecules within the interior of a cell.

Trans fat: Trans fats are mainly synthetic in origin and were once widely used in commercial cooking. They are unsaturated fats where the long fatty acid chains are attached in opposing directions, in contrast with the *cis* (natural-type) fat, where the fatty acid chains are arranged in parallel with each other.

Translocase: A generic class of enzymes that assist in the transfer of molecules across membranes.

Transporters: Substances that assist in the transport of molecules across membranes.

Triacylglycerol: Triacylglycerol is an ester (an organic compound) formed from glycerol and three long-chained fatty acids.

Very-low-density lipoprotein (VLDL): VLDL is a form of lipoprotein formed in the liver; it is converted in the blood stream to low-density lipoprotein (one of the 'bad' lipids).

Key Points

1. Fat mobilization depends essentially on the intensity of exercise. During moderate exercises (<40%–50% maximal oxygen intake), fats are the main energy source, but their contribution to overall metabolism diminishes progressively as the intensity of exercise is increased.

2. Trained athletes metabolize a higher proportion of fat than sedentary subjects.
3. The oxidation of fat is increased as the availability of fat is augmented.
4. There seems no direct relationship between the size of fat stores and aerobic performance.
5. The technique of indirect calorimetric can define crossover and maximal fat oxidation points.
6. Ramadan observance and other forms of fasting increase fat oxidation both at rest and during exercise, both in sedentary individuals and in trained subjects, probably with improved endurance performance.
7. Ramadan observance combined with aerobic exercise reduces body mass and body fat content, but has little effect upon fat-free mass. Despite greater fat metabolism, performance does not seem to be modified, at least in events lasting less than 10 minutes.

Questions for Discussion

1. What mechanisms affect fat oxidation at rest under non-fasting conditions?
2. What mechanisms modify the metabolic contribution of fat when exercising under non-fasting conditions?
3. What parameters influence fat oxidation in a resting subject under fasting conditions?
4. What parameters influence fat oxidation when a person is exercising under fasting conditions?
5. What are the assumptions inherent in indirect calorimetry, and what could lead to inaccuracies in use of this technique?
6. What is the likely value of the respiratory gas exchange ratio when the metabolic contribution of fat predominates?
7. What dietary regimen would you recommend during Ramadan? Do you think fat supplementation would enhance an athlete's physical performance?

References

1. Achten J, Gleeson M, Jeukendrup AE. Determination of the exercise intensity that elicits maximal fat oxidation. *Med Sci Sports Exerc* 2002;34:92–97.
2. Achten J, Jeukendrup AE. Maximal fat oxidation during exercise in trained men. *Int J Sports Med* 2003;24:603–608.
3. Achten J, Jeukendrup AE. Optimizing fat oxidation through exercise and diet. *Nutrition* 2004;20:716–727.
4. Adlouni A, Ghalim N, Benslimane A et al. Fasting during Ramadan induces a marked increase in high-density lipoprotein cholesterol and decrease in low-density lipoprotein cholesterol. *Ann Nutr Metab* 1997;41:242–249.
5. Adlouni A, Ghalim N, Saile R et al. Beneficial effect on serum apo AI, apo B and Lp AI levels of Ramadan fasting. *Clin Chim Acta* 1998;23:179–189.

6. Aksungar FB, Eren A, Ure S et al. Effects of intermittent fasting on serum lipids levels, coagulation status and plasma homocysteine levels. *Ann Nutr Metab* 2005;49:77–82.
7. Arepally A, Barnett BP, Patel TT et al. Catheter-directed gastric artery chemical embolization suppresses systemic ghrelin levels in porcine model. *Radiology* 2008;249(1):127–133.
8. Bean A. *The Complete Guide to Sport Nutrition*. A & C Black, London, U.K., 2013.
9. Beltaifa L, Bouguerra R, ben Slama C et al. Food intake and anthropometrical and biological parameters in adult Tunisians during fasting at Ramadan. *East Mediterr Health J* 2002;63:497–501.
10. Berg AH, Combs TP, Du X et al. aCRP30/adiponectin: An adipokine regulating glucose and lipid metabolism. *Trends Endocrinol Metab* 2002;13:84–89.
11. Bergman BC, Brooks GA. Respiratory gas exchange ratios during graded exercise in fed and fasted trained and untrained men. *J Appl Physiol* 1999;86:479–487.
12. Bistrian BR. Clinical use of protein-sparing modified fast. *JAMA* 1978;240(21):2299–2302.
13. Brandou F, Dumortier M, Garandeau P et al. Effects of two-month rehabilitation program on substrate utilization during exercise in obese adolescents. *Diabetes Metab* 2003;29:20–27.
14. Brinkworth GD, Noakes M, Buckley JD et al. Long-term effects of a very-low-carbohydrate weight loss diet compared with an isocaloric low-fat diet after 12 mo. *Am J Clin Nutr* 2009;90(1):23–32.
15. Bouhlel E, Salhi Z, Bouhlel H et al. Effect of Ramadan fasting on fuel oxidation during exercise in trained male rugby players. *Diabetes Metab* 2006;32(6):617–624.
16. Bouhlel E, Zaouali M, Miled A et al. Ramadan fasting and the GH/IGF-1 axis of trained men during submaximal exercise. *Ann Nutr Metab* 2008;52:261–266.
17. Bouhlel E, Denguezli M, Zaouali M et al. Ramadan fasting's effect on plasma, leptin, adiponectin concentrations, and body composition in trained young men. *Int J Sport Nutr Exerc Metab* 2008;18:617–627.
18. Brisswalter J, Bouhlel E, Falola JM et al. Effects of Ramadan intermittent fasting on middle distance running performance in well-trained runners. *Clin J Sport Med* 2011;21:422–427.
19. Brooks GA, Mercier J. Balance of CHO and lipid utilization during exercise: The "crossover" concept. *J Appl Physiol* 1994;76:2253–2261.
20. Cannon B, Nedergaard J. Brown adipose tissue: Function and physiological significance. *Physiol Rev* 2004;84(1):277–359.
21. Cardoso Saldaña GC, Hernández de León S, Gonzalez Zamora GJ et al. Lipid and lipoprotein levels in athletes in different sports disciplines. *Arch Inst Cardiol Mex* 1995;65:229–235.
22. Chennaoui M, Desgorces F, Drogou C et al. Effects of Ramadan fasting on physical performance and metabolic, hormonal, and inflammatory parameters in middle-distance runners. *Appl Physiol Nutr Metab* 2009;34:587–594.
23. Christensen EH, Hansen O. Zur Methodik der respiratorischen Quotient-Bestimmungen in Ruhe und bei Arbeit (methodology for the respiratory quotient determinations at rest and at work). *Skand Arch Physiol* 1939;81(1):137–171.
24. Claus TH, Lowe DB, Liang Y et al. Specific inhibition of hormone-sensitive lipase improves lipid profile while reducing plasma glucose. *J Pharmacol Exp Ther* 2005 Dec;315(3):1396–1402.
25. Cnop M, Havel PJ, Utzschneider KM et al. Relationship of adiponectin to body fat distribution, insulin sensitivity and plasma lipoproteins: Evidence for independent roles of age and sex. *Diabetologia* 2003;46:459–469.
26. Coyle EF, Jeukendrup AE, Oseto MC et al. Low-fat diet alters intramuscular substrates and reduces lipolysis and fat oxidation during exercise. *Am J Physiol Endocrinol Metab* 2001;280:E391–E398.
27. de Garine I, Pollock N. *Social Aspects of Obesity*. Routledge, Abingdon, U.K., 2014.
28. Diller KD. Modelling of bioheat transfer processes at high and low temperatures. In: Cho YI (ed.), *Bioengineering Heat Transfer*. Academic Press, New York, 1992, pp. 157–348.

29. Dohm GL, Tapscott EB, Barakat HA et al. Influence of fasting on glycogen depletion in rats during exercise. *J Appl Physiol* 1983;55:830–833.
30. El Ati J, Beji C, Danguir J. Increased fat oxidation during Ramadan fasting in healthy women: An adaptive mechanism for body-weight maintenance. *Am J Clin Nutr* 1995;62:302–307.
31. FAO/WHO. Joint FAO/WHO expert consultation on fats and fatty acids in human nutrition, Geneva, Switzerland, November 10–14, 2008. WHO, Geneva, Switzerland, 2008.
32. Filaire E, Maso F, Degoutte F et al. Food restriction, performance, psychological state and lipid values in judo athletes. *Int J Sports Med* 2001;22:454–459.
33. Food and Nutrition Board, Institute of Medicine of the National Academies. *Dietary Reference Intakes for Energy, Carbohydrate, Fiber, Fat, Fatty Acids, Cholesterol, Protein, and Amino Acids (Macronutrients)*. National Academies Press, Washington, DC, 2005.
34. Foster W, Larsen K. *Williams Textbook of Endocrinology*, 9th ed. WB Saunders Company, Philadelphia, PA, 2000, pp. 940–943.
35. Friedlander AL, Casazza GA, Horning MA et al. Effects of exercise intensity and training on lipid metabolism in young women. *Am J Physiol* 1998;275:E853–E863.
36. Gleeson M, Greenhaff PL, Maughan RJ. Influence of a 24 h fast on high intensity cycle exercise performance in man. *Eur J Appl Physiol Occup Physiol* 1988;57:653–659.
37. Greenberg AS, Egan JJ, Wek SA et al. Perilipin, a major hormonally regulated adipocyte-specific phosphoprotein associated with the periphery of lipid storage droplets. *J Biol Per Chem* 1991;266(17):11341–11346.
38. Hallak MH, Nomani MZ. Body weight loss and changes in blood lipid levels in normal men on hypo-caloric diets during Ramadan fasting. *Am J Clin Nutr* 1988;48:1197–1210.
39. Helge JW, Richter EA, Kiens B. Interaction of training and diet on metabolism and endurance during exercise in man. *J Physiol* 1996;492(Pt 1):293–306.
40. Horowitz JF, Klein S. Lipid metabolism during endurance exercise. *Am J Clin Nutr* 2000;72:558S–563S.
41. Horowitz JF, Kaufman AE, Fox AK et al. Energy deficit without reducing dietary carbohydrates alters resting carbohydrate oxidation and fatty acid availability. *J Appl Physiol* 2005;98:1612–1618.
42. Howlett KF, Spriet LL, Hargreaves M. Carbohydrate metabolism during exercise in females: Effect of reduced fat availability. *Metabolism* 2001;50:481–487.
43. Ibrahim WH, Habib HM, Jarrar AH et al. Effect of Ramadan fasting on markers of oxidative stress and serum biochemical markers of cellular damage in healthy subjects. *Ann Nutr Metab* 2008;53:175–181.
44. Jeukendrup AE, Saris WH, Wagenmakers AJ. Fat metabolism during exercise: A review—Part II: Regulation of metabolism and the effects of training. *Int J Sports Med* 1998;19:293–302.
45. Kelly DE, Mandarino LJ. Fuel selection in human skeletal muscle in insulin resistance: A reexamination. *Diabetes* 2000;49:677–683.
46. Kiens B, Kristiansen S, Jensen P et al. Membrane associated fatty acid binding protein (FABPpm) in human skeletal muscle is increased by endurance training. *Biochem Biophys Res Commun* 1997;231:463–465.
47. Kiens B, Helge JW. Adaptations to a high fat diet. In: Maughan RJ (ed.), *Nutrition in Sport*. Blackwell Publishing, Oxford, U.K., 2005; pp. 192–202.
48. Klok MD, Jakobsdottir S, Drent ML. The role of leptin and ghrelin in the regulation of food intake and body weight in humans: A review. *Obes Rev* 2007;8(1):21–34.
49. Malenfant P, Joanisse DR, Thériault R et al. Fat content in individual muscle fibers of lean and obese subjects. *Int J Obes Relat Metab Disord* 2001;25(9):1316–1321.
50. Manetta J, Brun JF, Perez-Martin A et al. Fuel oxidation during exercise in middle-aged men: Role of training and glucose disposal. *Med Sci Sports Exerc* 2002;33:423–429.
51. Manetta J, Brun JF, Maimoun L et al. Effect of training on the GH/IGF-1 axis during exercise in middle-aged men: Relationship to glucose homeostasis. *Am J Physiol* 2002;283:E929–E936.

52. Manetta J, Brun JF, Prefaut C et al. Substrate oxidation during exercise at moderate and hard intensity in middle-aged and young athletes vs sedentary men. *Metabolism* 2005;54:1411–1419.

53. Matisson FH, Grundy SM. Comparison of effects of dietary saturated, monounsaturated and polyunsaturated fatty acids on plasma lipids and lipoproteins in man. *J Lipid Res* 1985;26:194–202.

54. Montain SJ, Hopper MK, Coggan AR et al. Exercise metabolism at different time intervals after a meal. *J Appl Physiol* 1991;70:882–888.

55. Muoio DM, Leddy JJ, Horvath PJ et al. Effect of dietary fat on metabolic adjustments to maximal VO_2 and endurance in runners. *Med Sci Sports Exerc* 1994;26:81–88.

56. O'Hara WJ, Allen G, Shephard RJ. Loss of body weight and fat during exercise in a cold chamber. *J Appl Physiol* 1977;37:205–218.

57. Oliver JM, Lambert BS, Martin SE et al. Predicting football players' dual-energy x-ray absorptiometry body composition using standard anthropometric measures. *J Athl Training* 2012;47(3):257–263.

58. Otvos L, Haspinger E, La Russa F et al. Design and development of a peptide-based adiponectin receptor agonist for cancer treatment. *BMC Biotechnol* 2011;11:90.

59. Perello M, Scott MM, Sakata I et al. Functional implications of limited leptin receptor and ghrelin receptor coexpression in the brain. *J Comp Neurol* 2012;520(2):281–294.

60. Pérez-Martin A, Dumortier M, Raynaud E et al. Balance of substrate oxidation during submaximal exercise in lean and obese people. *Diabetes Metab (Paris)* 2001;27:466–474.

61. Péronnet F, Massicotte D. Table of nonprotein respiratory quotient: An update. *Can J Sports Sci* 1991;16:23–29.

62. Phillips SM, Green HG, Tarnopolsky MA et al. Effects of training duration on substrate turnover and oxidation during exercise. *J Appl Physiol* 1996;81:2182–2191.

63. Phinney SD. Ketogenic diets and physical performance. *Nutr Metab* 2004;1:2 (on-line publication).

64. Pincivero DM, Bompa TO. A physiological review of American football. *Sports Med* 1997;23(4):247–260.

65. Rahman M, Rashid M, Basher S et al. Improved serum HDL cholesterol profile among Bangladeshi male students during Ramadan fasting. *East Mediterr Health J* 2004;10:131–137.

66. Ramadan J, Telahoun G, Al-Zaid NS et al. Responses to exercise, fluid, and energy balances during Ramadan in sedentary and active males. *Nutrition* 1999;15:735–739.

67. Randle PJ, Garland PB, Hales CN et al. The glucose fatty-acid cycle: Its role in insulin sensitivity and the metabolic disturbances of diabetes mellitus. *Lancet* 1963;1(7285):785–789.

68. Roepstorff C, Steffensen CH, Madsen M et al. Gender differences in substrate utilization during submaximal exercise in endurance-trained subjects. *Am J Physiol* 2002;282:E435–E447.

69. Roky R, Houti I, Moussamih S et al. Physiological and chronobiological changes during Ramadan intermittent fasting. *Ann Nutr Metab* 2004;48:296–303.

70. Romijn JA, Klein S, Coyle EF et al. Strenuous endurance training increases lipolysis and triglyceride-fatty acid cycling at rest. *J Appl Physiol* 1993;75:108–113.

71. Romijn JA, Coyle EF, Sidossis LS et al. Relationship between fatty acid delivery and fatty acid oxidation during strenuous exercise. *J Appl Physiol* 1995;79:1939–1945.

72. Saltin B, Gollnick B. Skeletal muscle adaptability: Significance for metabolism and performance. In: Peachy LD, Adrian RH, Geiger SR (eds.), *Handbook of Physiology*, Section 10. American Physiological Society, Bethesda, MD, 1983; pp. 555–631.

73. Satabin P, Portero P, Defer G et al. Metabolic and hormonal responses to lipid and carbohydrate diets during exercise in man. *Med Sci Sports Exerc* 1987;19:218–223.

74. Shephard RJ. The impact of Ramadan performance upon athletic performance. *Nutrients* 2012;4:491–505.

75. Shephard RJ, Johnson N. Effects of physical activity upon the liver. *Eur J Appl Physiol* 2015;115(1):1–46.

76. Sidossis LS, Wolfe RR. Glucose and insulin-induced inhibition of fatty acid oxidation: The glucose-fatty acid cycle reversed. *Am J Physiol* 1996;270:E733–E738.
77. Stannard SR, Thompson MW. The effect of participation in Ramadan on substrate selection during submaximal cycling exercise. *J Sci Med Sport* 2008;11:510–517.
78. van Loon LJC, Koopman R, Stegen JHCH et al. Intramyocellular lipids from an important substrate source during moderate intensity exercise in endurance-trained males in a fasted state. *J Physiol* 2003;553:611–625.
79. Weltman A, Pritzlaff CJ, Wideman L et al. Intensity of acute exercise does not affect serum leptin concentrations in young men. *Med Sci Sports Exerc* 2000 Sep;32(9):1556–1561.
80. Ziaee V, Razaei M, Ahmadinejad Z et al. The changes of metabolic profile and weight during Ramadan fasting. *Singapore Med J* 2006;47:409–414.
81. Ziegler PJ, Nelson JA, Jonnalagadda SS. Nutritional and physiological status of U.S. national figure skaters. *Int J Sport Nutr* 1999;9(4):345–360.

Further Reading

Berg JM, Tymoczo JL, Stryer L. *Biochemistry*, 5th edn. W.H. Freeman, New York, 2002.
Jeukendrup A, Gleeson M. Dehydration and its effects on performance. In: *Sport Nutrition. An Introduction to Energy Production*. 2nd edn., Jeukendrup A, Gleeson M (eds.). Human Kinetics, Champaign, IL, 2010; pp. 397–488.
Shephard RJ. *Physiology and Biochemistry of Exercise*. Praeger, New York, 1982.

5

Protein Metabolism during Dietary Restriction

Roy J Shephard

Learning Objectives

1. To review the normal protein needs of the body
2. To understand mechanisms regulating anabolic and catabolic activity
3. To learn the impact of dietary restrictions upon protein intake and serum levels of protein, urea, uric acid and glucose
4. To consider what changes in body composition develop over the course of dietary restrictions
5. To determine practical implications for athletes, coaches and trainers

Normal Protein Needs of the Body

The body normally needs good quality protein (containing an appropriate proportion of the 'essential' amino acids that the body cannot synthesize) in an amount that depends on many factors, including the person's size, their level of habitual physical activity, the ability to satisfy the energy demands of such activity from carbohydrate and fat stores, and the added energy demands of normal growth, pregnancy, lactation, and the hypertrophy of muscle during athletic training and tissue repair following illness or injury [41,63,64,96,94].

Nutritional Recommendations

The standard U.S. and Canadian nutritional recommendation for adults aged 19–70 years is a daily protein intake of 0.8 g/kg of body mass [15]. This quantity of protein is adequate for a sedentary person, but is insufficient for competitive athletes [96]. Their needs are particularly great if the individual concerned is undergoing vigorous athletic training and/or protein is being metabolized to maintain energy balance [15,64,96]. Since protein is essentially the only source of nitrogen in the diet, the precise body requirement can be assessed by undertaking nitrogen balance studies in the laboratory. If the protein intake is meeting the requirements of the body, then the amount of nitrogen ingested in the food equals that excreted from the body; account must be taken not only of nitrogen losses in the urine and feces but also of substantial quantities of urea excreted in the sweat [31]. Lemon has suggested that endurance athletes need about 1.2–1.4 g/kg of protein per day and that strength athletes require about 1.4–1.8 g/kg [63,64]. Such requirements do not pose a major problem for the average North American, even during moderate dietary restriction, including the intermittent fasting of Ramadan, since the typical normal diet contains a substantial excess of protein. However, care must be undertaken to get an appropriate balance of foods if reliance is placed on vegetable sources of protein either habitually (as in those following a vegan diet) or during a specific type of religious fast that excludes animal protein [102]. Those arranging the diet of an athlete should also guard against an excessive protein intake. An excess of dietary protein increases the loss of calcium in the urine and also predisposes a person to kidney stones. The maximum daily intake probably should not exceed 2.5 g/kg [15].

Nutritional Deficiency

If the diet provides insufficient energy to meet metabolic expenditures, the body will draw upon its own store of nutrients, with a progressive depletion of body fat and a wasting of the muscles. Such a situation is likely during severe dietary restriction or total fasting. During the observance of Ramadan, a sedentary person can usually meet any daytime energy deficit by drawing upon body fat stores. This could be more difficult for athletes. They have much higher energy requirements than sedentary people, and their initial reserves of body fat are much smaller; in events where they must sustain a high rate of energy expenditure for long periods, they may thus be unable to maintain their energy balance simply by an increase of fat metabolism.

Dietary Timing

The timing of protein intake may also be a critical issue, particularly during intermittent fasting, as in the observance of Ramadan. There are growing indications that an increased appropriately-timed peak of blood levels of amino acids is important to maximize the response to a given training regimen. The ingestion of 20 g of good quality protein or amino acids immediately before or up to 3 hours after a bout of strength training seems to facilitate the development of a positive nitrogen balance [21,47,73,83,85,97,98]. Some authors have suggested that the protein is best taken immediately following exercise [48,97], although others have reported benefit if food has been ingested either before or as late as 3 hours following training [73,99]. The muscle glycogen depletion that is likely in a fasting athlete can also compromise expression of the genes needed for hypertrophy in the active muscles [29]. If feeding is only permitted at certain times of the day, as during Ramadan, the timing of training sessions may thus need to be changed to mesh with feeding schedules [49]. For those who are observing Ramadan, training is best undertaken either in the evening (before or after sunset) or following the morning meal (around sunrise) [21,22,56,88].

Essential Amino Acids

As many as 21 amino acids are required for the synthesis of body proteins, but some of the 21 can be manufactured from other substrates. An 'essential' or 'indispensible' amino acid is one that cannot be synthesized in the body and thus must be provided in the diet in adequate quantities in order for protein synthesis to proceed. Adults have traditionally been said to require 10 such amino acids, with growing children also requiring cysteine- and/or sulphur-containing amino acids, tyrosine and/or aromatic amino acids, and arginine. One recent assessment by Dr. Vernon Young set the respective daily needs of a sedentary adult (per kg of body mass) as follows: phenylalanine and/or tyrosine (39 mg), valine (20 mg), threonine (15 mg), tryptophan (6 mg), isoleucine (23 mg), methionine and/or cystine (13 mg), leucine (40 mg), and lysine (30 mg). The needs of athletes have not been quantified, but seem likely to be about twice as large as those of sedentary individuals.

Dietary proteins are ascribed a nutritional quality, based on their ability to provide an appropriate mix of amino acids. Meat generally has a high nutritional quality, and athletes from developed countries who eat large quantities of meat are unlikely to be deficient in essential amino acids. Problems are more likely in those from poor countries, where meat is in short supply, and among those who are vegetarians. Many vegetable products fail to provide all of the necessary amino acids, but as Wolff and associates have emphasized, combinations such as corn and beans, soybeans and rice, or red beans and rice can offer an appropriate balance of the needed amino acids.

Mechanisms Regulating Anabolic and Catabolic Activity

Hormonal Regulators

A multiplicity of hormones regulates the processes of anabolism and catabolism, including glucagon, catecholamines, cortisol, growth hormone (GH), thyroid hormones and atrial natriuretic peptide (ANP). GH, catecholamines and the thyroid hormones all have an anabolic effect, contributing to the hypertrophy of skeletal muscle, boosting the size of existing fibres, and stimulating the accretion of protein in the satellite precursor cells.

Training Response

Training often requires some remodeling of existing tissues, but given an appropriate physical stimulus such as resistance training and an adequate concentration of amino acids in the blood, the synthesis of new protein exceeds the rate of protein degradation involved in tissue remodeling, and muscle hypertrophy occurs. The primary regulators of anabolism are insulin and insulin-like growth factor 1 (IGF-1), and the addition of glucose to a protein meal helps anabolic activity by increasing the secretion of insulin. Cortisol has a negative impact upon anabolism and favours catabolism. The cortisol/insulin ratio has to be less than 4 for protein synthesis to occur; this explains the importance of ensuring that amino acid and glucose concentrations peak around the time of training [84]. Commonly, the cortisol/insulin ratio is optimal in the period 3–7 hours following a meal [66].

Energy Deficiency during Exercise

The muscle, liver and other organs can detect the decline in energy availability that occurs when a person is exercising, and the immediate response is an increased breakdown of glycogen stored in the muscle and the liver (glycogenolysis) and depot fat (lipolysis). Glucagon and catecholamines stimulate glycogenolysis in the liver and muscle; glucagon is the more effective stimulus at rest, but norepinephrine levels are the most important regulating factor during exercise [60]. Lipolysis is also increased during exercise, through a combination of the stimulation of beta-adrenoreceptors by catecholamines and a suppression of the action of insulin and alpa-2 adrenoreceptors [59]. If the combined effects of glycolysis and lipolysis fail to meet the energy demands of exercise as activity continues, then the process of gluconeogenesis begins, with the hepatic formation of glucose from amino acids, lactate, pyruvate and glycerol. The breakdown of protein and amino acids is stimulated by the actions of glucagon, cortisol and catecholamines, and the suppression of insulin activity [42].

Severe Dietary Restriction

Severe dieting or total fasting depletes glycogen stores, so that the body begins to meet glucose needs by gluconeogenesis early during a bout of exercise. However, the demand for glucose and thus the rate of depletion of lean tissue mass depends on the individual's training status; well-trained individuals have a higher capacity for meeting their metabolic needs by lipid metabolism. The intensity of exercise is another important variable; the proportion of energy met from fat oxidation is maximal when exercising at about 70% of maximal oxygen intake (Chapter 4).

Regulation during Ramadan Observance

Changes in blood levels of the metabolic regulators seem to be quite small during Ramadan observance [86]. Bogdan et al. [16] observed no change in either

circulating concentrations or diurnal rhythm of GH secretion in a group of physicians during Ramadan [16]. Perhaps because of alterations in the timing of meals
and/or patterns of sleeping, a study of non-athletes in contrast showed a displacement of the normal circadian rhythm of cortisol secretion (with peak blood levels of this hormone shifting from morning toward evening). Nevertheless, the
response of cortisol secretion to corticotropin remained unaltered [13]. Our empirical data from rugby players who were observing Ramadan showed no changes
in concentrations of plasma GH, IGF or insulin-like growth factor binding protein 3 during Ramadan observance [18]. Likewise, we saw no change in resting concentrations of the fat-regulating hormones leptin and adiponectin during
Ramadan [19]. Middle-distance runners might be thought relatively vulnerable to
glycogen depletion and gluconeogenic catabolism, but a study of such a population showed an unaltered testosterone/cortisol ratio during Ramadan [27], implying that there had been no change in the stability of their lean tissue. However, the
runners did show a doubling of interleukin-6 (IL-6) concentrations, perhaps in
an attempt to mobilize muscle carbohydrate from diminishing muscle stores [27].
There were significant increases in blood levels of thyroid-stimulating hormone
and free thyroxine (T4) in a group of judokas during Ramadan [25].

Prolonged Energy Deficit

Prolonged periods of energy deficit are well recognized as leading to reductions
in basal levels of insulin, leptin, IGF-1 and triiodothyronine (T3) (the active form
of the thyroid hormone) [78]. Conservation of lean tissue is more likely if an
energy deficit is created by an increase of physical activity and moderate dietary
restriction than if it is based on dieting alone (Chapter 2).

Dietary Restrictions, Protein Intake and Catabolism

Dietary Composition during Prolonged Dieting

If a sedentary person is seeking to reduce body fat by restricting the daily energy
intake, it might be thought helpful to increase the percentage of carbohydrate that
is ingested, in order to minimize the use of protein in maintaining blood glucose
levels. However, carbohydrate ingestion stimulates the secretion of insulin and thus
appetite, making it difficult to adhere to the proposed diet, and it also encourages
the muscles to consume carbohydrate when exercising. Thus, some nutritionists find
advantages in a high-fat diet. This encourages the activation of fat-metabolizing
enzymes in muscle. It also suppresses insulin secretion, encouraging lipolysis (the
breakdown of fat stores), and because fat is digested more slowly than carbohydrate, it seems easier to adhere to a restricted diet with a high fat content.

Controversy regarding this approach continues. Some authors find it effica-
cious [89–65,40], but others question its long-term efficacy [8,51], and some have
condemned it as increasing the secretion of C-reactive protein and thus predisposing to future cardiovascular disease [52].

Dietary Options during Ramadan Observance

The sedentary person who is observing Ramadan can usually ingest sufficient food during the hours of darkness to maintain a positive energy balance, and unless they are planning to use Ramadan as a help to fat loss, there is no specific need to change their normal food choices.

Some athletes may also find it possible to maintain an energy balance during Ramadan (Chapter 2), but those with very high daily energy expenditures (such as participants in the Tour de France, where requirements reach 23–26 MJ/day [100]) would find it very difficult to ingest this amount of food at night. In theory, a reduction of food intake during Ramadan could deplete the athlete's glycogen stores. Thus, to maintain a normal performance during very prolonged exercise, the competitor would need to increase fat metabolism and/or boost blood glucose levels through gluconeogenesis, with a progressive depletion of tissue protein [75]. There would then be a decrease in body and lean tissue mass, potentially an increase in blood urea, and a shift in the balance of activity between anabolic and catabolic hormones. As lean tissue mass was decreased, one would also anticipate some deterioration of performance, particularly in events requiring muscular strength, and there would be a poorer response to any resistance training that was undertaken.

Determining Dietary Composition

Both the amount and the composition of dietary intake can be estimated by having subjects record the food that they eat and the sizes of individual portions over a period of at least a week, preferably with the help of a nutritionist. A computer program such as Microsoft's Bilnut is then used to convert this information into estimates of the quantities of protein, carbohydrate and fat ingested. Observers must rely on subjects remembering to record all food, drinks and snacks that they have consumed and assessing accurately the portion sizes that are assumed by the computer program. The absolute accuracy of data is questionable, but comparisons between Ramadan and non-fasting periods in the same individual are likely to have a reasonable validity.

Empirical Data for Ramadan

Table 5.1 summarizes available information on modifications of food intake adopted by sedentary and athletic subjects during Ramadan. In general, observations made during Ramadan have been compared with data obtained before and/or after the celebration, without recruitment of any control comparison group. A few studies have compared data between individuals who observed Ramadan and others who did not, but where the non-fasters have been drawn from the same athletic milieu, this is not entirely satisfactory as a basis of comparison, since the feeding arrangements for an entire athletic team may have been changed to accommodate the needs of those who were engaged in daytime fasting.

TABLE 5.1 Influence of Ramadan Observance on Total Energy Intake and Percentage Attributable to Protein, Carbohydrate and Fat in Sedentary and Athletic Subjects

Subjects	Total Energy Intake	Protein	CHO	Fat	Author
Sedentary					
32 healthy men	No significant change	+0.4%	+1.4%	−0.7%	Adlouni et al. [1]
163 male, 102 female university students	No change in 50%, loss in 32%, increase in 14%	Increased			Afifi et al. [2]
38 hyperlipidemic men	Decreased 1.2 MJ/day (about 12%)				Afrasiabi et al. [3]
57 university women	Decreased 6.5% (not significant)	No change	No change	No change	Al-Hourani and Atoum [5]
Adult men	Decreased				Angel and Schwarz [6]
19 men, 6 women	Decreased 5.3% (not significant)	−28%	−5.7%	No significant change	Barkia et al. [11]
20 adults	Decreased 10%	+12%	−8.3%	+13.7%	Beltaifa et al. [12]
9 sedentary men	Decreased 4%	−13%	−13%	No significant change	Chiha [28]
16 women	No change	+3%	+8.1%	−8.8%	El Ati et al. [32]
91 men and women dieters	Decreased 15.7% (M), 28.4% (F)				Fakhrzadeh et al. [33]
15 young men	Increased	Small increase	Small increase	Small increase	Frost and Pirani [38]
34 men, 96 women	Increased 20% in those aged 18–25 years, no significant increase in older subjects	+32% (young), +15% (older subjects)	+9% (young), no change (older subjects)	+34% (young), +14% (older subjects)	Gharbi et al. [43]
42 young men	Decreased 7% (not significant)	No change	No change	No change	Grantham et al. [44]
12 men, 9 women	Decreased				Husain et al. [50]
10 healthy men	Decreased 3.6 MJ/day (about 36%)				Khan and Kharzak [54]
67 men, 48 women	Decreased 19%				Larijani et al. [58]

(Continued)

TABLE 5.1 (*Continued*) Influence of Ramadan Observance on Total Energy Intake and Percentage Attributable to Protein, Carbohydrate and Fat in Sedentary and Athletic Subjects

Subjects	Total Energy Intake	Protein	CHO	Fat	Author
24 male, 31 female adolescents	No change in males, increased 21% in females	+11.2%	+36.5%	−17.6%	Morilla et al. [74]
51 boys, 66 girls	Decreased 19% (boys), 23% (girls)	No change	Decreased	Decreased	Poh et al. [81]
Athletes					
9 male rugby players	Decreased 4.8 MJ/day (−28%)	+0.2% (not significant)	−8.8%	+8.1%	Bouhlel et al. [18,17]
15 elite judokas	No change	No significant change	No significant change	No significant change	Chaouachi et al. [23]
8 middle-distance runners	No change				Chennaoui et al. [27]
12 soccer players	Decreased 14%	Decreased 7%, also decreased % of total energy intake	No change	Tendency to 13% increase, increased percentage of total energy intake	Chiha [28]
59 male soccer players	No significant change	+2.5%	−3%	No change	Maughan et al. [69]
19 male adolescent soccer players	Increased energy intake during final week of Ramadan	−1.8%	−8.8%	+10.6%	Meckel et al. [71]
12 female taekwondo athletes	Decreased 30%				Memari et al. [72]
8 cyclists	Decreased			Increased lipid oxidation	Stannard and Thompson [93]
4 male soccer teams (64 fasting, 36 non-fasting controls)	No changes relative to controls	Small increase of protein intake in experimental and control groups			Zerguini et al. [105]

Sedentary Subjects

In general, sedentary subjects have shown a trend to small decreases of total energy intake during Ramadan, although often these changes have not been statistically significant. Five studies showed large decreases of food intake, but in some if not all of these trials, this was the result of deliberate dieting [1,2,43,74]. In three trials food intake was increased [52,54], with a particularly large surge in younger adults [74]; possibly, this reflects communal feasting during and toward the end of Ramadan. In studies where the relative proportions of protein, carbohydrate and fat intake were reported, changes were generally small and varied considerably from one study to another; no evidence of a common pattern of dietary adaptation was apparent.

Athletes

Information on the eating behaviour of athletes during Ramadan is quite limited, and it is unclear how far any of the reported changes reflect personal choices and how far specific nutritional advice was given by coaches and trainers. Four studies reported a lower total energy intake during Ramadan, and in three of these trials, the decrease was quite large [17,18,72,75]. However, in four other reports, there was no change in total energy intake, and in one study, food consumption was increased during the final week of Ramadan. Possible factors leading to these divergent results include the level of competition, the total magnitude of energy expenditures during events and training, and cultural differences in the way Ramadan is celebrated in different parts of the world. Changes of protein intake during Ramadan were generally small and statistically insignificant, but in the three studies where this was reported, there was a decreased intake of carbohydrate, with an increased consumption of fat in two of these studies. Bouhlel et al. [17] reported that the daily protein intake of their 9 rugby players decreased from an initially satisfactory value of 1.45 to 1.05 g/kg during Ramadan; although the contribution of protein ingestion to total energy intake remained unchanged at about 11.6%, the latter value would be undesirably low, even if the group remained in energy balance. In another group of 12 junior soccer players and 8 sedentary individuals, the contribution of ingested protein to total energy intake decreased by 7.6% during Ramadan, and the total daily protein intake dropped slightly, from an initially low value of 1.04 g/kg to an even less satisfactory 0.97 g/kg [28]. In contrast, a third group of 59 competitive soccer players tended to increase their protein intake by 2.5% during Ramadan, reaching an average intake of 1.76 g/kg/day [69], a figure that would be sufficient to sustain both anabolism and some gluconeogenesis.

In some studies, it is difficult to reconcile the estimated changes of energy intake with changes in body composition, emphasizing the difficulty in drawing conclusions from simple dietary records. Thus, in our study of rugby players [17], the cumulative decrease of energy intake over the 29 days of Ramadan averaged 136 MJ. Other factors being equal, this should have equated to a 3.5 kg loss of fat, but perhaps because of some slackening of training or an underreporting of food intake, the actual decrease in body fat content was only 1.8 kg, with no significant change in the estimated lean tissue mass. Likewise, a group of 12 female tae-kwondo players reported a 30% decrease of energy intake over Ramadan, but the decrease of body mass was only 2.9% [72].

Changes in Plasma Amino Acid and Protein Concentrations

A decrease of plasma protein concentration during fasting might be thought to offer an early warning of a developing negative nitrogen balance, but this measure is somewhat fallible during a fast such as Ramadan, where water intake is also restricted, particularly if data are collected in the afternoon, since short-term haemoconcentration could mask a decrease in the total circulating volume of protein [70].

Studies of subjects who had fasted for 24–36 hours showed decreased plasma levels of the branch-chained amino acids leucine, isoleucine and valine [68], and infusion of radioactively marked leucine in subjects fasted for 4 days demonstrated an increased metabolism of this amino acid [37]. If glycogen stores are compromised by a combination of fasting and lactation, there is also evidence of an increased metabolism of amino acids, particularly alanine and glutamine [80,94]. Any effect of this type from the repeated 12–15 hours fasts of Ramadan seems quite limited. Two studies of sedentary subjects found no significant change of plasma protein concentrations during Ramadan [12,82]. Another study of healthy but non-athletic individuals (12 men and 12 women) found no change in total protein, but for reasons that were not explained, blood levels of homocysteine (an amino acid on the pathway linking methionine and cysteine) showed an 11% decrease in men and a 21% decrease in women [4]. Another study of 32 women and 7 men found a 15% decrease of serum protein concentrations by the 28th day of Ramadan [39].

In athletes, plasma proteins may decrease, particularly if athletes do not take the precaution of sustaining total energy and protein intake during Ramadan. Our observations on a small group of rugby players who reported decreased intakes of both protein and total energy demonstrated a small increase of serum protein during the first week of Ramadan (7%), but a substantial decrease (19%) by the fourth week [17,18]. Studies of blood chemistry in judoka also showed a progressive decrease of serum protein, with a statistically significant diminution of 8% by the second week of Ramadan and slightly greater decrease by the fourth week of fasting [23]; in this group, neither the reported overall energy intake nor protein intake was decreased during Ramadan. This paper also noted a host of small changes in individual serum constituents; although statistically significant, most figures remained within clinical limits, and it is difficult to discern any consistent pattern in responses [23]. Ramadan et al. [82] found no changes of plasma protein levels in a small group of moderately active individuals during Ramadan observance.

Changes in Serum of Urea and Uric Acid

As proteins and amino acids are metabolized, increased concentrations of the nitrogen-containing breakdown products urea and uric acid are found in the serum. Increases as large as 10% have sometimes been seen during Ramadan [35,46,77,79,86], but this is not always the case. A study of 32 women and 7 men found no significant change in serum uric acid levels [39], and Ramadan et al. found no changes in serum urea or uric acid in either sedentary or active individuals during the intermittent fasting of Ramadan [82]. Any increases of urea and uric acid concentration could certainly imply an increase of gluconeogenesis, but the dehydration and alterations of renal function associated with fasting seem more likely causes [86,79].

Changes in Blood Glucose

A final indication of the need for gluconeogenesis would be a decrease of serum glucose readings (see Chapter 3). Some reports have indeed noted a decrease of fasting glucose concentrations during Ramadan [58,35,39], but such observations seem to have been more common in sedentary individuals than in athletes [10]. In our study of 9 rugby players, we collected blood samples in the afternoon, at least 12 hours after the previous meal. Nevertheless, both resting and immediate post-exercise serum glucose concentrations remained unchanged during Ramadan [18]. Likewise Beltaifa et al. [12] reported no Ramadan-related change of resting blood glucose levels in 20 non-athletic adults.

Changes in Body Composition with Dietary Restriction

Sedentary subjects have little practical difficulty in ingesting the amounts of food needed for energy balance during the hours of darkness, so no changes of body composition would be anticipated from the intermittent fasting of Ramadan observance unless the individual concerned was using the celebration in a deliberate attempt to reduce body fat. In contrast, athletes often increase their metabolism of body fat during Ramadan in order to meet the energy needs of the body [11,58], and there is also a possibility of an increase in gluconeogenesis, with a decrease in lean tissue mass [11,18,19], particularly among participants in ultraendurance sports. Such changes are exacerbated with longer periods of dieting.

Sedentary Subjects

Relatively few empirical studies of diet and body composition have focused specifically upon changes induced by endogenous protein metabolism during Ramadan observance and other types of dieting [87,90]. Available data for Ramadan are summarized in Table 5.2.

TABLE 5.2 Changes of Body Composition during Ramadan, as Seen in Sedentary and Athletic Subjects

Subjects	Body Mass	Body Fat	Lean Mass	Author
Sedentary				
32 healthy men	Decreased 2.6%			Adlouni et al. [1]
38 hyperlipidemic men	No change	No change	No change	Afrasiabi et al. [3]
57 university women	Decreased 1.0%	No change except the first week of Ramadan	No change	Al-Hourani and Atoum [5]
20 adults	No change		No change	Beltaifa et al. [12]
11 fighter pilots	Decreased 2.7%			Bigard et al. [14]
9 men	Decreased 1.6%	No change	No change	Chiha [28]
18 healthy men	Decrease in 11/18			Ch'ng et al. [30]
16 women	No change	No change	No change	El Ati et al. [32]
50 men and 41 women	Decrease 1.8% in men No change in women	No change of waist circumference in men, decrease in women		Fakhrzadeh et al. [33]
15 men, 26 women	No change			Finch et al. [36]
15 young men	Increase			Frost and Pirani [38]
7 men, 32 women	No change			Furuncuoglu et al. [39]
42 young men	No change	No change	No change	Grantham et al. [44]
12 men, 9 women	Decreased, females > males	Decreased, females > males		Husain et al. [50]
10 healthy men	Decreased 3.2 kg (4%)			Khan and Kharzak [54]
20 healthy adults	No change			Krifi et al. [57]
16 men, 8 women	No change			Maislos et al. [67]
7 sedentary men	No change	No change		Ramadan et al. [82]
46 young men	Small increase of body mass after Ramadan			Siddiqui et al. [92]
7 men, 1 woman	Decrease 2.7%	Decreased 2.33 kg (10%)	Decreased 0.5 kg (not significant)	Sweileh et al. [95]
21 men, 17 women	No change	No change		Yucel et al. [104]
81 medical students	Decrease			Ziaee et al. [106]

(*Continued*)

TABLE 5.2 (*Continued*) Changes of Body Composition during Ramadan, as Seen in Sedentary and Athletic Subjects

Subjects	Body Mass	Body Fat	Lean Mass	Author
Athletes				
9 rugby players	Decreased 2.2%	Decreased 7.5%	Decreased 1.8% (not significant)	Bouhlel et al. [17]
18 runners (9 fasting)	No change	No change		Brisswalter et al. [20]
15 male judokas	Decreased 2%	Decreased 0.65 kg		Chaouachi et al. [23]
8 male middle-distance runners	No change	No change		Chennaoui et al. [27]
12 athletes	Decreased 1.4%	Decreased 8.8%	No change	Chiha [28]
18 power and sprint athletes	No change			Karli et al. [53]
59 soccer players	Decreased 0.7 kg			Maughan et al. [69]
12 female taekwondo athletes	Decreased 2.9%			Memari et al. [72]
6 active men	No change	No change		Ramadan et al. [82]
15 athletic men	No change	No change	No change	Asl [7]
8 cyclists	Decreased 1.8%	No significant change	No change	Stannard and Thompson [93]
64 fasting, 36 non-fasting male soccer players	Decreased 0.7%			Zerguini et al. [105]

Methods of Assessing Lean Body Mass

The simplest method of assessing body mass, often used in dietary studies, is to estimate body fat either by underwater weighing or the measurement of skinfold thicknesses and then to determine lean tissue mass as the difference between total body mass and fat mass. However, this approach may cause problems if dehydration causes a decrease in total body mass. The volume of lean tissue in the limbs can also be determined anthropometrically, from measurements of limb circumferences, bone diameters and skinfold estimates of the thickness of the superficial layer of fat. Another simple approach is the use of bio-impedance equipment to estimate body fat; this method is also vulnerable to changes in body hydration. Other more sophisticated options include dual-photon absorptiometry and computed tomography. Dual-photon absorptiometry uses two low-dose x-ray beams with differing levels of energy; after computerized analysis, a detailed image is provided of body structures in the path of the beam. Computed tomography is also based upon x-irradiation; a computer program reconstructs a cross-sectional image of the underlying structures, based upon the absorption of x-rays; this approach was used by Yucel and colleagues in their studies of changes in body composition during Ramadan [104].

Many groups of sedentary subjects have shown no change of body mass; where body mass has decreased, this has typically reflected a desire to decrease body fat rather than an inability to eat sufficient food to maintain energy balance. Fighter pilots were one group showing a 2.7% decrease of body mass [14]; possibly, these men were more active than many of the other populations that were examined. Only two sedentary groups reported a consistent decrease in body fat content [50,95], and none of seven trials found any significant decrease in lean tissue mass. Perhaps the most reliable information came from a computed tomography study of 38 non-athletic volunteers; this found no changes of body mass or body fat content during Ramadan [104].

Athletes

Among the studies of athletes, several investigators have examined teams of soccer and rugby players, but none have examined participants in ultraendurance events; 7 of 12 trials found a decrease of body mass during Ramadan, but only 3 of 8 studies found a statistically significant decrease of body fat, and none showed any significant change of lean tissue mass. Judoka ingested a consistent 1.6 g/kg of protein over the course of Ramadan, but nevertheless trended to a 0.6 kg decrease of lean tissue mass [23,26].

Practical Implications

With any form of dieting, the potential for loss of lean tissue is a concern. Sedentary individuals who restrict their energy intake in order to lose body fat should ensure that a part of their energy imbalance is created by physical activity, should initiate regular resistance activity to maintain their muscle mass and should see that their diet still contains at least the minimum recommended amount of protein. Anorexia nervosa is potentially dangerous to life, with a heavy protein loss, and it requires psychiatric treatment.

Competitors who are 'making weight' or attempting to improve their physical appearance also need to ensure that they are ingesting the protein requirement appropriate to their athletic discipline. Burke [21] and Shephard [91] have offered a number of practical suggestions to maintain the health and performance of Muslim athletes who find themselves competing during the month of Ramadan, although the benefits of many of the proposed tactics have yet to be tested experimentally. Some of the immediate effects of Ramadan observance can be countered by arranging training sessions and competitions early in the morning or after sunset, when the interval between feeding and activity is similar to that for an athlete who is not observing Ramadan. This solution is often adopted when competitions involve predominantly athletes from Arab nations, but it has not been accepted for international competitions.

Because of dehydration and thus a decrease of blood volume, the circulatory load imposed by a given training plan may be increased slightly during Ramadan [105]. Other disincentives to maintaining a full training regimen at this season include increased sleepiness, feelings of fatigue and higher ratings of perceived exertion [61]. Many of the general sedentary population and their employers see a reduction in their work load and (or) daytime napping as appropriate tactics to counteract the effects of hunger and thirst [27]. Some athletes also opt to reduce the duration [101], intensity, or volume of their training programme [24], although this choice may not only lead to a loss of peak performance but also exacerbate any loss of lean tissue during Ramadan. The desire to reduce the demands of training can sometimes be incorporated into a planned 'tapering' of an athlete's regimen, or a learning of tactics (Chapter 11), but such an approach plainly carries a risk of losing some of the gains of muscle strength that have previously been achieved. Because of disincentives to daytime effort, one potential alternative is to train during the night [99,101]. However, the competitor is then not exercising at the peak of his or her circadian rhythm [101], sleep patterns are further disrupted, and nighttime training sessions may be unacceptable to other team members who are not observant Muslims.

Despite various disincentives, the maintenance of training during Ramadan is an important component of counteracting the tendency to muscle catabolism. Most experienced competitors seem able to sustain their normal volume of training during Ramadan, without significant adverse effects [23,24,26,53,55,62,65]. For example, 79 adolescent soccer players maintained their normal intensity of training (62% of their heart rate reserve) during Ramadan observance [62]. However, less experienced competitors are frequently tempted to slacken their routine. One group of 14–16-year-old soccer players decreased the time allocated to intensive physical activity from an average of 6.4 to 4.5 h/week; in consequence, they showed a decrease in their running speed and vertical jump height and greater fatigue over a series of sprints [71].

In terms of muscle mass, the observance of Ramadan generally seems to have little impact upon athletes, but there are two areas of continuing concern. Does the altered timing of meals hamper the anabolic process, and are participants in marathon and ultraendurance sports vulnerable to increased gluconeogenesis and a cumulative depletion of lean tissue? More evidence is needed on these specific issues, as well as in other situations where protein needs are likely to be challenged by any form of added dietary restriction (growing athletes, vegetarians and those from poor countries with a low initial protein intake). Where possible, all athletes should rearrange their training schedules to ensure that plasma protein levels are high during and immediately following conditioning sessions.

The stimulus to conservation of muscle mass should also be maximized by continued training. The likelihood of an increase in protein gluconeogenesis should be minimized. Possible tactics include encouraging the metabolism of fat at high intensities of exercise (through a combination of aerobic training and adoption of a high-fat diet in the weeks leading up to Ramadan) and eating of a high-carbohydrate diet at night to maximize glycogen stores immediately before competition. In the morning before an event, eating of a fatty meal may slow gastric emptying, and minimizing extraneous activity in the hours prior to competition will also help to conserve carbohydrate reserves.

Conclusions

In theory, any form of dietary restriction can challenges an athlete's protein metabolism and competitive performance. The combination of a reduced protein intake and increased gluconeogenesis could potentially lead to a progressive loss of lean tissue, with adverse effects, particularly in strength events. Moreover, a decrease in blood levels of amino acids could compromise the immediate response to resistance training. More research is needed in situations where the protein supply is challenged (for instance, participants in ultraendurance events, adolescent competitors, those from poor countries and those following vegetarian diets). Nevertheless, empirical data obtained to date suggest that although such problems may develop with sustained dieting, Ramadan observance has surprisingly little adverse affect upon protein metabolism, body composition, training response or competitive performance.

Key Terms

Adiponectin: Adiponectin is a hormone produced and secreted by fat cells. It increases the sensitivity of cells to insulin and encourages the metabolism of circulating free fatty acids by the muscles, with a decrease of body fat stores.

Amino acids: Compounds containing an amino (NH_2) and a carboxyl (COOH) grouping that are the chief constituents of plant and animal protein.

Anabolism: The metabolic process by which living cells convert simple compounds (such as amino acids) into more complex compounds (such as muscle protein).

Atrial natriuretic peptide (ANP): ANP is a powerful hormone, secreted mainly by the heart muscle cells. Its primary effect is upon blood vessels in the kidneys, increasing the glomerular excretion of sodium and water. However, it also increases the release of fatty acids from adipose tissue.

Bioimpedance: Bioimpedance is a measure of the opposition to passage of an electrical current through living tissues (the opposite of conductance). Fat and membranes have a high bioimpedance, whereas fluid containing lean tissue has a low impedance; the measurement of bioimpedance can thus be used to estimate the composition of tissues interposed between the measuring electrodes.

Catabolism: The breakdown of complex tissue components to simpler elements (for instance, the conversion of muscle protein to its constituent amino acids).

Catecholamines: A family of neurotransmitters that includes epinephrine, norepinephrine and dopamine.

Computed tomography: Computed tomography (or CT scan) is a widely used medical imaging procedure. A computer processing of x-rays passed through a given body region is used to generate a cross-sectional image; it can be used, for instance, to assess lean tissue dimensions.

Cortisol: Cortisol, or hydrocortisone, is a hormone produced by the adrenal cortex. Its primary function is to increase blood sugar through gluconeogenesis; catabolism is associated with increased cortisone/insulin and cortisone/testosterone ratios.

Dual-photon absorptiometry: This technique uses two x-ray beams of differing energy levels to produce an image of a body region. It is most commonly employed to evaluate bone density, but it can also be used for assessments of lean tissue.

Epinephrine: Epinephrine is a neurotransmitter released by the adrenal medulla and by some nerve endings. In terms of metabolism, it stimulates the processes of glycolysis, gluconeogenesis and the mobilization of fat.

Glucagon: Glucagon is a hormone secreted by alpha cells in the pancreatic islets of Langerhans. It increases blood sugar levels by stimulating glycogen breakdown in the liver.

Gluconeogenesis: Gluconeogenesis is the synthesis of glucose from molecules such as amino acids, lactate and glycerol; it occurs mainly in the liver.

Glycolysis: Glycolysis is the process of breakdown of glucose to pyruvate or lactate, with the release of energy.

Growth hormone (GH): The GH is produced by the adenohypophysis of the anterior pituitary gland. Among other actions, GH increases muscle mass and stimulates protein synthesis. It also promotes gluconeogenesis, reduces the uptake of glucose by the liver and triggers the secretion of IGF-1.

Hormone: A hormone is a chemical messenger, produced in one part of the body, and after transport via the blood stream, it elicits a response elsewhere within the organism.

Hypertrophy: Hypertrophy is the increase in volume of an organ such as muscle through the enlargement of its component cells. It must be distinguished from hyperplasia, where the number of cells in the organ is increased.

Insulin: Insulin is a hormone produced by the beta cells of the pancreas. Insulin is concerned primarily with the regulation of blood glucose levels, but its actions also include a stimulation of glycogen and lipid synthesis, an inhibition of protein breakdown, and a stimulation of amino acid uptake by muscle cells.

Insulin-like growth factor 1 (IGF-1): IGF-1 is also called somatomedin C. It is produced by the liver in response to GH secretion. The chemical structure of IGF-1 is similar to insulin, and it has a potent action in stimulating anabolism.

Interleukin-6 (IL-6): IL-6 is a cytokine, a chemical messenger that operates over shorter distances than hormones. It has pro- and anti-inflammatory actions, and in the metabolic context, it is released from the active muscle, contributing to the maintenance of a stable blood glucose concentration by the breakdown of intramuscular glycogen stores.

Joule: The Joule is the standard international unit for the measurement of energy intake or usage. It should replace the calorie, which is sometimes still used in U.S. texts. One Joule equals the work done in applying a force of 1 N over a distance of 1 m. 1 kcal = 4.18 J.

Leptin: Leptin is a hunger-regulating hormone. It is synthesized in body fat and acts on the hypothalamus to inhibit food intake and increase energy expenditures.

Norepinephrine: Norepinephrine is a catecholamine synthesized in the adrenal medulla and at some nerve endings. Along with epinephrine, it triggers the release of glucose from stored glycogen.

Satellite cells: Satellite cells are the precursors of developed muscle cells. They are found in skeletal muscle and can develop under the influence of resistance or endurance training, with GH and IGF-1 contributing to their differentiation.

Substrate: A substrate is a molecule that is acted upon by an enzyme.

Testosterone: Testosterone is produced mainly in the Leydig cells of the testes, but smaller amounts are also produced in women, in their ovaries. Testosterone and synthetic analogs are potent stimulants of muscle development and are frequently abused by strength athletes.

Thyroid hormones: T3 and T4 are hormones produced by the thyroid gland that stimulate metabolism.

Urea: Urea is a nitrogen-containing compound, produced in the liver by the breakdown of amino acids during gluconeogenesis. It is excreted in the urine and in sweat.

Uric acid: Uric acid is a compound formed by the breakdown of the purine nucleotides found in proteins. It is excreted in the urine, but it can occasionally cause problems of gout and kidney stones.

Key Points

1. With the intermittent fasting of Ramadan, sedentary individuals can normally meet all of their requirements of food energy by eating during the hours of darkness, and unless they engage in deliberate weight loss, they show little disturbance of protein metabolism.

2. Athletes with high rates of daily energy expenditure may show some reduction of their total food intake during Ramadan, sometimes with a small increase in the fractional contribution of proteins. This can cause small reductions of plasma protein and plasma amino acids, exacerbated during longer periods of dieting.

3. Some athletes show no change of body composition during Ramadan. In many, there is some decrease in both total body mass and fat mass, but there have been no reports of significant decreases of lean tissue mass to date. Longer periods of fasting are likely to reduce lean tissue mass, with associated decreases in muscular strength.

4. Further studies are needed to examine the ability of ultraendurance athletes to satisfy their energy requirements even during the short-duration fasts of Ramadan.

5. Several studies have shown that athletes can maintain normal training schedules during Ramadan, but further study is needed of the optimal timing of conditioning sessions when meals are taken at night.

Questions for Discussion

1. How would you set about assessing the protein needs of an athlete?
2. What changes in the hormones regulating protein anabolism and catabolism would you expect to observe in an athlete during a period of dieting?
3. How would you determine whether the nutritional needs of an athlete were being satisfied during Ramadan?
4. What recommendations would you make to minimize any adverse impact of dieting upon protein metabolism in a high-performance athlete?

References

1. Adlouni A, Ghalim N, Benslimane A et al. Fasting during Ramadan induces a marked increase in high-density lipoprotein cholesterol and decrease in low-density lipoprotein cholesterol. *Ann Nutr Metab* 1997;41:242–249.
2. Afifi Z-M. Daily practices, study performance and health during the Ramadan fast. *J R Soc Health* 1997;117:231–235.
3. Afrasiabi A, Hassanzadeh S, Sattarivand R et al. Effects of Ramadan fasting on serum lipid profiles on 2 hyperlipidemic groups with or without diet pattern. *Saudi Med J* 2003;24:23–26.
4. Aksungar FB, Eren A, Ure S et al. Effects of intermittent fasting on serum lipid levels, coagulation status and plasma homocysteine levels. *Ann Nutr Metab* 2005;49:77–82.
5. Al-Hourani HM, Atoum MF. Body composition, nutrient intake and physical activity patterns in young women during Ramadan. *Singapore Med J* 2007;48:906–910.
6. Angel J, Schwarz N. Metabolic changes resulting from decreased meal frequency in adult male Muslims during Ramadan fast. *Nutr Rep Int* 1975;11:29–38.

7. Asl NS. The effects of Ramadan fasting on endurance running performance in male athletes. *Int J Sport Studies* 2011;1:18–22.
8. Astrup A, Larsen TM, Harper A. Atkins and other low-carbohydrate diets: Hoax or an effective tool for weight loss? *Lancet* 2004;364(9437):897–899.
9. Aziz AR, Wahid MF, Png W et al. Effects of Ramadan fasting on 60 min of endurance running performance in moderately trained men. *Br J Sports Med* 2010;44:516–521.
10. Ba A, Samb A, Seck D et al. Etude comparative de l'effet du jeûne pendant le Ramadan sur la glycémie au repos chez les sportifs et les sédentaires (Comparative study of the effect of fasting during Ramadan on the glycaemia at rest in sportsmen and sedentaries). *Dakar Med* 2005;50:22–25.
11. Barkia A, Mohammed K, Smaoui M et al. Change of diet, plasma lipids, lipoproteins and fatty acids during Ramadan: A controversial association of the considered Ramadan model with atherosclerosis risk. *J Health Pop Nutr* 2011;29:486–493.
12. Beltaifa L, Bouguerra R, Ben Slama C et al. Food intake, and anthropometrical and biological parameters in adult Tunisians during fasting at Ramadan. *East Med Health J* 2002;8:603–611.
13. Ben Salem L, B'chir S, Bchir F et al. Circadian rhythm of cortisol and its responsiveness to ACTH during Ramadan. *Annales d'Endocrinologie* 2002;63:497–501.
14. Bigard AX, Boussif M, Chalabi H et al. Alterations in muscular performance and ortho-static tolerance during Ramadan. *Aviat Space Environ Med* 1998;69:341–346.
15. Bilsborough S, Mann N. A review of issues of dietary protein intake in humans. *Int J Sports Nutr Exerc Metab* 2006;16:129–152.
16. Bogdan A, Bouchareb B, Touitou Y. Ramadan fasting alters endocrine and neuroendocrine circadian patterns. Meal-time as a synchronizer in humans? *Life Sci* 2001;68:160–167.
17. Bouhlel E, Salhi Z, Bouhlel H et al. Effect of Ramadan fasting on fuel oxidation during exercise in trained male rugby players. *Diabetes Metab* 2006;32:617–624.
18. Bouhlel E, Zaouali M, Miled A et al. Ramadan fasting and the GH/IGF-I axis of trained men during submaximal exercise. *Ann Nutr Metab* 2008;52:261–266.
19. Bouhlel E, Zaouali M, Dengezueli M et al. Effects of Ramadan fasting on plasma leptin and adiponectin concentrations, biochemical parameters and body composition in trained young men. *Int J Sport Nutr Metab* 2008;18:617–627.
20. Brisswalter J, Bouhlel E, Falola JM et al. Effects of Ramadan intermittent fasting on middle-distance running performance in well-trained runners. *Clin J Sport Med* 2011;21:422–427.
21. Burke L. Fasting and recovery from exercise. *Br J Sports Med* 2010;44:502–508.
22. Burke LM, King C. Ramadan fasting and the goals of sports nutrition around exercise. *J Sports Sci* 2012;30(Suppl. 1):S21–S31.
23. Chaouachi A, Chamari K, Roky R et al. Lipid profiles of judo athletes during Ramadan. *Int J Sports Med* 2008;29:282–288.
24. Chaouachi A, Leiper JB, Souissi N et al. Effects of Ramadan intermittent fasting on sports performance and training: A review. *Int J Sports Physiol Perform* 2009;4:419–434.
25. Chaouachi A, Coutts AJ, Wong dP et al. Haematological, inflammatory, and immunologi-cal responses in elite judo athletes maintaining high training loads during Ramadan. *Appl Physiol Nutr Metab* 2009;34:907–915.
26. Chaouachi A, Coutts AJ, Chamari K et al. Effect of Ramadan intermittent fasting on aerobic and anaerobic performance and perception of fatigue in male elite judo athletes. *J Strength Cond Res* 2009;23:2702–2709.
27. Chennaoui M, Desgorces F, Drogou C et al. Effects of Ramadan fasting on physical performance and metabolic, hormonal, and inflammatory parameters in middle-distance runners. *Appl Physiol Nutr Metab* 2009;34:587–594.
28. Chiha F. *Variations du métabolisme énergétique à l'effort des footballeurs lors du jeûne de Ramadan* (Changes of exercise metabolism during Ramadan fasting). University of Algiers, Algiers, Algeria, 2008/2009.

29. Churchley EG, Coffey VG, Pedersen DJ et al. Influence of preexercise muscle glycogen content on transcriptional activity of metabolic and myogenic genes in well-trained humans. *J Appl Physiol* 2007;102:1604–1611.

30. Ch'ng SL, Cheah SH, Husain R et al. Effect of altered eating pattern on serum fructosamine: Total protein ratio and plasma glucose level. *Ann Acad Med Singapore* 1989;18:326–327.

31. Consolazio CF, Nelson RA, Matoush LO et al. Nitrogen excretion in sweat and its relation to nitrogen balance requirements. *J Nutr* 1963;79:399–406.

32. El Ati J, Beji C, Danguir J. Increased fat oxidation during Ramadan fasting in healthy women: An adaptative mechanism for body-weight maintenance. *Am J Clin Nutr* 1995;62:302–307.

33. Fakhrzadeh H, Larihani B, Sanjari M et al. Effect of Ramadan fasting on clinical and biochemical parameters in healthy adults. *Ann Saudi Med* 2003;23:223–226.

34. Faye J, Fall A, Badji L et al. Effets du jeûne du ramadan sur le poids, la performance et de la glycémie lors de l'entraînement à la résistance (Effects of Ramadan fast on weight, performance and glycemia during training for resistance). *Dakar Med* 2005;50:146–151.

35. Fedail SS, Murphy D, Salib SY et al. Changes in certain blood constituents during Ramadan. *Am J Clin Nutr* 1982;36:350–353.

36. Finch GM, Day JEL, Welch DA et al. Appetite changes under free living conditions during Ramadan: A pilot study. *Appetite* 1998;31:159–170.

37. Frexes-Steed M, Warner ML, Bulus N et al. Role of insulin and branch-chained amino acids in regulating protein metabolism. *Am J Physiol* 1990;258:E907–E917.

38. Frost G, Pirani S. Meal frequency and nutritional intake during Ramadan: A pilot study. *Hum Nutr Appl Nutr* 1987;41:47–50.

39. Furuncuoglu Y, Karaca E, Aras S et al. Metabolic, biochemical and psychiatric alterations in healthy subjects during Ramadan. *Pakist J Nutr* 2007;6:209–211.

40. Gardner CD, Kiazand A, Alhassan S et al. Comparison of the Atkins, Zone, Ornish, and LEARN diets for change in weight and related risk factors among overweight premenopausal women. The ATOZ weight loss study: A randomized trial. *JAMA* 2007;297(9):969–977.

41. Genton L, Melzer K, Pichaud C. Energy and macronutrient requirements for physical fitness in exercising subjects. *Clin Nutr* 2010;29:413–423.

42. Gerich GE. Glucose counterregulation and its impact on diabetes mellitus. *Diabetes* 1988;37:1608–1617.

43. Gharbi M, Akrout M, Zouari B. Food intake during and outside Ramadan. *East Med Health J* 2003;9:131–140.

44. Grantham JR, Belhaj J, Balasekaran J. The effect of four weeks' fasting during Ramadan on body composition in Muslim Arab males. *Med Sci Sports Exerc* 2007;37(Suppl. 5):293 (abstract).

45. Gueye L, Samb A, Seck D et al. Influence of a 12-hour fast on maximal exercise. *Scripta Med* (Brno). 2005;77:271–276.

46. Gumaa KA, Mustafa KY, Mahmoud NA et al. The effects of fasting in Ramadan. 1. Serum uric acid and lipid concentrations. *Br J Nutr* 1978;40:573–581.

47. Hartman ML, Veldhuis JD, Johnson ML et al. Augmented growth hormone (GH) secretory burst frequency and amplitude mediate enhanced GH secretion during a two day fast in normal men. *J Clin Endocrinol Metab* 1992;74:757–764.

48. Hartman JW, Tang JE, Wilkinson SB et al. Consumption of fat-free milk after resistance exercise promotes greater lean mass accretion than does consumption of soy or carbohydrate in young, novice, male weightlifters. *Am J Clin Nutr* 2007;86:373–381.

49. Hawley JA, Gibala MJ, Bermon S. Innovations in athletic preparation: Role of substrate availability to modify training adaptation and performance. *J Sport Sci* 2007;25 (Suppl. 1): S115–S124.

50. Husain R, Duncan MT, Cheah SH et al. Effects of fasting in Ramadan on tropical Asiatic Moslems. *Br J Nutr* 1987;58:41–48.

51. Johnston CE, Sherrie L, Tjonn SL et al. Ketogenic low-carbohydrate diets have no metabolic advantage over nonketogenic low-carbohydrate diets. *Am J Clin Nutr* 2006;83(5):1055–1061.
52. Kappagoda CT, Hyson DA, Amsterdam EA. Low-carbohydrate–high-protein diets: Is there a place for them in clinical cardiology? *JAMA* 2004;43(5):725–730.
53. Karli U, Guvenc A, Aslan A et al. Influence of Ramadan fasting on anaerobic performance and recovery from short high intensity exercise. *J Sport Sci Med* 2007;6:490–497.
54. Khan A, Kharzak A. Islamic fasting: An effective strategy for prevention of obesity. *Pakist J Nutr* 2002;1:185–187.
55. Kirkendall DT, Leiper JB, Bartagi Z et al. The influence of Ramadan on physical performance measures in young Muslim footballers. *J Sports Sci* 2008;26(Suppl. 3):S15–S27.
56. Kirkendall DT, Chaouachi A, Aziz A-R et al. Strategies for maintaining fitness and performance during Ramadan. *J Sports Sci* 2012;30(Suppl. 1):S10–S108.
57. Krifi M, Ben Salem M, Ben Rayana MC et al. Food intake, and anthropometrical and biological parameters in adult Tunisians in Ramadan. *J Méd Nutr* 1989;25:223–228.
58. Larijani B, Zahedi F, Sanjari M et al. The effect of Ramadan fasting on fasting serum glucose in healthy adults. *Med J Malaysia* 2003;58:678–680.
59. Lafontan M, Langin D. Lipolysis and lipid mobilization in human adipose tissue. *Progr Lipid Res* 2009;48:275–297.
60. Lavoie C, Ducros F, Bourque J et al. Glucose metabolism during exercise in man: The role of insulin and glucagon in the regulation of hepatic glucose production and gluconeogenesis. *Can J Physiol Pharmacol* 1997;75:26–35.
61. Leiper JB, Junge A, Maughan RJ et al. Alteration of subjective feelings in football players undertaking their usual training and match schedule during the Ramadan fast. *J Sports Sci* 2008;26(Suppl. 3):S55–S69.
62. Leiper JB, Watson P, Evans G et al. Intensity of a training session during Ramadan in fasting and non-fasting Tunisian youth football players. *J Sports Sci* 2008;26(Suppl. 3):571–579.
63. Lemon PW. Protein and amino acid needs of the strength athlete. *Int J Sport Nutr* 1991;1:127–145.
64. Lemon PW. Do athletes need more dietary protein and amino acids? *Int J Sports Nutr* 1995;5:S39–S51.
65. Linda Stern L, Nayyar Iqbal N, Prakash Seshadri P et al. The effects of low-carbohydrate versus conventional weight loss diets in severely obese adults: One-year follow-up of a randomized trial. *Ann Int Med* 2004;140(10):778–785.
66. Loucks AB. The endocrine system: Integrated influences on metabolism, growth and reproduction. In: Tipton CM, Sawka MN, Tate CA, Terjung RL (eds.), *ACSM's Advanced Exercise Physiology*. Lippincott, Williams & Wilkins, Philadelphia, PA, 2006.
67. Maislos M, Khamayi N, Assali A. Marked increase in plasma high-density lipoprotein cholesterol after prolonged fasting during Ramadan. *Am J Clin Nutr* 1993;57:640–642.
68. Maughan RJ, Gleeson M. Influence of a 36 h fast followed by refeeding with glucose, glycerol or placebo on metabolism and performance during prolonged exercise in man. *Eur J Appl Physiol* 1988;57:570–576.
69. Maughan RJ, Bartagi Z, Dvorak J et al. Dietary intake and body composition of football players during the holy month of Ramadan. *J Sports Sci* 2008;26(Suppl. 3):S20–S38.
70. Maughan RJ, Leiper JB, Bartagi Z et al. Effect of Ramadan fasting on some biochemical and haematological parameters in Tunisian youth soccer players undertaking their usual training and competition schedule. *J Sports Sci* 2008;26(Suppl. 3):539–546.
71. Meckel Y, Ismael A, Eliakim A. The effect of the Ramadan fast on physical performance and dietary habits in adolescent soccer players. *Eur J Appl Physiol* 2008;102:651–657.
72. Memari A-H, Kordh R, Panahl N et al. Effect of Ramadan fasting on body composition and physical performance in female athletes. *Asian J Sports Med* 2011;2:161–166.
73. Moore DR, Robinson MJ, Fry JL et al. Ingested protein dose response of muscle and albumin protein synthesis after resistance exercise in young men. *Am J Clin Nutr* 2009;89:161–168.

74. Morilla RG, Rodrigo JR, Caravaca AS et al. Modificaciones dietéticas, en jóvenes Musulmanes que practican el ayuno del Ramadán (dietary modifications in young Muslims practicing the fast of Ramadan). *Nutrición Hospitalaria* 2009;24:738–743.

75. Mujika I, Chaouachi A, Chamari K. Precompetition taper and nutritional strategies: Special reference to training during Ramadan intermittent fast. *Br J Sports Med* 2010;44:495–501.

76. Murphy R, Shipman KH. Hyperuricaemia during total fasts. *Arch Int Med* 1963;112:954–959.

77. Mustafa KY, Mahmoud NA, Gumaa KA et al. The effects of fasting in Ramadan. 2. Fluid and electrolyte balance. *Br J Nutr* 1978;40:583–589.

78. Nindl BC, Pierce JR. Insulin-like growth factor I as a biomarker of health, fitness and training status. *Med Sci Sports Exerc* 2010;42:39–49.

79. Nomani MZA, Hallak MH, Nomani S et al. Changes in blood urea and glucose and their association with energy containing nutrients in men on hypocaloric diet during Ramadan. *Am J Clin Nutr* 1989;49:1141–1145.

80. Prentice AM, Prentice A, Lamb WH et al. Metabolic consequences of fasting during Ramadan in pregnant and lactating women. *Hum Nutr Clin Nutr* 1983;37(4):283–294.

81. Poh B, Zawiah H, Ismail M, Henry C. Changes in body weight, dietary intake and activity pattern of adolescents during Ramadan. *Malaysian J Nutr* 1996;2:1–10.

82. Ramadan J, Telahoun G, Al-Zaid NS et al. Responses to exercise, fluid, and energy balances during Ramadan in sedentary and active males. *Nutrition* 1999;15:735–739.

83. Rasmussen BB, Tipton KD, Miller SL et al. An oral essential amino acid-carbohydrate supplement enhances muscle protein anabolism after resistance exercise. *J Appl Physiol* 2000;88:386–392.

84. Rasmussen BB, Phillips DM. Contractile and nutritional regulation of human muscle growth. *Exerc Sport Sci Rev* 2003;31:127–131.

85. Rodriguez NR, Vislocky LM, Gaine PC. Dietary protein, endurance exercise, and human skeletal muscle protein turnover. *Curr Opin Clin Nutr Metab Care* 2007;10:40–45.

86. Roky R, Houti I, Moussamih S et al. Physiological and chronobiological changes during Ramadan intermittent fasting. *Ann Nutr Metab* 2004;48:296–303.

87. Roky R. Les variations physiologiques et comportementales pendant le Ramadan (Physiological and behavioural changes during Ramadan). *Biomatec Echo* 2007;2(5) On-line publication.

88. Roy J, Ooi CH, Singh R et al. Self-generated coping strategies among Muslim athletes during Ramadan fasting. *J Sports Sci Med* 2011;10:137–144.

89. Shai I. Weight loss with a low-carbohydrate, Mediterranean, or low-fat diet. *N Engl J Med* 2008;359(3):229–241.

90. Shephard RJ. Physical performance and training response during Ramadan observance, with particular reference to protein metabolism. *Br J Sports Med* 2012;46:477–484.

91. Shephard RJ. The impact of Ramadan observance upon athletic performance. *Nutrients* 2012;4:491–505.

92. Siddiqui QA, Sabir S, Subhan MM. The effect of Ramadan fasting on spirometry in healthy subjects. *Respirology* 2005;10:525–528.

93. Stannard SR, Thompson MW. The effect of participation in Ramadan on substrate selection during submaximal cycling exercise. *J Sci Med Sport* 2008;11:510–517.

94. Sukker MY, El-Munshid HA, Ardawi MSM. *Concise Human Physiology.* Blackwell Science, Abingdon, U.K., 2000, p. 149.

95. Sweileh N, Schnitzler A, Hunter GR et al. Body composition and energy metabolism in resting and exercising Muslims during Ramadan fast. *J Sports Med Phys Fitness* 1992;32:156–163.

96. Tarnopolsky MA, Atkinson SA, MacDougall JD et al. Evaluation of protein requirements for trained strength athletes. *J Appl Physiol* 1992;73:1986–1995.

97. Tipton KD, Elliot TA, Cree MG et al. Stimulation of net muscle protein synthesis by whey protein ingestion before and after exercise. *Am J Physiol* 2007;292:E71–E76.

98. van Loon LJC, Gibala MJ. Dietary protein to support muscle hypertrophy. In: Maughan RJ, Burke LM (eds.), *Sports Nutrition: More than Just Calories—Triggers for Adaptation.* Karger Publications, Basel, Switzerland, 2012.

99. Waterhouse J. Effects of Ramadan on physical performance: Chronobiological considerations. *Br J Sports Med* 2010;44:509–515.

100. Westerterp KR, Saris WHM, vanEs M, ten Hoor F. Use of the doubly labeled water technique in humans during heavy sustained exercise. *J Appl Physiol* 1986;61:2162–2167.

101. Wilson D, Drust B, Reilly T. Is diurnal lifestyle altered during Ramadan in professional Muslim athletes? *Biol Rhythm Res* 2009;40:385–397.

102. Woolf PJ, Fu LL, Basu A. Protein: Identifying optimal amino acid complements from plant-based foods. *PLoS ONE* 2011;6(4):e18836.

103. Young VR. Adult amino acid requirements: A case for revision of current recommendations. *J Nutr* 1994;124(8 Suppl.):1517S–1523S.

104. Yucel A, Degirmenci B, Acar M et al. Effect of fasting month of Ramadan on the abdominal fat distribution: Assessment by computed tomography. *Tohoku J Exp Med* 2004;204:179–187.

105. Zerguini Y, Dvorak J, Maughan RJ et al. Influence of Ramadan fasting on physiological and performance variables in football players: Summary of the F-MARC 2006 Ramadan fasting study. *J Sports Sci* 2008;26(Suppl. 3):S3–S6.

106. Ziaee V, Razaei M, Ahmadinejad Z et al. The changes of metabolic profile and weight during Ramadan fasting. *Singapore Med J* 2006;47:409–414.

Further Reading

Borer KT. *Advanced Exercise Endocrinology.* Human Kinetics, Champaign, IL, 2013.

Constantini N, Hackney AC. *Endocrinology of Physical; Activity and Sport.* Humana Press, New York, 2013.

Cruz-Jentoft AJ, Morley JE. *Sarcopenia.* Wiley-Blackwell, Chichester, U.K., 2012.

Lamprecht, M. *Acute Topics in Sports Nutrition.* Karger, Basel, Switzerland, 2012.

Tipton KT, van Loon LJC. *Nutritional Coaching Strategy to Modulate Training Efficiency.* Karger, Basel, Switzerland, 2013.

6

Hydration and Fluid Restriction in Athletes

Roy J Shephard

Learning Objectives

1. To understand mechanisms for the normal regulation of fluid balance in humans and to distinguish total from 'free' body water
2. To understand methods of assessing dehydration
3. To discover the limits of adaptation to dehydration
4. To review the extent of fluid challenges for sedentary individuals during Ramadan
5. To understand how the challenges of a restricted fluid intake are exacerbated in various classes of athlete
6. To consider practical implications for the athlete who chooses to restrict fluid intake

Introduction

Total water deprivation may arise during certain emergencies such as a shipwreck or becoming lost in the desert and as a political manifestation or as a desire to end one's life [54]. Short-term water deprivation may be imposed by various means such as sauna exposure, exercising in extreme heat or the administration of diuretics in an attempt to qualify for a particular weight category in weight-classified sports. Finally, during Ramadan observance, fluid intake is prohibited during daylight hours, leading to a progressive dehydration over the course of the day, and if unusually large volumes of fluid are not ingested at night, a cumulative dehydration may develop over the 29 days of Ramadan. Some authors distinguish simple fluid loss (which can increase plasma sodium ion concentrations) from fluid loss with salt depletion.

117

Functional and Total Water Volumes

The functional water volume of the body must be distinguished from the total water, which includes water bound to glycogen molecules, osmolytes such as sodium in the extracellular space and organic osmolytes within cells [8]. From the viewpoint of body physiology, the functional water volume is more important than the total body water. During voluntary dehydration, there can be a decrease of both body mass and total body water but no change in the functional water volume.

Normal Regulation of Fluid Balance in Human Subjects

Water comprises some 70% of the human body mass (i.e. 40–60 L). The body of a sedentary individual normally loses about 2.5 L of water per day, due to the excretion of 1.2–1.5 L as urine, a percutaneous transpiration of 0.5 L as 'insensible' water loss at the skin surface, the loss of 0.4 L of water in saturating expired air at body temperature and a further 150–200 mL in the feces. In exercising athletes, there can be additional sweat losses of up to 2 L/hours, and depending upon the humidity of the inspired air, respiratory water losses can also increase greatly during vigorous exercise [49].

In the United States, the reference daily fluid intake from all sources is 3.7 L for men and 2.7 L for women. Hydration is normally maintained by the ingestion of water and other fluids (at least 1 L/day, but commonly much more), the presence of water as a major constituent of many foods (providing about 1.2 L of water per day), and the production of water during the metabolism of carbohydrates, lipids, proteins and alcohol (providing about 0.3 L of water per day). A significant additional resource is the water of hydration associated with the glycogen molecule (about 2.7 g/g); it is liberated as glycogen reserves are depleted during metabolism, and given a normal intramuscular and hepatic store of about 500 g, this can yield about 1.4 L of water during sustained aerobic exercise [48].

The output of urine can be reduced somewhat if fluids are in short supply or water losses are increased, but the minimum volume of fluid needed to accommodate urinary function and transpiration can only be reduced by about 1 L, to around 1.5 L/day. Maintenance of hydration within fairly close limits is important to the regulation of chemical reactions in the body, for instance, plasma sodium concentrations normally fall within a 3.5% range around a mean value of 140 mmol/L. A tight balance of plasma sodium and potassium concentrations is important to the maintenance of cell volume and function [42,45].

The main basis of regulation is a change in the output of two hormones (Table 6.1). The antidiuretic hormone (ADH) secreted by the pituitary gland encourages fluid retention, and aldosterone secreted by the adrenal cortex encourages sodium retention, potassium secretion and water retention. The secretion of these hormones is increased in the face of dehydration, whether caused by heat

TABLE 6.1 Hormonal Regulation of Urinary Output

Hormone	Site of Secretion	Mechanism of Action	Body Responses
Antidiuretic hormone	Neurohypophysis	Increases retention of fluid in the collecting tubules of the kidney	Water retention and vascular constriction
Aldosterone	Outer part of the adrenal cortex	Acts on distal tubules and collecting ducts of the kidney, causing sodium retention, potassium secretion and water retention	Increases blood volume and blood pressure

exposure or prolonged exercise [19,56], leading to a reduction in urinary output; an excessive antidiuretic response is believed to have contributed to occasional cases of hyponatraemia in endurance athletes [39]. Adaptive changes in the output of ADH and aldosterone may also occur with repeated exposure to heat stress [21,28].

Methods of Assessing Dehydration

Methods of assessing dehydration have included a review of changes in body mass, haemoglobin, haematocrit and plasma sodium concentrations, the measurement of urinary volume and specific gravity, and bioimpedance determinations of body water. With the intermittent water deprivation of Ramadan observance, it is necessary to look both at acute changes of hydration over the course of daylight hours, and chronic, cumulative trends developing over the month of water deprivation. Given the cyclic nature of Ramadan dehydration, it is important to make measurements at a fixed time of day, preferably each evening, immediately before breaking the fast.

Any changes seen during a communal period of water deprivation such as Ramadan must be interpreted cautiously relative to control subjects, since the overall social environment at this season can create substantial changes in the blood picture and fluid balance even among those who do not observe Ramadan [15]. Unfortunately, many of the published studies lack information on non-fasting controls.

Body Mass

The determination of changes in body mass is the simplest approach. If a subject is dried carefully before weighing and allowance is made for any food ingested and the passage of urine and feces, the decrease of nude body mass offers a fairly clear picture of the decrease in total body water over a single day, although as noted earlier, it does not necessarily reflect the free body water. Over a longer period of water deprivation, such as the entire month of Ramadan, cumulative changes in body mass could also be caused by the breakdown of fat and lean tissue to sustain metabolism and meet the energy costs of physical activity. Sedentary individuals sometimes exploit the observance of Ramadan to induce a deliberate decrease in body fat content. Sometimes, the communal feasts of Ramadan may also lead to an increase of body fat (Chapter 2). Thus, if body mass is to be used to examine cumulative dehydration, it is necessary to associate findings with estimates of changes in lean tissue and body fat.

Haemoglobin and Haematocrit

Over short periods, changes in the haemoglobin concentration provide a convenient measure of haemoconcentration and thus overall decreases in the free body water. However, over a period as long as a month, these values could alter due to a change in red cell count rather than dehydration. An increase in red cell count that is independent of haemoconcentration is particularly likely in athletes who are training hard (or who are engaging in autotransfusion or abuse of erythropoietin).

Measuring Changes in Blood Volume

Physiologists commonly assess changes in blood volume using the formula of Dill and Costill [16]:

Blood volume (2) = Blood volume (1) × [Hb (1)/Hb (2)]
Red cell volume (2) = Blood volume (2) × Haematocrit (2)
Plasma volume (2) = Blood volume (2) − Red cell volume (2)
Δ Blood volume (%) = 100 (BV$_2$ − BV$_1$)/BV$_1$
Δ Red cell volume (%) = 100 (RCV$_2$ − RCV$_1$/RCV$_1$
Δ Plasma volume (%) = 100 (PV$_2$ − PV$_1$)/PV$_1$

The haemoglobin concentration is measured by lysing the red cells, oxidizing to methaemoglobin and treating with cyanide to form cyanmethaemoglobin; this end product is then determined by absorption of light at 540 nm. The haematocrit was originally measured by centrifuging blood samples in graduated tubes. A correction factor of 0.96 was applied for trapped plasma and a further factor of 0.91 was used to convert venous into whole body packed cell volume. Electronic determination of the haematocrit is now possible, based on the change of voltage observed when blood is passed through a special transducer.

Serum Sodium Concentrations

Serum sodium concentrations are increasingly used to test athletes for dehydration following prolonged events such as marathon races. However, measurements are subject to an appreciable measurement error, particularly when using portable monitors in a field environment [57]. One hospital laboratory reported serum sodium levels of 125–152 mE/L (a range from serious hyponatraemia to hypernatraemia) on a sample that was known to contain a very normal sodium concentration of 141 mE/L [14]. More recent evaluations have set the precision of laboratory data at 1.0%–1.5%, but field measurements using the portable i-STAST device show a standard deviation of at least 2 mE/L [17,22], implying that some reports of hyper- or hyponatraemia will be erroneous. Changes in electrolyte concentrations over the course of the day may also underestimate the extent of fluid depletion in athletes who have been sweating hard, since sweat normally contains a lower concentration of sodium ions than the plasma.

Urinary Volumes and Specific Gravity

The collection of 24-hour urine samples is a cumbersome procedure, but it is possible to compare changes of the specific gravity of the urine over the course of a day. If specialized laboratory facilities are available, it is also possible to follow fluid exchanges by examining the dilution of small volumes of deuterated water within the body.

Bioimpedance Data

The bioimpedance of the limbs is influenced by the cross-sectional dimensions of the lean tissues interposed between the measuring electrodes. In the short term, increased impedance would imply a dehydration of lean tissue, but in a longer-term perspective, an increase in readings could reflect either cumulative dehydration or a reduction in lean tissue mass.

Effects of Water Deprivation

A safe level of dehydration is still debated. In a temperate climate, temporary losses amounting to 7%–8% of body mass (i.e. as much as 5 L or 10% of total body water) can be tolerated [46], although if the dehydration is caused by exercising, some of the loss may have been compensated by a release of bound water [48]. Moreover, physiological capacity and the resulting aerobic performance become suboptimal as body fluids are depleted; Saltin argued that during aerobic exercise in a hot environment (where the water of hydration of glycogen was probably mobilized), maximal oxygen intake and cardiac output decreased if water losses exceeded 5% of body mass (about 3.5 L) [17]. Under such conditions, the capacity to perform aerobic exercise was reduced as much as 30%.

Armstrong and associates tested the effects of furosemide-induced reductions in plasma volume of 10%–12% (corresponding to a much smaller 1.6%–2.1% decrease of body mass). Although this amount of dehydration was insufficient to reduce maximal oxygen intake, track performances were decreased in 1,500, 5,000 and 10,000 m running events [5].

Participants in weight-categorized events such as wrestling often engage in substantial dehydration prior to their 'weigh-in'. Once they have been categorized, they attempt a rapid rehydration, but if this is incomplete prior to competition, there are decreases of maximal isometric strength and circulatory function. Sometimes, quite small fluid deficits (2% of body mass, perhaps 2 L in a heavy wrestler) can have such effects [4,25,40,53]. The physical performance and skill of soccer players has also shown some improvement with the provision of fluids at half-time, although gains have been slight when correcting fluid losses of up to 2.5% of body mass (1.5 L) [41], and it has not always been clear whether the source of benefit was the water or the glucose content of the beverage that was provided [23,34].

Perhaps more seriously, as body fluid reserves are depleted, sweating diminishes (reducing evaporative cooling), and the blood flow to the skin is restricted, reducing conductive and convective heat loss; this leaves an individual more vulnerable to various forms of heat stress [47].

Under resting conditions, symptoms begin to appear with more than 2% dehydration, and complaints become more marked with 5%–6% dehydration. A severe depletion of body fluids is accompanied by thirst, headache, tiredness, irritability, a small volume of dark, concentrated urine, constipation, postural hypotension, insomnia and a loss of skin elasticity. The blood volume is decreased, and in an attempt to compensate for this, the heart rate and breathing rate are increased. If symptoms are ignored, there is ultimately a loss of consciousness and death. With 10%–15% dehydration, muscle spasms may appear and urination becomes painful, and if fluid loss exceeds 15%, there is a progressive failure of the body organs, beginning with the kidneys, which progresses to death [6].

Effects of Repeated Moderate Fluid Restriction in Sedentary Individuals

Ramadan observance exposes sedentary individuals to repeated moderate fluid restriction for each of 29 days, but in general, the impact upon fluid balance is small. Although there may be some changes of dietary composition during Ramadan, the total energy intake generally shows little change during this celebration [50] (Chapter 2), so that the water contained in food and derived from its metabolism (1.5 L/day) is likely to remain unchanged. This, in itself, is almost enough to meet the minimum fluid needs of a sedentary individual. Furthermore, it is quite possible to ingest at least the normal daily fluid intake of 1 L during the hours of darkness [43], leaving 500 mL or more of fluid in the stomach as the day dawns. Because of a large night-time intake, many people gain the subjective impression that their daily fluid intake actually increases during Ramadan [52]. There may be a slight haemoconcentration during the afternoons if the duration of the daily fast is long and the weather is warm, but there is no inherent reason why a sedentary person should develop a cumulative fluid deficit during the month of Ramadan. Empirical data support this viewpoint (Table 6.2).

TABLE 6.2 Empirical Evidence on Changes in the Hydration of Sedentary Individuals during Ramadan

Author	Subjects	Methodology	Changes during Ramadan
Body mass change			
See Table 2.3	29 studies	Body mass	19 studies show decrease of body mass, 9 no change, 2 an increase
Haemoglobin and haematocrit changes			
Al-Hourani et al. [2]	57 healthy females	Haematocrit	No change of haematocrit
Bigard et al. [9]	11 male fighter pilots	Haematocrit	7% decrease of plasma volume over Ramadan
Chiha [14]	9 sedentary subjects	Body mass, body fat, and haematocrit	No significant decrease of plasma volume at rest or after lab exercise, but volume of water ingested decreased by 0.46 L/day
Farshidfar et al. [18]	62 M and F students	Haematocrit and haemoglobin	No significant change of haematocrit, but decrease of haemoglobin, also decrease of body mass
Furuncuoglu et al. [20]	7 males, 32 females	Body mass, haematocrit and blood chemistry	No significant changes (but trend to decrease of haematocrit)
Serum electrolyte changes			
Ramadan et al. [44]	7 sedentary Kuwaitis	Body mass, serum osmolarity, serum sodium	Decrease of body mass <1.3% increased plasma sodium concentration
Sweileh et al. [55]	7 healthy men, 1 healthy woman	Body mass, body fat, serum electrolytes	Decrease of fluids in the first week, increase of plasma sodium, but recovery by the end of Ramadan
Urinary volumes			
Cheah et al. [12]	13 sedentary Malaysians	Urinary volume, osmolality and solute excretion	No change in total daily urine volume, although during daytime tendency to decrease during Ramadan, with more concentrated urine
Chiha [14]	9 sedentary subjects	Body mass, body fat and haematocrit, water ingestion	No significant decrease of plasma volume at rest or after lab exercise, but volume of water ingested decreased by 0.46 L/day (16%) during Ramadan
Leiper and Prastowow [30]	Sedentary Muslims	Isotope tracer	No change of water turnover; decrease of non-renal water loss
Miladipour et al. [36]	57 males aged 30–55 years, including 37 with recurrent calculi	Urinary volume and urinary composition	0.16 L/day (10%) decrease of urinary volume during Ramadan

(*Continued*)

TABLE 6.2 (*Continued*) Empirical Evidence on Changes in the Hydration of Sedentary Individuals during Ramadan

Author	Subjects	Methodology	Changes during Ramadan
Mustafa et al. [38]	16 sedentary Sudanese men	Body mass, fluid intake, urinary volume and electrolytes	2.7% decrease of body mass at the beginning of the second week, recovery by the fourth week of Ramadan; 2 L/day fluid balance deficit at the beginning of Ramadan, compensated by the end of the month by urinary concentration and salt retention
Prentice et al. [43]	20 lactating Gambian women	Body mass, body fat, urine volume and osmolality	7.6% depletion of total body water over the day, but made good at night; no chronic loss
Sweileh et al. [55]	7 males, 1 female	Body mass, body fat, serum electrolytes	Decrease of body mass and fluids in the first week, with no change of body fat. Recovery by the end of Ramadan, but water intake reduced 0.8 L (36%)
Waterhouse et al. [59]	20 healthy males	Urinary osmotic pressure	Afternoon rise of osmotic pressure during Ramadan, not seen on control days

Body Mass

A decrease in body mass of up to 3.6 kg was seen in 19 of 29 studies of sedentary subjects over the course of Ramadan (Table 2.3), but on the other hand, 8 studies reported no significant change of body mass, and 2 other investigations noted an increase of body mass during and following Ramadan; the gain was attributed to an increased consumption of carbohydrates and fats during Ramadan [7] and group festivities associated with the celebration.

Even in studies were there a decrease of body mass during Ramadan, this cannot necessarily be equated with the development of chronic dehydration. In some cases, there was also a substantial associated fat loss [18,24,26], and in at least one study, quite large changes of body mass occurred without any alteration of urinary output [26].

Haemoglobin and Haematocrit

Of five studies in sedentary individuals, four showed no significant change in the plasma volume as estimated from haemoglobin and haematocrit values during Ramadan. The one exception was a group of fighter pilots [9], who probably led a more active lifestyle than the remaining groups.

Serum Biochemistry

Two studies of sedentary individuals [44,55] showed increased sodium ion concentrations early during Ramadan, but values tended to normalize as the fast continued.

Urinary Volumes and Fluid Balance

Most published studies of sedentary subjects have reported some decrease of daytime urinary volumes during Ramadan, but there has been little [36] or no significant change of urinary output on a 24-hour basis [26,30,38,43,59,60]. Any overall change was certainly insufficient to have an adverse effect on health, even in individuals with a high risk of urinary calculi [31]. One report found daytime urinary concentrations rising close to the maximal renal concentrating ability, but unfortunately, this study included no data on the osmolality of night urine specimens [60]. Another study found a small decrease in urinary output, although this began before there had been a significant change in body mass [37].

Conclusions

Sedentary individuals show at most some small increase of haematocrit and serum sodium and secretion of more concentrated urine during the afternoons of Ramadan observance, but any fluid deficiency is usually made good before the next dawn. Often, the initial daily disturbances of fluid balance tend to diminish as the month continues, although it is unclear how far this is due to physiological adaptations and how far it reflects alterations of dietary behaviour.

Effects of Intermittent Fluid Restriction in Athletes

The situation of the distance athlete or team competitor is less favourable than that of a sedentary person during intermittent fluid restriction, as during Ramadan observance, given that the competitor is likely to have a much greater respiratory water loss and may well secrete 3–4 L of sweat during a 90-minute team game or an endurance run. A deuterated water comparison of water turnover between sedentary middle-aged men and peers who ran an average of 14.8 km/day concluded that the fluid requirements of the runners were even greater than suggested by the summing of anticipated respiratory and sweat losses [29], because they also had a greater urinary output than sedentary individuals. Up to 2 L of water may be derived from the breakdown of glycogen during endurance exercise [48], but if 3–4 L of sweat is produced, there will still remain a fluid deficit of 1–2 L at the end of a match or a distance race. In theory, the observance of Ramadan could thus cause short-term dehydration (over the course of a day of fasting), and unless this deficit is made good at night, cumulative effects could develop over the month of intermittent fluid restriction. Empirical data certainly show some evidence of dehydration. Few of the studies have been on athletes who engage in prolonged endurance events (Table 6.3), and in this group, the effects of a Ramadan fast upon both performance and safety during the event could be considerably greater than in the studies yet published.

TABLE 6.3 Empirical Evidence on Changes in Body Fluids of Athletes and Active Individuals during Ramadan

Changes in body mass			
See Table 2.4	16 studies	Body mass	Small decrease in 8 studies, no change in 8 studies
Changes in haemoglobin and haematocrit			
Aloui et al. [3]	12 active males	Haematocrit and haemoglobin	Readings for both haematocrit and haemoglobin increased in afternoon during Ramadan, implying decrease of plasma volume
Bigard et al. [9]	11 male fighter pilots	Body mass and haematocrit	2 kg (2.7%) decrease of body mass over Ramadan
Bouhlel et al. [10]	9 male rugby players	Body mass, body fat, haematocrit	Increase of haematocrit, decrease of afternoon plasma volumes both early and late during Ramadan, similar effect upon post-exercise values
Chaouachi et al. [11]	15 male Tunisian Judokus	Body mass, body fat and haematocrit	Variable changes in morning plasma volumes over the course of Ramadan (−4% to +4%)
Chiha [14]	12 male soccer players	Body mass, body fat and haematocrit	Increase of haemoglobin at rest and post-exercise, non-significant trend to increase of haematocrit during Ramadan. Volume of water ingested decreased by 1.07 L/day
Maughan et al. [32]	79 male soccer players	Body mass, body fat, haematocrit	Loss of body mass, no loss of fat; no significant change in haematocrit but puzzling *decrease* in haemoglobin, particularly during the fourth week of Ramadan
Shireffs and Maughan [51]	55 observant male soccer players, 37 non-observant	Body mass, haemoglobin and haematocrit	Decrease of haemoglobin and haematocrit during Ramadan, seen also in controls. Study appears to overlap with [52]
Trabelsi et al. [58]	12 male recreational rugby players	Haematocrit, haemoglobin	Increase of resting haematocrit and haemoglobin, with decrease of blood volume but not total body water, particularly at the beginning of Ramadan; not exacerbated by Rugby match
Serum biochemistry, impedance			
Karli et al. [27]	10 elite power athletes	Toe-to-toe body impedance	No change in this measure of total body water
Maughan et al. [32]	59 fasting and 32 not fasting male football players	Dietary intake and body composition	Decrease in daily sodium intake during Ramadan Decrease in dietary iron in the fasting group

(Continued)

TABLE 6.3 (*Continued*) Empirical Evidence on Changes in Body Fluids of Athletes and Active Individuals during Ramadan

Maughan et al. [33]		Body mass	Reduction of body water of 1% in rested individuals exposed to a temperate environment, during a day fast
Ramadan et al. [44]	6 active Kuwaitis	Body mass, serum osmolarity, serum sodium	Decrease of body mass <1.4% trend to increase of plasma sodium not significant
Shirreffs and Maughan [51]	55 junior soccer players	Body mass, serum biochemistry and urinary specific gravity	2% change of body mass during exercise, but no chronic effect; plasma sodium did not differ from controls throughout (but some samples collected in the morning)
Urinary volumes and specific gravity			
Al-Hadramy [1]	Males	Urinary stone colic	No significant increase in urinary stone colic during Ramadan fasting
Chiha [14]	12 soccer players	Body mass, body fat and haematocrit	No significant decrease of plasma volume at rest or after laboratory exercise, but volume of water ingested decreased by 1.07 L/day (31%) during Ramadan
Karli et al. [27]	10 power athletes	Body mass, urinary specific gravity, bioimpedance	No change of body mass, but increase of afternoon urinary specific gravity during Ramadan
Shirreffs and Maughan [51]	55 junior soccer players	Body mass, serum biochemistry and urinary specific gravity	2% change of body mass during training session, not seen in controls, but no chronic effect on body mass or urinary specific gravity (some of urine samples collected in the morning)

Body Mass

In athletes, any decrease in body mass that develops over the course of Ramadan could reflect not only a progressive dehydration but also the breakdown of fat and lean tissue to meet metabolic needs. Empirical data (Table 2.4) show nine studies where there was a small decrease of body mass and nine where there was no significant change. Unfortunately, many studies of active individuals did not document associated changes in lean tissue and fat. However, two studies specifically concerned with athletes saw no changes of body mass, body composition, fluid volumes or sweat rates [13,35].

Haemoglobin and Haematocrit

Among six studies of haemoglobin and haematocrit in active individuals, four found an increase of afternoon readings during Ramadan, suggesting that some dehydration developed over the course of the day [1,3,11,14]; however, no reports suggested a cumulative effect.

Bouhlel et al. [10] observed haemoconcentration both at rest and following 30 minutes of submaximal cycle ergometer exercise; in the study of Aloui et al. [3], the afternoon-resting haematocrit was increased, but following repeated sprint exercise, the data showed little change from pre-Ramadan values. A group of judoka showed no consistent changes of daily water intake over Ramadan (probably because blood samples were collected in the morning), and the changes of haematocrit and haemoglobin seen in this study showed no consistent pattern of change [11]. Maughan and associates collected blood samples on some subjects during the morning and some during the afternoon, but perhaps because of changes in the living environment during Ramadan, they saw a decrease of haemoglobin and haematocrit levels in both fasting and non-fasting subjects over the course of Ramadan [32,51].

Serum Biochemistry and Bioimpedance

One study of active individuals [36] showed an insignificant trend to increased sodium ion concentrations during Ramadan. A second study evaluated soccer players prior to training sessions; this found no change of serum electrolytes, but some of the blood samples were apparently collected in the morning rather than the afternoon [3].

Foot-to-foot bioimpedance data were obtained during the afternoon on a small group of elite power athletes (two wrestlers, seven sprinters and one thrower) [11]. No significant change was seen in this estimate of total body water.

Urinary Volumes and Specific Gravity

Most published studies of urinary volumes and specific gravity have involved sedentary subjects. Two studies of athletes concerned soccer players [2,3], and the third involved power athletes [55]. There were no chronic changes in body mass [3,11] or plasma volume [14]. The power athletes showed some increase in the specific gravity of their afternoon urine samples during Ramadan. No such change was seen in one group of soccer players [51], although apparently some of the measurements on this group were apparently made in the morning. Training sessions nevertheless caused a temporary 2% decrease of body mass that was not seen when a similar volume of training was performed in control periods with free access to water [51]. The second study of soccer players recorded the total daily intake of water and reported a substantial decrease during Ramadan (1.07 L/day) [37].

In many groups of athletes, the intermittent fluid deprivation of Ramadan observance apparently induces a moderate haemoconcentration during the late afternoon, but in general, this appears to be made good by an increased fluid intake at night. Even in one study where a decreased fluid intake was reported [14], the amount of the decrease (1 L/day) was probably at the upper limit of the body's ability to adjust by a reduction of urine output.

Practical Implications for the Muslim Athlete

Both theoretical considerations and empirical data support the view that the restrictions on fluid intake imposed by Ramadan observance have little effect upon sedentary individuals. If the fluid intake is increased during the hours of darkness, there is little evidence of either short-term afternoon dehydration or accumulation of a fluid deficit over the course of Ramadan. Even individuals with clinical problems such as repeated episodes of urinary calculi do not seem to be adversely affected [51].

Available data suggest that the observance of Ramadan has somewhat greater import for competitors, particularly if they engage in team sports or sustained bouts of endurance activity. Observations in power athletes [27], rugby [10] and soccer [14] players have all shown evidence of afternoon haemoconcentration, although this appeared to be corrected by an increased intake of fluid during the hours of darkness. Further, the athletes observing Ramadan showed a weight loss during a training session that was not duplicated in controls with access to fluid [51]. No research has yet examined the effects of Ramadan in events such as a marathon or ultramarathon run, but it seems likely that the effects would be even greater than those associated with team sports. The resulting temporary decrease of blood volume seems likely to reduce maximal cardiac output, thus impairing both aerobic performance and thermoregulation. A lesser blood flow to the brain could also reduce various aspects of cognitive performance, particularly vigilance, and cause irritation, decreasing cooperation in team sports.

Since the effects of fluid deprivation are mainly acute in nature and limited to the afternoon and early evening, if possible, the timing of training and competition should be adjusted until after the athlete has had opportunity to rehydrate. Other potential tactics to minimize the adverse effects of Ramadan include maximizing the night-time intake of fluid, beginning the hours of daylight with at least 500 mL of fluid in the stomach, maximizing glycogen reserves (with their substantial associated store of water), remaining in a cool room away from sunlight until the time of competition and possibly wetting the clothing, so that body cooling comes from the drying of clothing rather than sweating. There remains a need for research on events such as the marathon and the ultramarathon, and officials should certainly watch particularly carefully for evidence of hcat stress in such events.

Other Patterns of Fluid Depletion in Athletes

Details of the effects of deliberate dehydration by athletes 'making weight' are given in Chapter 2. In terms of aerobic performance, the maximal oxygen intake is decreased, and there is a substantial shortening of the tolerance of submaximal effort. Strength is also substantially reduced, with larger effects upon power and endurance than upon isometric strength. Effects upon anaerobic power and capacity seem smaller. Heat tolerance and cerebral function are both impaired, and there is an increase of oxidant stress. Finally, recovery from such dehydration can require as long as 36 hours.

In the event of total fluid deprivation, the limiting loss of 10%–15% (5–7.5 L) is reached within 3–4 days, given a minimum daily fluid requirement in the range of 2.0–2.5 L.

Conclusions

The intermittent fluid deprivation associated with Ramadan observance poses no serious physiological threats to fluid balance in the sedentary individuals. Athletes are likely to show some decrease of plasma volumes during the afternoons and evenings of Ramadan observance. Adverse consequences for both performance and safety are likely to be greatest in prolonged events where considerable sweating occurs, and there is a need for further research examining performance and safety in such competitions.

Key Terms

Antidiuretic hormone: This hormone is also known as arginine vasopressin. It is produced by the neurohypophysis and causes vascular constriction and water retention.

Bioimpedance: Bioimpedance is a measure of the opposition to passage of an electrical current through living tissues (the opposite of conductance). Fat and membranes have a high bioimpedance, whereas fluid containing lean tissue has a low impedance; the measurement of bioimpedance can thus be used to estimate the composition of tissues interposed between the measuring electrodes.

Deuterated water: Deuterium is an isotope of hydrogen with a molecular mass of two rather than one. Thus, it is possible to estimate body water by ingesting a small quantity of water containing the deuterium isotope and seeing how it is diluted after equilibrating it with body fluids.

Haematocrit: The percentage volume of a blood sample attributable to packed red cells.

Haemoconcentration: A reduction in the fluid component of the blood, leading (for example) to an increase of haematocrit.

Haemoglobin: The oxygen-carrying pigment in red cells.

Hyponatraemia: A low plasma level of sodium ions. Biochemical hyponatraemia is diagnosed if the plasma sodium concentration falls below 135 mmol/L and clinical hyponatraemia (with symptoms and signs of ill-health) if the plasma sodium is less than 130 mmol/L.

Neurohypophysis: The posterior (neural) lobe of the pituitary gland.

Osmolarity: The concentration of a solution in terms of osmoles of solute per litre of solution.

Osmole: A unit of osmotic pressure equivalent to the amount of a solute that dissolves in solution to form 1 mol.

Osmotic pressure: The pressure required to prevent passage of a solution through a semipermeable membrane.

Percutaneous transpiration: An unperceived loss of water from the tissues that occurs continually across the skin.

Postural hypotension: A sudden drop of blood pressure on standing that can cause dizziness and fainting.

Specific gravity: The mass of a substance relative to that of an equal volume of distilled water at a specified temperature.

Key Points

1. The minimum fluid need of a sedentary adult is about 1.5 L/day. Greater volumes are needed by athletes, particularly if their sport induces much sweating.
2. Dehydration is best assessed by repeated measures of haemoglobin and haematocrit.
3. Athletic performance is adversely affected when total body water loss exceeds about 2%, but health is unlikely to be endangered until losses exceed 10%.
4. Sedentary individuals show little evidence of dehydration during the intermittent fluid deprivation of Ramadan.
5. Athletes sweat less and typically show some haemoconcentration during the afternoons of Ramadan observance.
6. There is no evidence of cumulative dehydration during Ramadan observance; rather, body adaptations seem to diminish acute reductions in body fluids as Ramadan continues.
7. Substantial fluid depletion in attempts to make a specific athletic weight category substantially reduces muscular strength and other aspects of performance.

Questions for Discussion

1. What tactics can an athlete adopt during Ramadan to minimize the effects of fluid restriction while continuing to observe the requirements of fasting?
2. Why is a decrease of body mass an unreliable indication of dehydration during some forms of fasting?
3. Which aspects of performance and health are likely to be affected adversely by dehydration?
4. How do sedentary individuals compensate for the fluid restrictions imposed by Ramadan observance?
5. Which groups of athlete are most vulnerable to the effects of dehydration?

References

1. Al-Hadramy MS. Seasonal variations of urinary stone colic in Arabia. *J Pak Med Assoc* 1997;47:281–284.
2. Al-Hourani HM, Atoum MF. Body composition, nutrient intake and physical activity patterns in young women during Ramadan. *Singapore Med J* 2007;48:906–910.
3. Aloui A, Chaouchi A, Chtourou H et al. Effects of Ramadan on the diurnal variations of repeated sprint performances. *Int J Sports Physiol Perf* 2013;8:254–263.
4. American College of Sports M. Position stand on weight loss in wrestlers. *Med Sci Sports* 1976;8(2):xi.
5. Armstrong LE, Costill DL, Fink WJ. Influence of diuretic-induced dehydration on competitive running performance. *Med Sci Sports Exerc* 1985;17:456–461.
6. Ashcroft F. *Life without Water in Life at the Extremes*. University of California Press, Berkeley, CA, 2000, pp. 134–138.
7. Bakhotmah B. The puzzle of self-reported weight gain in a month of fasting (Ramadan) among a cohort of Saudi families in Jeddah, Western Saudi Arabia. *Nutr J* 2011;10:84.
8. Bauernschmitt HG, Kinne RK. Metabolism of the 'organic osmolyte' glycerophosphocholine in isolated rat inner medullary collecting duct cells. II. Regulation by extracellular osmolality. *Biochim Biophys Acta* 1993;1150:25–34.
9. Bigard AX, Boussif M, Chalabi H et al. Alterations in muscular performance and orthostatic tolerance during Ramadan. *Aviat Space Environ Med* 1998;69:341–346.
10. Bouhlel E, Salhi Z, Bouhlel H et al. Effect of Ramadan fasting on fuel oxidation during exercise in trained male rugby players. *Diabetes Metab* 2006;32:617–624.
11. Chaouachi A, Chamari K, Roky R et al. Lipid profiles of judo athletes during Ramadan. *Int J Sports Med* 2008;29:282–288.
12. Cheah SH, Ch'ng SL, Husain R et al. Effects of fasting during Ramadan on urinary excretion in Malaysian Muslims. *Br J Nutr* 1990;63:329–337.
13. Chennaoui M, Desgorces F, Drogou C et al. Effects of Ramadan fasting on physical performance and metabolic, hormonal, and inflammatory parameters in middle-distance runners. *Appl Physiol Nutr Metab* 2009;34:587–594.
14. Chiha F. Variations du métabolisme énergétique à l'effort des footballeurs lors du jeûne de Ramadan (Changes in exercise metabolism of soccer players during Ramadan fasting). University of Algiers, Algiers, Algeria, 2008/09.
15. Dewanti L, Watanabe C, Sulistiawati, Ohtsuka R. Unexpected changes in blood pressure and hematological parameters among fasting and nonfasting workers during Ramadan in Indonesia. *Eur J Clin Nutr* 2006;60:877–881.
16. Dill DB, Costill DL. Calculation of percentage changes in volumes of blood, plasma and red cells in dehydration. *J Appl Physiol* 1974;37:247–248.
17. Erickson KA, Wilding P. Evaluation of a novel point-of-care system, the i-STAT portable clinical analyzer. *Clin Chem* 1993;39:283–287.
18. Farshidfar G, Yousfi H, Vakili M et al. The effect of Ramadan fasting on hemoglobin, hematocrit and blood biochemical parameters. *J Res Health Sci* 2006;6:21–27.
19. Freund BJ, Shizuru EM, Hashiro GM et al. Hormonal, electrolyte and renal responses to exercise are intensity dependent. *J Appl Physiol* 1991;70:900–906.
20. Furuncuoglu Y, Karaca E, Aras S et al. Metabolic, biochemical and psychiatric alterations in healthy subjects during Ramadan. *Pak J Nutr* 2007;6:209–211.
21. Glaser EM, Shephard RJ. Simultaneous experimental acclimatization to heat and cold in man. *J Physiol* 1963;169:592–602.
22. Green RP, Landt M. Home sodium monitoring in patients with diabetes insipidus. *J Pediatr* 2002;141:618–624.
23. Guerra I, Chaves R, Barros T et al. The influence of fluid ingestion on performance of soccer players during a match. *J Sports Sci Med* 2004;3:198–202.
24. Hallack MH, Nomani MZ. Body weight loss and changes in blood lipid levels in normal men on hypocaloric diets during Ramadan fasting. *Am J Clin Nutr* 1988;48:1197–1210.

25. Herbert WG, Ribisl PM. Effect of dehydration upon physical working capacity of wrestlers under competitive conditions. *Res Q* 1972;43:416–422.
26. Husain R, Duncan MT, Cheah SH et al. Effects of fasting in Ramadan on Tropical Asiatic Moslems. *Br J Nutr* 1987;58:41–48.
27. Karli U, Guvenc A, Aslan A et al. Influence of Ramadan fasting on anaerobic performance and recovery from short high intensity exercise. *J Sport Sci Med* 2007;6:490–497.
28. Kirby CR, Convertino VA. Plasma aldosterone and sweat sodium concentrations after exercise and heat acclimation. *J Appl Physiol* 1985;61(3):967–970.
29. Leiper JB, Carnie A, Maughan RJ. Water turnover rates in sedentary and exercising middle aged men. *Br J Sports Med* 1996;30:24–26.
30. Leiper JB, Prastowow S-M. Effects of fasting during Ramadan on water turnover in men living in the tropics. *J Physiol* 2000;528:43.
31. Leiper JB, Molla AM, Molla AM. Effects on health of fluid restriction during fasting in Ramadan. *Eur J Clin Nutr* 2003;57(Suppl. 2):S30–S38.
32. Maughan RJ, Bartagi Z, Dvorak J et al. Dietary intake and body composition of football players during the holy month of Ramadan. *J Sports Sci* 2008;26(Suppl. 3):S20–S38.
33. Maughan RJ, Shirrefs SM. Hydration and performance during Ramadan. *J Sports Sci* 2012;30(Suppl. 1):S33–S41.
34. McGregor SJ, Nicholas CW, Lakomy HKA et al. The influence of intermittent high-intensity shuttle running and fluid ingestion on the performance of a soccer skill. *J Sports Sci* 1999;17:895–903.
35. Meckel Y, Ismael A, Eliakim A. The effect of the Ramadan fast on physical performance and dietary habits in adolescent soccer players. *Eur J Appl Physiol* 2008;102:651–657.
36. Miladipour AH, Shakhssalim N, Parvin M et al. Effect of Ramadan fasting on urinary risk factors for calculus formation. *Iran J Kidney Dis* 2012;6:33–38.
37. Muazzam MG, Khaleque KA. Effect of fasting in Ramadhan. *J Trop Med Hygiene* 1959;62:292–294.
38. Mustafa KY, Mahmoud NA, Gumaa KA et al. The effects of fasting in Ramadan. 2. Fluid and electrolyte balance. *Br J Nutr* 1978;40:583–589.
39. Noakes TD, Sharwood K, Speedy D et al. Three independent biological mechanisms cause exercise-associated hyponatremia: Evidence from 2,135 weighed competitive athletic performances. *Proc Natl Acad Sci USA* 2005;102(51):18550–18555.
40. Opplinger RA, Case HD, Horswell CA et al. American College of Sports Medicine Position Stand. Weight loss in wrestlers. *Med Sci Sports Exerc* 1996;28(6):1x–xii.
41. Owen JA, Kehoe SJ, Oliver SJ. Influence of fluid intake on soccer performance in a temperate environment. *J Sports Sci* 2013;31:1–10.
42. Pollock AS, Arieff AI. Abnormalities of cell volume regulation and their functional consequences. *Am J Physiol* 1980;239:F195–F205.
43. Prentice AM, Lamb WH, Prentice A et al. The effect of water abstention on milk synthesis in lactating women. *Clin Sci* 1984;66:291–298.
44. Ramadan J, Telahoun G, Al-Zaid NS et al. Responses to exercise, fluid, and energy balances during Ramadan in sedentary and active males. *Nutrition* 1999;15:735–739.
45. Rose BD, Post TW. *Clinical Physiology of Acid–Base and Electrolyte Disorders*. McGraw Hill, New York, 2001, pp. 285–296.
46. Saltin B. Circulatory responses to submaximal and maximal exercise after thermal dehydration. *J Appl Physiol* 1964;19:1125–1132.
47. Sawka M, Montain SJ. Fluid and electrolyte supplementation for exercise heat stress. *Am J Clin Nutr* 2000;72(2 Suppl.):564S–572S.
48. Shephard RJ, Kavanagh T. Biochemical changes with marathon running. Observations on post-coronary patients. In: Howald H, Poortmans J (eds.), *Metabolic Adaptations to Prolonged Exercise*. Birkhauser Verlag, Basel, Switzerland, 1975, pp. 245–252.
49. Shephard RJ. *Physiology and Biochemistry of Exercise*. Praeger Publications, New York, 1982.
50. Shephard RJ. The impact of Ramadan observance upon athletic performance. *Nutrients* 2012;4:491–505.

51. Shirreffs SM, Maughan RJ. Water and salt balance in young male football players in training during the holy month of Ramadan. *J Sports Sci* 2008;26(Suppl. 3):S47–S54.
52. Singh R, Hwa OC, Roy J et al. Subjective perceptions of sports performance, training, sleep and dietary patterns of Malaysian junior Muslim athletes during Ramadan intermittent fasting. *Asian J Sports Med* 2011;2:167–176.
53. Sproles CB, Smith DP, Byrd RJ et al. Circulatory responses to submaximal exercise after dehydration and rehydration. *J Sports Med Phys Fitness* 1976;16:98–105.
54. Sullivan RJ. Accepting death without artificial nutrition or hydration. *J Gen Int Med* 1993;8(4):220–224.
55. Sweileh N, Schnitzler A, Hunter GR, Davis B. Body composition and energy metabolism in resting and exercising Muslims during Ramadan fast. *J Sports Med Phys Fitness* 1992;32:156–163.
56. Takamata A, Mack GW, Stachenfeld MS et al. Body temperature modification of osmotically induced vasopressin secretion and thirst in humans. *Am J Physiol* 1995;269:R874–R880.
57. Thompson GS, Jones ES. Errors in the measurement of serum electrolytes. *J Clin Pathol* 1965;18:443–445.
58. Trabelsi K, Rebai H, el-Abed K et al. Effect of Ramadan fasting on body water status markers after a Rugby sevens match. *Asian J Sports Med* 2011;2:186–194.
59. Waterhouse J, Alabed H, Edwards B et al. Changes in sleep, mood and subjective and objective responses to physical performance during the daytime in Ramadan. *Biol Rhythm Res* 2009;40:367–383.
60. Zebidi A, Rachel S, Dhidah M et al. The effect of Ramadan fasting on some plasmatic and urinary parameters. *Tunisie Méd* 1990;68:367–372.

Further Reading

Andersson B. Regulation of body fluids. *Ann Rev Physiol* 1977;39:185–200.
Jeukendrup A, Gleeson M. Dehydration and its effects on performance. In: *Sport Nutrition*, 2nd edn. Jeukendrup A, Gleeson, M. (eds.), Human Kinetics, Champaign, IL, 2010.

7

Changes in Hormone Levels and Circadian Rhythms during Fasting

Ezdine Bouhlel, Zouhair Tabka and Roy J Shephard

Learning Objectives

1. To understand hormonal and metabolic adaptations to exercise and training
2. To comprehend the general effects of fasting upon hormonal responses
3. To determine specific features of the hormonal changes associated with Ramadan observance, both at rest and during exercise
4. To explore changes of circadian rhythm associated with Ramadan observance, to consider their implications for determinations of hormone concentrations, and to evaluate their impact upon physical and psychomotor performance

Introduction

We have discussed previously some of the hormones involved in the metabolic regulation of carbohydrates, fat and protein (Chapters 3 through 5). We will now review this information in more detail, looking at the adaptations to exercise, training and fasting, and specifically at the influence of the intermittent fasting of Ramadan and its disturbances of meal times and sleep patterns upon mean values and circadian variations in hormone levels.

Hormonal Adaptations to Exercise and Training

The maintenance of a consistent blood glucose level and fluid volume is important to optimal human performance. The blood glucose is regulated on the one hand by insulin, the only hormone that reduces blood glucose concentration, and on the other hand by a substantial group of hormones that boost blood glucose (growth hormone [GH], cortisol, catecholamines, glucagon and thyroxine) (Table 7.1). Fat stores are increased indirectly by an opposing pair of satiety hormones, leptin (reducing appetite) and ghrelin (increasing appetite). More directly, catecholamines mobilize depot fat, and various hormones including insulin, glucagon, cortisol and adiponectin all increase fat storage. Protein stores are also regulated by opposing hormones; cortisol increases the catabolism of lean tissue, and pituitary GH, thyroxine, insulin-like growth factors (IGF-1) and steroids all increase anabolic activity. Fluid balance is controlled by antidiuretic hormone (ADH) and by aldosterone. Changes in the activity of these various hormones are seen with exercise, training and fasting, and many hormones also show distinct circadian rhythms.

Insulin

Insulin is an anabolic hormone, secreted by the beta cells of the pancreatic islets of Langerhans. The metabolic effects of this hormone are exerted on three main target tissues, liver, muscle and adipose tissue. Insulin regulates glucose

TABLE 7.1 Hormonal Responses to an Acute Bout of Exercise

Endocrine Gland	Hormone	Response to Acute Exercise
Anterior pituitary	Growth hormone	Increases with increasing work intensity
	Thyrotropin	Increases with increasing work intensity
	Adrenocorticotropin	Increases with increasing intensity and duration
	Prolactin	Increases with exercise intensity
Posterior pituitary	Antidiuretic hormone (vasopressin)	Increases with increasing work intensity
Thyroid	Thyroxine (T4) and triiodothyronine (T3)	Free T3 and T4 increase with increasing work intensity
Parathyroid	Parathyroid hormone	Increases with prolonged exercise
Adrenal medulla	Epinephrine	Increases with increasing work, starting at about 75% of $\dot{V}O_{2max}$
	Norepinephrine	Increases with increasing rates of work, starting at about 50% of $\dot{V}O_{2max}$
Adrenal cortex	Aldosterone	Increases with increasing intensity
	Cortisol	Increases only with high-intensity exercise
Pancreas	Insulin	Decreases with increasing work intensity
	Glucagon	Increases with increasing work intensity

Source: Galbo, H, *Hormonal and Metabolic Adaptation to Exercise*, Thieme-Stratton, New York, 1983.

homeostasis, capturing glucose molecules, and storing them as glycogen in liver and muscle as blood sugar is reduced to its target value.

Insulin also inhibits the hepatic production of glucose, whether by glycogenolysis or gluconeogenesis. Further, it regulates fat metabolism, promoting fatty acid synthesis from the products of glycolysis; it activates the enzyme *lipoprotein lipase*, causing a hydrolysis of circulating triglycerides. In addition, insulin plays an antilipolytic role, protecting fat stores by inhibiting the adipocyte hormone-sensitive lipase.

Respective Roles of Neural and Hormonal Regulation

Physiological responses are regulated by two main systems acting in close coordination: the nervous system and the endocrine system. The amplitude of these responses is related to immediate metabolic needs, such as satisfying the 10–20-fold increase of metabolism that occurs during vigorous exercise. One important objective for the body is to maintain a consistent blood glucose concentration in the face of increasing tissue energy demands. A coordinated neurohormonal response regulates the metabolic flux and assures an adequate mobilization of energy stores. The sympathetic nervous system exerts two main effects, the inhibition of insulin secretion and the stimulation of glyco-genolysis, both increasing blood glucose. These effects are modulated by the various hormonal responses discussed in this chapter.

Physical exercise quickly reduces insulin secretion in proportion to the intensity and duration of effort [56,68], initially through a feed-forward action of the sympathetic nervous system that proceeds in parallel with the neural command to the muscles. The reduction of insulin output is sustained as exercise depletes blood glucose; this reverses the inhibition of hepatic gluconeogenesis, leads to a lesser capture and utilization of glucose molecules by insulin-sensitive tissues that are not directly involved in exercise, and increases adipocyte lipolysis and thus the supply of fat to the working muscles.

Growth Hormone

GH is an anabolic hormone, secreted by the anterior pituitary gland. Like many other hormones, it is active only when not combined with its binding protein (GH-binding protein). GH plays an important role in regulating bone and muscle growth and regeneration, but it is also involved in the metabolic regulation of liver, muscle and adipose tissue. It stimulates hepatic gluconeogenesis, and by an action upon lipase, it leads to a release of fatty acids from adipose tissue. GH levels increase during prolonged exercise, thus increasing both lipolysis and hepatic gluconeogenesis. The anabolic effects of GH are amplified as it stimulates the release of IGF-1 from the liver; the IGF-1 is also active only when it is not combined with its corresponding binding protein.

Cortisol

Cortisol has an important anti-inflammatory effect. It also plays a major role in the regulation of blood glucose and energy balance. It stimulates protein catabolism; this leads to the liberation of amino acids, particularly alanine, from lean tissue, facilitating hepatic gluconeogenesis. Cortisol also reduces the glucose uptake of some tissues, facilitates fatty acid mobilization, and may help the achievement of an energy balance by increasing the dietary intake of foodstuffs, particularly carbohydrate.

Physical exercise increases plasma cortisol in proportion to the intensity and duration of effort, and levels remain high during recovery following an intense or prolonged bout of exercise.

Catecholamines

Norepinephrine is rapidly released by the sympathetic nerve terminals at the outset of exercise. As activity continues, epinephrine and additional quantities of norepinephrine are also released from the adrenal medulla in amounts that increase with the intensity of effort. Both catecholamines play a major role in metabolic homeostasis. At rest, epinephrine secretion induces increases of lipolysis and glycogenolysis, and it inhibits insulin secretion [27,40]. Norepinephrine stimulates hepatic glucose production, and epinephrine stimulates muscle glycogenolysis during intensive exercise.

Glucagon

Glucagon is a hormone secreted by the alpha cells in the pancreatic islets of Langerhans. It acts directly on the liver, enhancing glucose release through a combination of increased glycogenolysis, gluconeogenesis and an inhibition of glycogen synthesis [91]. Glucagon also has a lipolytic effect on adipose tissue.

Glucagon secretion increases during exercise through the joint stimuli of sympathetic nerve activation and decreases in circulating levels of insulin and glucose.

Thyroid Hormones

There are two forms of thyroid hormone: thyroxine (T4), which is converted in the target cells to triiodothyronine (T3), and T3, which is the biologically active form. Both T3 and T4 facilitate the mobilization and usage of stored energy. They increase lipolysis and beta-oxidation of fatty acids. They also increase muscle glucose utilization, enhancing glycogenolysis and gluconeogenesis in the liver, and facilitating glucose uptake by the active tissues. Furthermore, the catabolism of proteins is enhanced by both T3 and T4.

The direct metabolic effects of thyroid hormones are similar at rest and during exercise. However, T3 also exerts a permissive effect on other hormones, increasing concentrations of the second messenger cyclic AMP.

Sex Hormones

The sex hormone steroids are important to muscle hypertrophy. Luteinizing hormone (LH) is produced in the anterior pituitary gland. In women, a surge of this hormone induces ovulation. In males, it stimulates the Leydig cells in the testes, with the secretion of testosterone. Testosterone is an anabolic steroid that promotes the hypertrophy of tissues, particularly the growth of muscle (Table 7.1).

Antidiuretic Hormone and Aldosterone

The output of ADH, secreted by the neurohypophysis, is increased when exercise-induced sweating and/or a restricted fluid intake causes haemoconcentration and dehydration. ADH acts by increasing water absorption in the collecting ducts of the kidneys. Aldosterone is secreted by the adrenal cortex. It also counters dehydration, although it acts by increasing sodium absorption in the distal tubules and collecting ducts of the kidneys. Prolonged exercise accompanied by substantial losses of water and/or sodium increases the release of both of these hormones.

Training Effects

The beneficial cardiovascular, respiratory and muscular effects of training are well documented, but much less is known about neurohormonal adaptations to a training regimen. The main response seems an increased ability to metabolize lipids. This is explained mainly by an enhanced activity of aerobic enzymes, an increase in the number and volume of the mitochondria and a hypertrophy of aerobic, slow-twitch type I muscle fibres. The increased capacity to metabolize fats during submaximal exercise plays a major role in augmenting a subject's endurance and aerobic capacity. The increased fat utilization conserves available muscle glycogen stores for use at the highest intensities of effort [23].

Hormonal Regulation of Metabolism

Plasma glucose levels during exercise depend on the balance that is struck between glucose uptake in the muscles and its release by the liver. The release of glucose is facilitated by glucagon, which promotes glycogenolysis and gluconeogenesis. Exercise increases glucagon levels and stimulates the release of catecholamines, both enhancing glycogenolysis. Exercise also increases cortisol levels, thus increasing protein catabolism and liberating amino acids that can to be used within the liver for gluconeogenesis. When carbohydrate stores are low, fat oxidation is enhanced by an increase of catecholamine concentrations. The triglycerides stored in fat cells and muscle are broken down to free fatty acids and glycerol by an enzyme called lipase; this is activated by at least four hormones: cortisol, epinephrine, norepinephrine and GH. For the same power output, trained athletes secrete less hormones for any given intensity of effort because their peripheral receptors have a greater sensitivity to hormones.

Carbohydrate metabolism is also modified; training increases muscle glucose transporters (GLUT-4).

There are associated changes in the neurohormonal response, including lesser reductions of insulin secretion and smaller increases of catecholamine and glucagon during physical activity [43,52]. These changes facilitate lipid oxidation and in consequence spare glycogen stores during prolonged exercise [97]. The lesser hormonal responses following training are explained in part by peripheral changes. For example, training increases the sensitivity of peripheral receptors to catecholamines, especially in adipose tissue. Moreover, training increases the sensitivity of muscle to insulin. Conversely, physical inactivity is a major factor inducing obesity, insulin resistance and type 2 diabetes mellitus. These pathologies are accompanied by abnormalities of muscle typology, microcirculation and metabolism [23,73]. Insulin resistance leads to a lesser capture, storage and utilization of glucose molecules. Moreover, high blood glucose levels reduce fat oxidation and encourage a hypersecretion of insulin that persists during exercise, exacerbating the normal exercise-induced decrease in blood glucose. The decreased oxidation of fatty acids leads to an accumulation of lipids in the muscle cytoplasm, and this further discourages glucose capture and storage.

Metabolic and Hormonal Responses to Fasting

Short-term fasting induces many changes in hormone secretion (Table 7.2). It increases GH and IGF-1 levels in subjects of normal body mass [2,13,50], with an accompanying increase in circulating levels of free fatty acids [78,88]. In contrast to this response, total fasting does not increase GH and IGF-1 levels in individuals who are obese [13,67].

Hormonal Responses to Fasting

Hormonal responses that help to maintain blood glucose levels and increase the mobilization of fat stores during fasting include a reduction in insulin secretion and increased circulating concentrations of glucagon, catecholamines, GH, thyroid-stimulating hormone (TSH) and corticosteroids.

Fasting inhibits leptin secretion. Grottoli et al. [44] found higher insulin levels in obese patients than in normal subjects after 36 h of fasting, suggesting that

TABLE 7.2 Hormonal Changes Observed in Sedentary Subjects during Fasting

Authors	Subjects	Changes during Fasting
Aimaretti et al. [2]	9 GH-deficient adults	36 hours fasting stimulates GH secretion
Aloi et al. [5]	6 healthy young men	Two 83 h fasting sessions induced decline in LH secretory burst mass/amplitude and frequency. GnRH infusion restores LH and serum total and free testosterone concentrations
Bang et al. [13]	Healthy subjects and obese	4 days of fasting depresses IGF-1 in healthy subjects but not in obese
Bergendahl et al. [16]	8 normal men	5 days of fasting increased serum cortisol concentrations
Bergendahl et al. [17]	8 healthy young versus 8 older men (average 67 years)	3.5 days fast induced similar increases in mean (24 h) serum cortisol concentrations in both groups (40% and 47%, respectively). 24 h endogenous LH secretion reduced in young, but not in older men. Reduced serum free testosterone concentrations in older men but not in younger. Testosterone levels did not decline further with fasting
Degoutte et al. [28]	20 male judoka	Energy intake reduced to 4 MJ/day for 1 week prior to competition reduced testosterone and testosterone/cortisol ratio
Gjedsted et al. [42]	10 healthy men	72 h fast did not alter insulin-/amino acid–stimulated regional phenylalanine flux in leg and forearm muscles
Grottoli et al. [44]	7 women with visceral obesity, 6 with Cushing's syndrome	Reduction of leptin and GH increase with 36 h fasting blunted by both simple obesity and Cushing's syndrome
Grottoli et al. [45]	7 normal women, 8 patients with acromegaly	Short-term fasting leads increased GH response in normal women but not in acromegaly
Hartman et al. [50]	9 normal men	2 days of fasting increased the 24 h endogenous GH production rate fivefold, with increases in the amplitude of GH secretory bursts
		Serum insulin-like growth factor I (IGF-1) concentrations were unchanged after 56 hours of fasting
Hartman et al. [51]	6 normal men	2 days of fasting increased GH secretion and decreased free IGF-1 concentrations
Langfort et al. [62]	8 healthy men	Low carbohydrate intake for 3 days enhanced activity of the sympathoadrenal system at rest and after exercise, accompanied by a reduction in 30-second anaerobic capacity
Maccario et al. [67]	9 patients with simple obesity	36 hours of fasting increased GH levels, but did not modify IGF-1 or IGFBP-3 responses
Moller et al. [75]	10 healthy men	37.5 hours of fasting reduced metabolic clearance of GH, decreased insulin sensitivity and reduced IGF-I bioactivity

(*Continued*)

TABLE 7.2 (*Continued*) Hormonal Changes Observed in Sedentary Subjects during Fasting

Authors	Subjects	Changes during Fasting
Nellemann et al. [77]	8 healthy male subjects	Both fasting (36 hours) and GH infusion promoted lipolysis, with an associated reduction of insulin sensitivity compared to the control day Significant reductions of active pyruvate dehydrogenase with both fasting and GH infusion
Salgin et al. [87]	7 female and 4 male normal weight subjects.	24 hours of fasting increased basal free GH, mean free GH, mean total GH and non-esterified fatty acid levels; I GHBP levels remained unchanged
Salgin et al. [88]	14 (8 female, 6 male) healthy young adults	24-hour but not overnight fasting increased of FFA levels, and decreased insulin sensitivity and the acute insulin response
Veldhuis et al. [99]	8 healthy young men	5-day (water only) fast attenuated the mass of LH secreted per burst without altering LH secretory event frequency or LH half-life
Zoladz et al. [107]	8 healthy non-smoking men	Overnight fasting did not change leptin and ghrelin concentrations, but plasma norepinephrine levels increased

GH, growth hormone; GHBP, growth hormone–binding protein; GnRH, gonadotropin-releasing hormone; IGF-1, insulin-like growth factor-1; IGFBP-3, insulin-like growth factor binding protein; LH, luteinizing hormone.

hyperinsulinism could play a role in altering leptin and GH responses to fasting in those who are overweight. Salgin et al. [87] found that a 24 hours fast induced decreases in insulin sensitivity and increased free fatty acids levels in healthy young adults. Gjedsted et al. [41] further found increased lipid oxidation, insulin resistance and decreased glucose oxidation in healthy subjects after 72 hours of fasting. Palmitate fluxes across the forearm and leg, leg muscle glycerol concentrations, and abdominal subcutaneous blood flow were all increased, indicating a stimulation of lipolysis. Hagström-Toft et al. [47] also found that 11 days of a very low-energy diet (2.2 MJ/day) increased fat mobilization in skeletal muscle.

Moller et al. [75] noted that 37.5 hours of fasting was associated with a slower clearance of an injected bolus of GH, an enhanced lipid response to this hormone, and a decrease in insulin sensitivity and IGF-1 activity. Nellemann et al. [77] also noted that both 36 hours of fasting and administration of GH promoted lipolysis in healthy subjects, with an associated reduction in insulin sensitivity. They concluded that a competition between the intermediates of glucose and fatty acids played a role in causing insulin resistance. Pyruvate dehydrogenase in its active form (PDHa) was significantly reduced by both GH and fasting [77].

An increase of GH secretion in fasting or malnourished subjects is mediated by an increased frequency of bursts of GH-releasing hormone [50]. Hartman et al. [50,51] found that 2 days of fasting induced a twofold increase in secretory burst amplitudes without changing the duration of bursts; the result was a fivefold increase in the 24 h GH production rate. However, serum IGF-1 concentrations were unchanged by the 2-day fast. These changes were associated with a decrease of rapid eye movement sleep, but no change in slow-wave (stages 3 and 4) sleep.

Cortisol

Cortisol levels are increased in fasted or malnourished subjects [16,17]. Five days of fasting increased the 24 h output of cortisol, with an increase in the amplitude of secretory bursts [16]. In addition, the mean (mesor) mass of glucocorticoid secreted over 24 hours was increased after 5 days of fasting. There was an inverse relationship between mean serum cortisol and GH concentrations in fasted men [16], suggesting a differential regulation of corticotropic and somatotropic axes during fasting and/or feedback interactions between these two axes when both are activated.

Sex Hormones

Five days of fasting or severe dietary restriction in healthy men decreased the daily secretion of LH, the mass of LH secreted per burst and the resulting output of testosterone. However, the administration of gonadotropin-releasing hormone restored the pre-fasting LH secretion and thus the total and free serum concentrations of testosterone [5,99]. Degoutte et al. [28] reduced the energy intake of 20 male judoka to 4 MJ/day for 1 week prior to competition; this induced a reduction in testosterone levels and the testosterone/cortisol ratio relative to matched competitors. In similar vein, Bergendahl et al. [17] found decreases in the 24 h endogenous LH production rate of young men after 3.5 days of fasting, although in their study, the daily LH secretion was unaffected in older men (where the testosterone response would in any event be much smaller).

Catecholamines

Zoladz et al. [107] examined alterations of response to an incremental cycle ergometer test (30 W stages to a ceiling of 150 W) after an overnight fast. No changes of leptin or ghrelin response were observed. However, plasma norepinephrine and IL-6 concentrations were both greater after fasting, helping to mobilize glucose and thus assure energy homeostasis. Langfort et al. [62] had their subjects follow a low (5%) carbohydrate diet for 3 days. The mean power output during a 30 s cycle ergometer exercise was decreased, but plasma norepinephrine and epinephrine concentrations reached higher values during the dietary restriction; they concluded that the activity of the sympathoadrenal system was increased both at rest and after exercise when dietary carbohydrate intake was limited.

Protein Metabolism

Prolonged fasting leads to a progressive loss of body proteins, with a suppression of anabolic mechanisms [100]. Vendelbo et al. [100] found an increased net phenylalanine release from skeletal muscle when healthy subjects underwent a 3-day fast. This was associated with a reduced activation of rapamycin (mTOR), a key regulator of cell growth. Likewise, Fryburg et al. [38] reported that a 60 h continuous fast increased urinary nitrogen loss, as well as whole body phenylalanine and leucine flux and oxidation. Despite this catabolic response and a marked impairment of insulin-mediated glucose storage, the muscles remained sensitive to insulin's antiproteolytic action. Gjedsted et al. [42] found unchanged insulin-stimulated phenylalanine fluxes in leg and forearm muscle of healthy subjects after a fast of 72 h, and they concluded that fasting did not induce insulin resistance as regards amino acid metabolism.

Hormonal Responses to the Intermittent Fasting of Ramadan

Hormonal responses in people observing Ramadan have shown some inconsistencies. This could reflect differences in dietary habits (particularly the exploitation of Ramadan to reduce body mass), month and latitudinal differences in the length of the required daily fast, and differences in the physical fitness of those evaluated. A further issue is limited blood sampling, since a circadian shift of hormone secretions relative to sampling times could give the impression of an increase or a decrease in plasma concentrations of a given hormone. Most studies have shown shifts in the circadian rhythm of most hormones during Ramadan observance (Table 7.3; [14,15,18]).

Melatonin

Melatonin, secreted by the pineal gland, is the main hormone regulating circadian rhythms. Bogdan et al. [18] found a decrease in nocturnal peak levels of melatonin during Ramadan observance, with associated displacements of the normal circadian rhythms of cortisol and testosterone secretion. BaHammam [10] also noted a flatter peak of melatonin concentrations during Ramadan, although the timing of the normal diurnal cycle was not displaced. Iraki et al. [55] found changes in the average 24 hours concentrations of most hormones except insulin (e.g. an increase in plasma gastrin, associated with a decrease in gastric pH, probably because of the altered meal times). These changes persisted one month after the end of Ramadan fasting.

Catecholamines and Thyroid Hormones

Chennaoui et al. [26] noted increases of epinephrine and norepinephrine levels in athletes during Ramadan observance. Bogdan et al. [18] also found an altered rhythm of TSH secretion. Sajid et al. [86] reported a gradual increase of TSH levels during Ramadan observance, although mean values remained within clinical limits, and the concentrations of triiodothyronine and thyroxine did not change.

TABLE 7.3 Hormonal Changes in Healthy Subjects during Ramadan Observance

Author	Sample	Changes during Ramadan
Sedentary subjects		
Ahmadinejad et al. [1]	81 students	Decrease in T4, increased TSH in male subjects, although TSH and T4 levels remained within the normal range, unchanged T3 levels
al-Hadramy et al. [3]	10 healthy subjects	Alteration of the cortisol rhythm
Alzoghaibi et al. [6]	8 healthy subjects	Reduction in leptin and unchanged ghrelin levels but significant changes of these hormones in the acrophases
Azizi et al. [8]	9 healthy men	No changes of FSH, LH, testosterone, prolactin, or TSH during Ramadan
Azizi et al. [9]	Healthy women	No change of thyroid hormones
BaHammam [10]	8 healthy subjects	No displacement of melatonin cycle, but flatter midnight peak
Ben Salem et al. [15]	11 healthy subjects	Reduction of cortisol at 8 hours but increase at 20 hours
Bogdan et al. [18]	10 healthy non-smoking males	Shift in the onset of cortisol and testosterone secretion, increase in evening peak of prolactin
		FSH and GH rhythms affected little or not at all
		Decrease in the mean 24 h level of FSH, unchanged LH levels, altered TSH rhythm
Bogdan et al. [19]	10 male subjects	Unchanged amplitude and mean 24 hours concentration of plasma leptin, but significant shifts of 5 hours 30 minutes in peak leptin levels by 23rd day of fasting
Cağlayan et al. [24]	30 women	Unchanged LH, FSH, estradiol and prolactin
Dwivedi et al. [32]	12 young students	Decrease of morning cortisol, increase of evening values
El-Migdadi et al. [34,35]	20 healthy male students living in the Jordan Valley 20 healthy males living in Ramtha City	Increase in serum LH levels only in students of the Jordan Valley, increase in serum testosterone levels in male students of Jordan Valley
Fedail et al. [37]	24 Muslims	Increase of thyroxine but not T3 by the end of Ramadan
Kassab et al. [58]	Lean and obese subjects	Increase in leptin levels in lean and obese subjects
Kassab et al. [59]	Healthy women	Increases in leptin and insulin levels, reduction of neuropeptide-y concentration
Mansi and Amneh [69]	42 healthy male students	Reduction of testosterone levels, increased FSH values, unchanged LH and T3 levels
Mesbahzadeh et al. [74]	52 students	Reduction of testosterone at the end of fasting, increase in FSH at the 20th day, unchanged LH levels

(Continued)

TABLE 7.3 (*Continued*) Hormonal Changes in Healthy Subjects during Ramadan Observance

Author	Sample	Changes during Ramadan
Sajid et al. [86]	41 men, 5 women	Gradual rise of TSH over Ramadan
Sulimani et al. [95]	28 healthy men	No change of thyroxine, TDSH, T3 or T4
Athletic subjects		
Bouhlel et al. [20]	Trained subjects	Unchanged GH, IGF-1 values
Bouhlel et al. [21]	Trained subjects	Unchanged leptin and adiponectin levels
Chennaoui et al. [26]	8 middle-distance runners	Unchanged testosterone/cortisol ratio Increase in epinephrine and norepinephrine levels
El Migdadi et al. [34]	Athletic students	Increase in ACTH and cortisol levels

ACTH, adrenocorticotropic hormone; FSH, follicle-stimulating hormone; GH, growth hormone; IGF-1, insulin-like growth factor 1; LH, luteinizing hormone; TSH, thyroid-stimulating hormone.

Fedail et al. [37] reported increases of serum thyroxine but not T4 by the end of Ramadan, and Sajid et al. [86] noted a gradual rise of TSH over the course of Ramadan. On the other hand, Azizi et al. [8] and Sulimani et al. [95] found no change in any of the thyroid hormones during Ramadan, and in one sample of women, there were even decreases in L-diiodothyronine (T2) and T4 [9]. Interpretation of these various findings is hampered by limited blood sampling and possible displacements of the normal circadian rhythm.

Cortisol and ACTH

Most investigators have seen changes in cortisol levels during fasting. Dwivedi et al. [32] found lower morning but higher evening cortisol values. Likewise, Ben Salem et al. [15] found that cortisol levels measured at 8:00 h were lower during than before Ramadan. On the other hand, cortisol levels measured at 20:00 h were higher during than before Ramadan. They suggested that the altered diurnal pattern reflected changes in feeding behaviour and sleep–wake rhythms, rather than a fundamental change in circadian rhythms [14]. al-Hadramy et al. [3] also found an altered cortisol rhythm in 4 of 10 subjects tested over the last two weeks of fasting. El-Migdadi et al. [34] found increases in both cortisol and adrenocorticotropic hormone values during fasting; however, they only collected a single afternoon blood sample, and their findings were thus vulnerable to effects from a shift of diurnal rhythm.

Bogdan et al. [18] found shifts in timing of the onset of cortisol and testosterone secretion in healthy subjects; they suggested that not only the intermittent fast but also the altered social habits and sleep schedules of Ramadan contributed to this response. Chennaoui et al. [26] reported an unchanged testosterone/cortisol ratio in middle-distance athletes.

In the study of Bogdan et al. [18], fasting had little effect on the rhythm of GH secretion. Bouhlel et al. [20] again found no change in GH, IGF-1 or IGFBP-3 secretion during Ramadan observance; in their subjects, plasma concentrations of glucose and insulin levels were also unchanged, either at rest or following exercise.

Leptin and Adiponectin

Most studies of Ramadan observance have reported changes in the magnitude or the phase of leptin levels. Bogdan et al. [19] found no changes in the mean leptin concentration, but they noted a shift in the timing of peak leptin levels. Kassab et al. [58] found increased leptin levels in both lean and obese subjects during fasting, with an increase in insulin and a decrease in neuropeptide-Y [59]. The adiponectin/leptin ratio provides an effective measure of insulin resistance [54]; Bouhlel et al. [21] found no change in leptin or adiponectin levels or their ratio in athletes during Ramadan observance, despite significant reductions of body mass and body fat.

Sex Hormones

Although a prolonged energy deficiency relative to exercise expenditures leads to depressed secretion of testosterone and oestrogen concentrations, with amen-orrhea in women [66] and depressed testicular function in men [46], reproductive hormones show few changes during the brief intermittent fasting periods of Ramadan [35]. Bogdan et al. [18] saw little alteration in the circadian rhythm of follicle-stimulating hormone (FSH) during Ramadan, although there was a shift in timing of the onset of testosterone secretion and the evening peak of prolactin secretion was increased. Cağlayan et al. [24] found unchanged LH, FSH, estradiol and prolactin levels during Ramadan observance. Mesbahzadeh et al. [74] found increases in FSH by the 20th day of Ramadan and a decrease of testosterone values toward the end of Ramadan fasting, but no change in LH levels.

Changes in Exercise Hormonal Responses during Ramadan Observance

There have been relatively few studies of hormonal responses during and follow-ing exercise in connection with Ramadan observance (Table 7.4).

Bouhlel et al. [20] found that during Ramadan, the levels of GH, IGF-1, IGFBP-3 and insulin maintained a normal pattern after undertaking a progres-sive exercise test to 60% of $\dot{V}O_{2max}$. Leptin and adiponectin levels and the leptin/adiponectin ratio of athletes also followed the usual pattern after this test exer-cise, despite significant reductions in body mass and body fat [20]. These authors suggested that the severity of food restriction and dehydration during Ramadan observance was insufficient to induce changes in either the GH/IGF-1 axis or

TABLE 7.4 Changes in Exercise Hormonal Responses during Ramadan Observance

Author	Subjects	Protocol	Changes during Ramadan Observance
Bouhlel et al. [20]	9 trained male rugby players	Progressive exercise to 60% of $\dot{V}O_{2max}$	No change in plasma concentrations of glucose, insulin, GH, IGF-1 or IGFBP-3
Bouhlel et al. [21]	9 male rugby players	Progressive exercise to 60% of $\dot{V}O_{2max}$	No significant changes in leptin or adiponectin levels
Chennaoui et al. [26]	8 middle-distance runners	Maximal aerobic velocity (MAV) test.	Testosterone/cortisol ratio unchanged before or after the MAV test, testosterone concentrations increased after the test
		Saliva samples, metabolic and hormonal parameters, mood state, and nutritional and sleep profiles	Cortisol concentrations increased only when subjects had performed the test on day 7 of fasting, increased catecholamine (epinephrine and norepinephrine) and IL-6 concentrations

GH, growth hormone; IGF-1, insulin-like growth factor-1; IGFBP-3, insulin-like growth factor binding protein; IL-6, interleukin-6.

the leptin/adiponectin ratio. Furthermore, fasting and dehydration could have had opposing effects upon hormones; food restriction would have reduced GH release, but dehydration and the resulting haemoconcentration would have increased the effective GH concentration, especially during exercise.

Despite increases in the catecholamine and IL-6 response to exercise, Chennaoui et al. [26] found a decrease in the maximal speed of medium-distance runners during Ramadan and an increase in testosterone concentrations post exercise, although the testosterone/cortisol ratio of their subjects remained unchanged.

Ramadan Observance, Sleep Patterns and Circadian Rhythms

Many biological functions such as body temperature, heart rate and wakefulness follow a circadian rhythm of fluctuation over a 24-hour cycle [76,79,80]. The magnitude and timing of these fluctuations is set not only by endogenous factors (genetic characteristics and the rhythm of a central circadian clock located in the hypothalamus) but also by exogenous factors (*zeitgebers or time signals*) that reinforce or run counter to the intrinsic rhythm (environmental factors such as the daily cycle of temperature and solar illumination, meal times, and required periods of physical activity) [93,94]. These fluctuations influence many aspects of human performance, particularly cyclic variations of hormone secretion that have an impact upon other parameters of physiological performance [90]. Many forms of fasting have little or no impact upon circadian rhythms but the need to cram two large meals and religious ceremonies into the hours of darkness, sometimes combined with daytime napping, can disturb circadian rhythms in the individual who is observing Ramadan.

Physical exercise is an important exogenous factor inducing changes in circadian rhythms and associated hormonal and metabolic responses. Fasting or dietary restriction removes an important zeitgeber that has the potential to disturb circadian rhythms of hormone secretion and metabolism [71,81,83], and a combination of physical exercise and altered feeding patterns can have a powerful effect upon regulatory processes. We will now explore these issues.

Sleep Duration

Sleep patterns are frequently disturbed during Ramadan (Table 7.5), particularly if the time of year and latitude require a prolonged daytime fast [85], and this can have a marked effect upon circadian rhythms [76]. Religious services, and the need to take a very late supper and an early breakfast, perhaps supplemented by the nighttime ingestion of fluids, occupy much of the time normally allocated to sleeping; normal patterns may be further disturbed by a delayed start to work or afternoon napping.

TABLE 7.5 Changes of Reported Sleep Duration during Observance of Ramadan

Author	Subjects	Change
Sedentary subjects		
BaHammam et al. [12]	71 healthy adults, 30 non-fasting controls	Bedtime delayed 60–90 minutes, but no sleep loss
Athletes		
Chennaoui et al. [26]	8 middle-distance athletes	88 min/day sleep loss during Ramadan
Herrera [53]	9 male soccer players	78 min/day loss of sleep
Karli et al. [57]	10 male power athletes	No significant change of sleep time
Leiper et al. [64]	54 male soccer players, 33 non-fasting controls	60 min/day sleep loss in those fasting, but 105 min/day loss in controls
Meckel et al. [72]	19 adolescent soccer players	No change of sleep pattern
Singh et al. [90]	734 junior athletes	No change of sleep pattern
Waterhouse et al. [102]	20 male university sports students	Bedtime delayed 171 minutes, 126 minutes sleep loss
Wilson et al. [104]	20 male professional soccer players	Bedtime delayed 199 minutes but sleep time increased 99 minutes
Zerguini et al. [106]	64 adolescent soccer players, 36 non-observant controls	Same findings as Leiper et al. [64]

Sedentary Subjects

One study of healthy non-athletic Saudi Arabians found that bedtime was delayed by 60–90 min during Ramadan, although in this study, the total duration of sleep was unchanged [11]; importantly, similar changes were observed in non-fasting controls, underlining a change in the total environment that complicates any comparison with control groups not observing Ramadan. In a sample of university sports students, bedtime was delayed by as long as 171 minutes [102]; their time of waking remained unchanged, but they took a compensatory daytime nap, reducing their sleep loss to an average of 126 minutes [101].

Athletes

Soccer players [71] and power athletes [57] both reported little change of sleep duration during Ramadan. The bedtime of 20 professional soccer players was delayed by an average of 199 minutes, but, because they were allowed to remain in bed after breakfast, their total sleeping time was actually increased by 99 minutes during Ramadan [104]. Most of 734 Malaysian male and female junior athletes also reported no disturbances of normal sleep [91]. In contrast, young Tunisian soccer players who normally slept for 9 hours lost 1 hours of sleep per night throughout Ramadan [64,106]; again, there was a large environmental effect, with players in a non-observant control group also losing 105 minutes of sleep per night during the first week of Ramadan. Other reports show a sleep loss of 88 minutes in middle-distance runners [26] and of 78 minutes in soccer players [53].

Sleep Quality

Sleep is normally triggered by a rapid decrease in core temperature. During Ramadan, this mechanism may be compromised by the eating of a large and late evening meal and (in the case of athletes) by a late-night training session following the meal [85]. The impact upon the quality of sleep has been variable, depending upon the methods used to record sleep patterns and differences in the local culture. In uncontrolled studies, it is important to exclude effects due to the excitement of competition rather than the changes of lifestyle associated with Ramadan [89]. Roky et al. [81,84] reported an increase of sleep latency, with a loss of slow-wave and rapid eye movements sleep. Algerian professional players complained of a poorer quality of sleep [105], and use of the Pittsburgh Sleep Quality Index suggested a deterioration of sleep quality in nine male soccer players [52]. Other changes during Ramadan included increased sleep latency and increased non-rapid eye movement sleep [11,103].

Daytime napping among those observing Ramadan seems more common in Libya, where observance of the fast is widely prevalent, than in the United Kingdom, where there are relatively few Muslims [101].

Circadian Rhythms

Given that both meal times and exercise bouts are mild zeitgebers [7], any changes in eating or training patterns associated with Ramadan are likely to disturb and/or displace normal circadian rhythms [81,83,103]. Changes of the acrophase for body temperature and metabolism may in turn modify the times of day when athletic performance and training responses reach their peak [31], although in practice, it is difficult to decide whether changes in performance are due to the immediate effects of hours of altered eating and sleeping and how far they reflect a more fundamental change in circadian rhythms [98,103].

Rhythms of Body Temperature and Metabolism

Most of the available information has been collected on sedentary people rather than on athletes; it shows a reduction of afternoon energy expenditures and some-times of total energy expenditures. Young women showed no change in their overall resting energy expenditure during Ramadan, but there was a dramatic drop in their oxygen consumption between 1100 and 1700 hours [33], presumably because of napping and/or a reduction of physical activity to compensate for fast-ing. The afternoon resting energy expenditure was also reduced in a second group of non-athletic adults who decreased their average energy intake to the very low figure of 5 MJ/day during Ramadan [96]. A third group of sedentary young men showed a 7% reduction of daily energy expenditure during Ramadan [12].

In keeping with these overall changes in metabolism, daytime oral tempera-tures were lower [80,84], and the peaks of skin temperature and physical activity as determined by an arm band sensor were displaced some 2 hours later into the evening during Ramadan [12].

Circadian Rhythms of Body Hormones

Many of the hormonal changes associated with Ramadan observance have been discussed earlier. Changes in hormonal patterns during Ramadan are generally small [83], although research has been hampered in many investigations because the number of blood samples has been insufficient to form a clear impression of any changes in diurnal patterns. Two hormones that are normally strongly linked to circadian rhythms are the metabolic regulator cortisol, and melatonin, the latter controlling wakefulness and synchronizing the body's internal clock with light/darkness cycles. Four-hour monitoring of 10 physicians showed a decrease, and possibly a delay, in the nocturnal peak of melatonin, a shift in the onset of cortisol and testosterone secretion, an enhanced evening peak in prolactin, little change in rhythmic patterns of FSH and GH, and a blunting of the serum TSH rhythm over Ramadan, with changes in meal times suggested as the main cause of these altered hormonal responses [81,18]. BaHammam [10] also noted a flattening of the mid-night peak of melatonin, but in his study, there was no displacement of the normal diurnal cycle of melatonin. Other studies of non-athletic adults have confirmed shifts in the magnitude and diurnal rhythm of cortisol during Ramadan [3,14,32].

Circadian Rhythms of Physical Performance

Under normal conditions, athletes show small circadian variations of performance [103], reflecting in part cyclic changes of body temperature and vigilance. Studies during Ramadan have been compromised by a small number of observations (only 2 or 3) over the course of the day. One report found impaired scores of sports school students on a Wingate 30 seconds cycle ergometer test in the afternoon and evening, but not in the morning [94]. These findings probably reflect Ramadan-related alterations in arousal rather than any change in the inherent circadian rhythm of physical performance. A study of physical education students found no changes of handgrip strength or vertical jump performances from initial control data [22].

Vigilance and Psychomotor Performance

A number of observers have reported a loss of daytime alertness and an increase of daytime sleepiness [29,61,63,80,82,84], although this was not seen by BaHammam [10] or Margolis and Reed [70]. In keeping with such changes, there have been impairments of memory and vigilance [36,48,49], altered perceptions of time and space [30,60] and increases in various types of reaction speed response time [29,30,80]. A decrease in one objective measure of arousal (the critical flicker fusion frequency) was seen by Ali and Amir [4], but not by Lofti et al. [65]. Issues concerning vigilance and athletic performance are discussed in more detail in Chapter 9.

Most of the studies cited have concerned sedentary young adults. Mental performance depends greatly upon the individual's motivation, and the impact of Ramadan is likely to be less dramatic in highly motivated and disciplined athletes who are encouraged to adopt optimal patterns of eating and sleeping during Ramadan [25]. Another important variable is the person's ability to take a compensatory daytime nap, which may be much easier to arrange when living or competing in the Muslim world than when fasting in a society where few people are observing Ramadan [70,101]. Finally, if the deterioration of cerebral performance is related to a low blood glucose, negative effects of Ramadan observance are much more likely to be observed toward the end of the day, immediately before breaking the fast.

Practical Implications

Fasting can disturb the hormonal balance, with adverse consequences for athletic performance. Equally, dehydration will impair performance. However, changes can be lessened by endurance training (which encourages the metabolism of fat rather than carbohydrate) and by maximizing carbohydrate stores prior to fasting. For those observing Ramadan, effects can be further minimized by an adequate intake of food and fluid at night. In those who are obese, the reduction of body fat associated with fasting has a favourable effect upon hormonal balance; in particular, increasing insulin sensitivity in individuals with type 2 diabetes mellitus. Moreover, the reduction of body mass will reduce the energy cost of activities that involve body displacement.

Conclusions

The body's hormones work in balanced fashion to conserve homeostasis through an appropriate balance of anabolic and catabolic activity, involving the storage and breakdown of carbohydrates, fats and proteins and an adjustment of body fluid levels. Fasting, fluid deprivation and prolonged exercise can all disturb this balance, calling forth adjustments of hormone concentrations in an attempt to restore a normal tissue environment. Changes of hormone balance can be seen even with the brief intermittent fasting of Ramadan, more commonly in sedentary individuals who are exploiting Ramadan to reduce body fat than in athletes, since the latter seek to counter the daytime fast by an increased intake of food and fluids during the hours of darkness. Many hormones show a diurnal fluctuation, and this may be modified by Ramadan observance, probably because of altered meal times and disturbances of sleep. This makes it difficult to determine alterations in the cumulative 24-hour secretion of hormones unless multiple blood samples are collected. The altered circadian rhythms can in turn affect both physical and psychomotor performance.

Key Terms

Acrophase: The acrophase is the time of day when a circadian rhythm peaks.

Adrenocorticotropic hormone (ACTH): ACTH is a hormone secreted by the anterior pituitary gland. Its main action is to increase the secretion and release of corticosteroids.

Antidiuretic hormone (ADH): ADH is produced by the neurohypophysis and causes vascular constriction and water retention.

Adrenocorticotropic hormone: Stimulates cortisol release from adrenal glands.

Circadian rhythm: A circadian rhythm is a fluctuation of a biological variable such as body temperature that occurs over a cycle of approximately 24 hours.

Cortisol: Cortisol is a hormone produced by the cortex of the adrenal gland, and it is involved in metabolic regulation, predisposing to catabolic reactions. It is released particularly in response to stress and low levels of blood glucose.

Cyclic AMP: cAMP or 3–5 cyclic adenosine monophosphate is a second messenger important to many biological reactions.

Epinephrine: Epinephrine is a hormone secreted by the adrenal glands and at the endings of the sympathetic nerves. It initiates the 'fight or flight' response in dangerous situations.

Follicle-stimulating hormone (FSH): FSH is secreted in the anterior pituitary gland. It regulates the growth and maturation of the reproductive system in both men and women.

Gonadotropin-releasing hormone: Gonadotropin-releasing hormone is synthesized within the hypothalamus, and it stimulates the release of FSH and LH.

Ghrelin: Ghrelin is a hormone that is secreted when the stomach is empty; it induces a sensation of hunger.

Homeostasis: Homeostasis is the ability of the body to maintain stable internal conditions.

IL-6: Interleukin-6 (IL-6) is a cytokine that in addition to having immune functions is now thought to be involved in regulating muscle glucose levels.

Insulin: Insulin is a hormone produced by the islets of Langerhans in the pancreas. It regulates blood sugar levels and is in inadequate supply in patients with diabetes mellitus.

Insulin-like growth factor 1: Insulin-like growth factor 1 has a structure similar to insulin. It is an important stimulant of anabolic metabolism.

Leptin: Leptin is a satiety hormone, produced by fat cells. It opposes the action of ghrelin.

Luteinizing hormone: Luteinizing hormone is produced in the anterior pituitary gland. It stimulates the Leydig cells of the testis to produce testosterone.

Melatonin: Melatonin is a hormone produced by the pineal gland; it regulates wakefulness and synchronizes the body clock with the light/darkness cycle; it also has antioxidant properties.

Neuropeptide-y: Neuropeptide-y is a neurotransmitter in the brain and the sympathetic nervous system.

Norepinephrine: Norepinephrine is a catecholamine that functions both as a neurotransmitter in the sympathetic nervous system and as a hormone. It increases blood pressure and contributes to vigilant concentration.

Prolactin: Prolactin is best known for its milk secreting function in women, but it is a hormone that has many other functions, including opposing the actions of testosterone and oestrogen.

Rapamycin (mTOR): Rapamycin (mTOR) is a regulator of cell growth.

Second messenger: A second messenger such as cAMP is important to the initiation of many biological processes.

Testosterone: Testosterone is an anabolic steroid produced in the testes; it promotes anabolic activity in tissues, particularly muscle building.

Thyroid-stimulating hormone: Controls thyroid hormone release from thyroid gland.

Zeitgeber: A zeitgeber is an external signal such as a meal that helps a person adjust the timing of his or her internal clock.

Key Points

1. The main action of insulin is to regulate glucose homeostasis. Insulin induces the capture of circulating glucose molecules and their utilization and storage as glycogen in liver and muscle.
2. The magnitude of hormonal responses to exercise declines after endurance training.

3. Fasting and the secretion of growth hormone both promote an increase of lipolysis in healthy subjects and they may also reduce insulin sensitivity.
4. Ramadan observance is associated with changes in the mean concentrations of many hormones and often with shifts in their circadian rhythm.
5. The GH/IGF-1 axis and leptin/adiponectin ratios do not appear to be changed during Ramadan observance.
6. Ramadan observance can have a significant impact upon sleep patterns and cerebral performance.

Questions for Discussion

1. How is blood glucose homeostasis maintained?
2. What sources of energy are responsible for maintaining a favourable muscle ATP/ADP ratio during exercise?
3. What changes would you anticipate in the concentrations of insulin, glucagon, cortisol, growth hormone, epinephrine, and norepinephrine during total fasting at rest and when exercising?
4. Do hormonal responses to exercise change during Ramadan observance?
5. Why do you think Ramadan observance modifies circadian rhythms?

References

1. Ahmadinejad Z, Ziaee V, Rezaee M et al. The effect of Ramadan fasting on thyroid hormone profile: A cohort study. *Pak J Biol Sci* 2006;9:1999–2002.
2. Aimaretti G, Colao A, Corneli G et al. The study of spontaneous GH secretion after 36-h fasting distinguishes between GH-deficient and normal adults. *Clin Endocrinol (Oxf)* 1999;51(6):771–777.
3. al-Hadramy MS, Zawawi TH, Abdelwahab SM. Altered cortisol levels in relation to Ramadan. *Eur J Clin Nutr* 1988;42(4):359–362.
4. Ali MR, Amir T. Effects of fasting on visual flicker fusion. *Percept Motor Skills* 1989;69:627–361.
5. Aloi JA, Bergendahl M, Iranmanesh A et al. Pulsatile intravenous gonadotropin-releasing hormone administration averts fasting-induced hypogonadotropism and hypoandrogen-emia in healthy, normal weight men. *J Clin Endocrinol Metab* 1997;82(5):1543–1548.
6. Alzoghaibi MA, Pandi-Perumal SR, Sharif MM et al. Diurnal intermittent fasting during Ramadan: The effects on leptin and ghrelin levels. *PLoS ONE* 2014;9(3):e92214.
7. Atkinson G, Edwards B, Reilly T et al. Exercise as a synchroniser of human circadian rhythms: An update and discussion of the methodological problems. *Eur J Appl Physiol* 2007;99:331–341.
8. Azizi F. Serum levels of prolactin, thyrotropin, thyroid hormones, TRH responsiveness and male reproductive function in intermittent Islamic fasting. *Med J Islam Repub Iran* 1991;5:145–148.
9. Azizi F, Nafarabadi M, Amini M. Serum thyroid hormone and thyrotropin concentrations during Ramadan in healthy women. *Emir Med J* 1994;12:140–143.
10. BaHammam A. Effect of fasting during Ramadan on sleep architecture, daytime sleepi-ness and sleep pattern. *Sleep Biol Rhythms* 2004;2:135–143.

11. BaHammam A. Assessment of sleep patterns, daytime sleepiness, and chronotype during Ramadan in fasting and non fasting individuals. *Saudi Med J* 2005;26:616–622.
12. BaHammam A, Alrajeh M, Albabtain M et al. Circadian pattern of sleep, energy expenditure, and body temperature of young healthy men during the intermittent fasting of Ramadan. *Appetite* 2010;54(2):426–429.
13. Bang P, Brismar K, Rosenfeld RG et al. Fasting affects serum insulin-like growth factors (IGFs) and IGF-binding proteins differently in patients with noninsulin-dependent diabetes mellitus versus healthy nonobese and obese subjects. *J Clin Endocrinol Metab* 1994;78:860–967.
14. Ben Salem L, B'chir S, Bchir F et al. Circadian rhythm of cortisol and its responsiveness to ACTH during Ramadan (article in French). *Ann Endocrinol (Paris)* 2002;63(6 Pt 1):497–501.
15. Ben Salem L, Bchir S, Bouguerra R et al. Cortisol rhythm during the month of Ramadan. *East Mediterr Health J* 2003;9(5–6):1093–1098.
16. Bergendahl M, Vance ML, Iranmanesh A et al. Fasting as a metabolic stress paradigm selectively amplifies cortisol secretory burst mass and delays the time of maximal nyctohemeral cortisol concentrations in healthy men. *J Clin Endocrinol Metab* 1996;81(2):692–699.
17. Bergendahl M, Aloi JA, Iranmanesh A et al. Fasting suppresses pulsatile luteinizing hormone (LH) secretion and enhances orderliness of LH release in young but not older men. *J Clin Endocrinol Metab* 1998;83(6):1967–1975.
18. Bogdan A, Bouchareb B, Touitou Y. Ramadan fasting alters endocrine and neuroendocrine circadian patterns. Meal-time as a synchronizer in humans? *Life Sci* 2001;68:1607–1615.
19. Bogdan A, Bouchareb B, Touitou Y. Response of circulating leptin to Ramadan day time fasting: A circadian study. *Br J Nutr* 2005;93:515–518.
20. Bouhlel E, Zaouali M, Miled A et al. Ramadan fasting and the CH/IGF-1 axis of trained men during submaximal exercise. *Ann Nutr Metab* 2008;52:261–266.
21. Bouhlel E, Denguezli M, Zaouali M et al. Ramadan fasting's effect on plasma leptin, adiponectin concentrations, and body composition in trained young men. *Int J sport Nutr Exerc Metab* 2008;18:1–12.
22. Bouhlel H, Shephard RJ, Gmada N et al. Effect of Ramadan observance on maximal muscular performance of trained men. *Clin J Sports Med* 2013;23:222–227.
23. Brooks GA, Mercier J. Balance of carbohydrate and lipid utilization during exercise: The "crossover" concept. *J Appl Physiol (1985)* 1994;76(6):2253–2261.
24. Cağlayan EK, Göçmen AY, Delibas N. Effects of long-term fasting on female hormone levels: Ramadan model. *Clin Exp Obstet Gynecol* 2014;41(1):17–19.
25. Chaouachi A, Coutts AJ, Chamari K et al. Effect of Ramadan intermittent fasting on aerobic and anaerobic performance and perception of fatigue in male elite judo athletes. *J Strength Cond Res* 2009;23(9):2702–2709.
26. Chennaoui M, Desgorces F, Drogou C et al. Effects of Ramadan fasting on physical performance and metabolic, hormonal, and inflammatory parameters in middle-distance runners. *Appl Physiol Nutr Metab* 2009;34:587–594.
27. Cryer PE. Adrenaline: A physiological metabolic regulatory hormone in humans? *Int J Obes Relat Metab Disord* 1993;17(Suppl. 3):S43–S46; discussion S68.
28. Degoutte F, Jouanel P, Bégue RJ et al. Food restriction, performance, biochemical, psychological, and endocrine changes in judo athletes. *Int J Sports Med* 2006;27:9–18.
29. Dolu N, Yüksek A, Sizer A et al. Arousal and continuous attention during Ramadan intermittent fasting. *J Basic Clin Physiol Pharmacol* 2007;18:315–322.
30. Doniger GM, Simon EY, Zivotofsky AZ. Comprehensive computerized assessment of cognitive sequelae of a complete 12–16 hour fast. *Behav Neurosci* 2006;120:804–816.
31. Drust B, Ahmed Q, Roky R. Circadian variation and soccer performance: Implications for training and match-play during Ramadan. *J Sports Sci* 2012;30(Suppl. 1):S43–S52.

32. Dwivedi S, Nalini K, Assim MO. Metabolic alterations during Ramadan fast. *Indian J Clin Biochem* 1996;11(2):171–172.
33. El Ati J, Beji C, Danguir J. Increased fat oxidation during Ramadan fasting in healthy women: An adaptive mechanism for body-weight maintenance. *Am J Clin Nutr* 1995;62:302–307.
34. El-Migdadi F, El-Akawi Z, Abudheese R et al. Plasma levels of adrenocorticotropic hormone and cortisol in people living in an environment below sea level (Jordan Valley) during fasting in the month of Ramadan. *Horm Res* 2002;58(6):279–282.
35. El-Migdadi F, Shotar A, El-Akawi Z et al. Effect of fasting during the month of Ramadan on serum levels of luteinizing hormone and testosterone in people living in the below sea level environment in the Jordan Valley. *Neuro Endocrinol Lett* 2004;25:75–77.
36. El Moutawakil B, Hassounr S, Sibai M et al. Effect of Ramadan fasting upon functions of attention (in French). *Rev Neurol* 2007;163(Suppl. 4):60.
37. Fedail SS, Murphy D, Salib SY et al. Changes in certain blood constituents during Ramadan. *Am J Clin Nutr* 1982;36:350–353.
38. Fryburg DA, Barrett EJ, Louard RJ et al. Effect of starvation on human muscle protein metabolism and its response to insulin. *Am J Physiol* 1990;259(4 Pt 1):E477–E482.
39. Galbo, H. *Hormonal and Metabolic Adaptation to Exercise*. Thieme-Stratton, New York, 1983.
40. Galster AD, Clutter WE, Cryer PE et al. Epinephrine plasma thresholds for lipolytic effects in man: Measurements of fatty acid transport with [l-13C]palmitic acid. *J Clin Invest* 1981;67(6):1729–1738.
41. Gjedsted J, Gormsen LC, Nielsen S et al. Effects of a 3-day fast on regional lipid and glucose metabolism in human skeletal muscle and adipose tissue. *Acta Physiol (Oxf)* 2007;191(3):205–216.
42. Gjedsted J, Gormsen L, Buhl M et al. Forearm and leg amino acid metabolism in the basal state and during combined insulin and amino acid stimulation after a 3-day fast. *Acta Physiol (Oxf)* 2009;197(3):197–205.
43. Green HJ, Jones S, Ball-Burnett M et al. Early adaptations in blood substrates, metabolites, and hormones to prolonged exercise training in man. *Can J Physiol Pharmacol* 1991;69(8):1222–1229.
44. Grottoli S, Gauna C, Tassone F et al. Both fasting-induced leptin reduction and GH increase are blunted in Cushing's syndrome and in simple obesity. *Clin Endocrinol (Oxf)* 2003;58(2):220–228.
45. Grottoli S, Gasco V, Mainolfi A et al. Growth hormone/insulin-like growth factor I axis, glucose metabolism, and lypolisis but not leptin show some degree of refractoriness to short-term fasting in acromegaly. *J Endocrinol Invest* 2008;31(12):1103–1109.
46. Hackney AC. Testosterone, the hypothalamic-pituitary-testicular axis and endurance exercise training. *Biol Sport* 1996;13:85–98.
47. Hagström-Toft E, Thörne A, Reynisdottir S et al. Evidence for a major role of skeletal muscle lipolysis in the regulation of lipid oxidation during caloric restriction in vivo. *Diabetes* 2001;50(7):1604–1611.
48. Hakkou F, Wast D, Jaouan C. Does Ramadan impair vigilance and memory? *Psychopharmacology* 1988;96:213.
49. Hakkou F, Iraki L, Tazi A. Ramadan, chronobiology and health. *Chronobiol Int* 1994;11:340–342.
50. Hartman ML, Veldhuid JD, Johnson ML et al. Augmented growth hormone (GH) secretory burst frequency and amplitude mediate enhanced GH secretion during a two day fast in normal men. *J Clin Endocrinol Metab* 1992;74:757–765.
51. Hartman ML, Pezzoli SS, Hellmann PJ et al. Pulsatile growth hormone secretion in older persons is enhanced by fasting without relationship to sleep stages. *J Clin Endocrinol Metab* 1996;81(7):2694–2701.

52. Helyar R, Green H, Zappe D et al. Blood metabolite and catecholamine responses to prolonged exercise following either acute plasma volume expansion or short-term training. *Eur J Appl Physiol Occup Physiol* 1997;75(3):268–273.
53. Herrera C. Total sleep time in Muslim football players is reduced during Ramadan: A pilot study on the standardized assessment of subjective sleep–wake patterns in athletes. *J Sports Sci* 2012;30(Suppl. 1):S85–S91.
54. Inoue M, Maehata E, Yano M et al. Correlation between the adiponectin-leptin ratio and parameters of insulin resistance in patients with type 2 diabetes. *Metabolism* 2005;54(3):281–286.
55. Iraki L, Bogdan A, Hakkou F et al. Ramadan diet restrictions modify the circadian time structure in humans. A study on plasma gastrin, insulin, glucose, and calcium and on gastric pH. *J Clin Endocrinol Metab* 1997;82:1261–1273.
56. Ivy JL. Role of exercise training in the prevention and treatment of insulin resistance and non-insulin-dependent diabetes mellitus. *Sports Med* 1997;24(5):321–336.
57. Karli U, Güvenç A, Aslan A et al. Influence of Ramadan fasting on anaerobic performance and recovery from short high intensity exercise. *J Sport Sci Med* 2007;6:490–497.
58. Kassab SE, Abdul-Ghaffar T, Nagalla DS et al. Serum leptin and insulin levels during chronic diurnal fasting. *Asia Pac J Clin Nutr* 2003;12(4):483–487.
59. Kassab S, Abdul-Ghaffar T, Nagalla DS et al. Interactions between leptin, neuropeptide-Y and insulin with chronic diurnal fasting during Ramadan. *Ann Saudi Med* 2004;24(5): 345–349.
60. Khazaie H, Tahmasian M, Ekhtiari H et al. Effects of Ramadan fasting on time perception task. *Neuroscience* 2009;14:196–197.
61. Lagarde D, Bategat D, Boussif M et al. Ramadan et vigilance (Ramadan and vigilance). *Méd Aéronaut Spa* 1996;35:175–182.
62. Langfort J, Zarzeczny R, Pilis W et al. The effect of a low-carbohydrate diet on performance, hormonal and metabolic responses to a 30-s bout of supramaximal exercise. *Eur J Appl Physiol Occup Physiol* 1997;76(2):128–133.
63. Laraqui S, Manar N, Laraqui O et al. Influence of Ramadan observance on wakefulness at work among health care workers in Morocco (in French). *Arch Mal Prof Environ* 2012;73(5):743–749.
64. Leiper JB, Junge A, Maughan RJ et al. Alteration of subjective feelings in football players undertaking their usual training and match schedule during the Ramadan fast. *J Sports Sci* 2008;26(Suppl. 3):S55–S69.
65. Lofti S, Madani M, Abassi A et al. CNS activation, reaction time, blood pressure and heart rate variation during Ramadan intermittent fasting and exercise. *World J Sports Sci* 2010;3:37–43.
66. Loucks AB. Physical activity, fitness, and female reproductive morbidity. In: Bouchard C, Shephard RJ, Stephens T (eds.), *Physical Activity, Fitness and Health*. Humqn Kinetics, Champaign, IL, 1994, pp. 943–954.
67. Maccario M, Aimaretti G, Grottoli S et al. Effects of 36 hour fasting on GH/IGF-I axis and metabolic parameters in patients with simple obesity. Comparison with normal subjects and hypo-pituitary patients with severe GH deficiency. *Int J Obes Relat Metab Disord* 2001;25:1233–1239.
68. Mann S, Beedie C, Balducci S et al. Changes in insulin sensitivity in response to different modalities of exercise: A review of the evidence. *Diabetes Metab Res Rev* 2014;30(4):257–68.
69. Mansi K, Amneh M. Impact of Ramadan fasting on metabolism and on serum levels of some hormones among healthy Jordanian students. *J Med Sci* 2007;7:755–761.
70. Margolis SA, Reed RL. Effect of religious practices of Ramadan on sleep and perceived sleepiness of medical students. *Teach Learn Med* 2004;16:145–149.
71. Maughan RJ, Fallah J, Coyle EF. The effects of fasting on metabolism and performance. *Br J Sports Med* 2010;44:490–494.

72. Meckel Y, Ismael A, Eliakim A. The effect of the Ramadan fast on physical performance and dietary habits in adolescent soccer players. *Eur J Appl Physiol* 2008;102:651–657.
73. Mercier J, Perez-Martin A, Bigard X, Ventura R. Muscle plasticity and metabolism: Effects of exercise and chronic diseases. *Mol Aspects Med* 1999;20(6):319–373.
74. Mesbahzadeh B, Ghiravani Z, Mehrjoofard H. Effect of Ramadan fasting on secretion of sex hormones in healthy single males. *East Mediterr Health J* 2005;11(5–6):1120–1123.
75. Moller L, Dalman L, Norrelund H et al. Impact of fasting on growth hormone signaling and action in muscle and fat. *J Clin Endocrinol Metab* 2009;94:965–972.
76. Montelpare WJ, Plyley MJ, Shephard RJ. Evaluating the influence of sleep deprivation upon circadian rhythms of exercise metabolism. *Can J Sport Sci* 1992;17(2):94–97.
77. Nellemann B, Vendelbo MH, Nielsen TS et al. Growth hormone-induced insulin resistance in human subjects involves reduced pyruvate dehydrogenase activity. *Acta Physiol* 2013;210(2):392–402.
78. Nørrelund H, Nielsen S, Christiansen JS et al. Modulation of basal glucose metabolism and insulin sensitivity by growth hormone and free fatty acids during short-term fasting. *Eur J Endocrinol* 2004;150(6):779–787.
79. Reilly T. Human circadian rhythms and exercise. *Crit Rev Biomed Eng* 1990;18(3):165–180.
80. Roky R, Iraki L, Haj Khilfla R et al. Daytime alertness, mood, psychomotor performances, and oral temperature during Ramadan intermittent fasting. *Ann Nutr Metab* 2000;44:101–107.
81. Roky R, Chapotot F, Hakkou F et al. Sleep during Ramadan intermittent fasting. *J Sleep Res* 2001;10:319–327.
82. Roky R, Chapotot F, Benchekroun MT et al. Daytime sleepiness during Ramadan intermittent fasting: Polysomnographic and quantitative waking EEG study. *J Sleep Res* 2003;12:95–101.
83. Roky R, Houti I, Moussamih S et al. Physiological and chronobiological changes during Ramadan intermittent fasting. *Ann Nutr Metab* 2004;48:296–303.
84. Roky R. Les variations physiologiques et comportementales pendant le Ramadan (Physiological and behavioural changes during Ramadan). *Biomatec Echo* 2007;2(5):8–16.
85. Roky R, Horrora CP, Ahmed Q. Sleep in athletes and the effects of Ramadan. *J Sports Sci* 2012;30(Suppl. 1):S75–S84.
86. Sajid KM, Akhtar M, Malik GQ. Ramadan fasting and thyroid hormone profile. *J Pak Med Assoc* 1991;41(9):213–216.
87. Salgin B, Marcovecchio ML, Humphreys SM et al. Effects of prolonged fasting and sustained lipolysis on insulin secretion and insulin sensitivity in normal subjects. *Am J Physiol Endocrinol Metab* 2009;296(3):E454–E461.
88. Salgin B, Marcovecchio ML, Hill N et al. The effect of prolonged fasting on levels of growth hormone-binding protein and free growth hormone. *Growth Horm IGF Res* 2012;22:76–81.
89. Samuels C. Sleep, recovery and performance: The new frontier in high performance athletics. *Neurol Clin* 2008;26:169–180.
90. Shephard RJ. Sleep, biorhythms and human performance. *Sports Med* 1984;1:11–37.
91. Shephard RJ, Johnson N. Physical activity and the liver. *Eur J Appl Physiol* 2015;1156(1):1–46.
92. Singh R, Hwa OC, Roy J et al. Subjective perceptions of sports performance, training, sleep and dietary patterns of Malaysian junior Muslim athletes during Ramadan intermittent fasting. *Asian J Sports Med* 2011;2:167–176.
93. Souissi N, Gauthier A, Sesboüé B et al. Circadian rhythms in two types of anaerobic cycle leg exercise: Force-velocity and 30-s Wingate tests. *Int J Sports Med* 2004;25(1):14–19.
94. Souissi N, Souissi H, Sahli S et al. Effect of Ramadan on the diurnal variation in short-term high power output. *Chronobiol Int* 2007;24(5):991–1007.
95. Sulimani RA. The effects of Ramadan fasting on thyroid functions in healthy male subjects. *Nutr Res* 1988;8:549–552.

96. Sweileh N, Schnitzler A, Hunter GR et al. Body composition and energy metabolism in resting and exercising Muslims during Ramadan fast. *J Sports Med Phys Fitness* 1992;32:156–163.
97. Talanian JL, Galloway SD, Heigenhauser GJ et al. Two weeks of high-intensity aerobic interval training increases the capacity for fat oxidation during exercise in women. *J Appl Physiol (1985)* 2007;102(4):1439–1447.
98. Taoudi Benchekroun M, Roky R, Toufiq J et al. Epidemiological study: Chronotype and daytime sleepiness before and during Ramadan. *Thérapie* 1999;54:567–572.
99. Veldhuis JD, Iranmanesh A, Evans WS et al. Amplitude suppression of the pulsatile mode of immunoradiometric luteinizing hormone release in fasting-induced hypoandrogenemia in normal men. *J Clin Endocrinol Metab* 1993;76(3):587–593.
100. Vendelbo MH, Møller AB, Christensen B et al. Fasting increases human skeletal muscle net phenylalanine release and this is associated with decreased mTOR signaling. *PLoS ONE* 2014;9(7):e102031.
101. Waterhouse J, Alkib L, Reilly T. Effects of Ramadan upon fluid and food intake, fatigue, and physical and mental, and social activities: A comparison between the UK and Libya. *Chronobiol Int* 2008;25:697–724.
102. Waterhouse J, Alabed H, Edwards B et al. Changes in sleep, mood and subjective and objective responses to physical performance during the daytime in Ramadan. *Biol Rhythm Res* 2009;40:367–383.
103. Waterhouse J. Effects of Ramadan on physical performance: Chronobiological considerations. *Br J Sports Med* 2010;44:509–515.
104. Wilson D, Drust B, Reilly T. Is diurnal lifestyle altered during Ramadan in professional Muslim athletes? *Biol Rhythm Res* 2009;40:385–397.
105. Zerguini Y, Kirkendall D, Junge A et al. Impact of Ramadan on physical performance in professional soccer players. *Br J Sports Med* 2007;41:398–400.
106. Zerguini Y, Dvorak J, Maughan RJ et al. Influence of Ramadan fasting on physiological and performance variables in football players: Summary of the F-MARC 2006 Ramadan fasting study. *J Sports Sci* 2008;26(Suppl. 3):S3–S6.
107. Zoladz JA, Konturek SJ, Duda K et al. Effect of moderate incremental exercise, performed in fed and fasted state on cardio-respiratory variables and leptin and ghrelin concentrations in young healthy men. *J Physiol Pharmacol* 2005;56(1):63–85.

Further Reading

Borer K. *Advanced Exercise Endocrinology*. Human Kinetics, Champaign, IL, 2013.
Constantini NW, Hackney AC. *Sports Endocrinology of Physical Activity and Sport*. Humana Press, New York, 2013.
Minors DS, Waterhouse JM. *Circadian Rhythms and the Human*. John Wright, Bristol, U.K., 2013.
Richter EA, Sutton JR. Hormonal adaptation to physical activity. In: Bouchard C, Shephard RJ, Stephens T (eds.), *Physical Activity, Fitness and Health: International Proceedings and Consensus Statement*. Human Kinetics, Champaign, IL, 1994, pp. 331–342.
Sutton, JR, Farrell PA. Endocrine responses to prolonged exercise. In: Lamb D, Murray R (eds.), *Perspectives in Exercise Science and Sports Medicine: Prolonged Exercise*, Vol. 1. Benchmark Press, Indianapolis, IN, 1988, pp.153–208.

8

Oxidative Stress and Fasting

Ezdine Bouhlel and Roy J Shephard

Learning Objectives

1. To review some characteristics of oxidative stress and its antidotes
2. To consider the balance between oxidative stress and the antioxidative response during physical activity
3. To compare the impact of fasting upon oxidative stress and the antioxidative response in sedentary individuals and athletes
4. To consider the effects of Ramadan observance upon oxidative stress and the antioxidative response in sedentary individuals and athletes
5. To determine practical implications for athletes, coaches and trainers

Introduction

Regular physical activity is a major factor in preventing metabolic diseases such as maturity-onset diabetes and atherosclerotic heart disease. However, intensive exercise increases the production of free radicals, and in theory, it could augment oxidative stress, with a worsening of the individual's long-term prognosis in terms of the metabolic syndrome, cardiac disease, cancer, Alzheimer's disease and other chronic conditions. The immune system may also be compromised, increasing the risk of developing acute upper respiratory infections [87]. The muscle soreness that develops in the limb muscles of athletes following a period of strenuous training (particularly if eccentric exercise has been involved) is due in part to the development of microscopic lesions and an associated increase in local oxidative stress. Athletes commonly ingest nutrients with antioxidative properties in order to limit the resulting inflammation and muscle soreness, and health conscious sedentary individuals may adopt a similar tactic to avert heart attacks and slow the course of aging, although there is little evidence that such supplements are helpful if a well-balanced diet is already being eaten.

Cell homeostasis depends on the body striking an appropriate balance between oxidative stress and its antioxidative responses. A small increase in oxidative stress may be an inevitable component of muscle or cardiac hypertrophy, but if the level of free radicals increases further, cellular damage occurs, with fatigue and the development of specific muscular lesions, and in a longer-term perspective, the risk of the metabolic syndrome, cardiac disease, cancer and accelerated aging is increased. The effects of dietary restriction and total fasting upon oxidative status seem to depend upon initial reserves of body fat. This chapter presents our current understanding of the effects of dietary restriction and exercise upon levels of oxidative stress in sedentary and athletic individuals.

Balance between Oxidative Stress and the Antioxidative Response

There is normally little evidence of oxidative stress in a young adult; although some free radicals are formed during normal metabolism, levels of enzymes such as peroxidase are adequate to prevent their accumulation [30]. However, manifestations of free radical activity can be seen in older individuals, particularly the formation of inappropriate cross-linkages between molecules that are one prominent manifestation of the aging process [86]. An imbalance between oxidative stress and the antioxidative response can also develop with exposure to tobacco, an excess of alcohol, air pollutants, unaccustomed exercise and the enzyme dysfunction that is associated with a diet that contains a high proportion of fat.

Controlling Oxidant Stress

What is oxidant stress? Oxidant stress arises when there is an imbalance between the generation of reactive oxygen species and the ability of the body to detoxify these products and repair any associated tissue damage. Disturbances in the redox state of the cell lead to an accumulation of peroxides and free radicals that can damage many components of a living cell.

How is oxidant stress measured? Many different techniques are used to assess the level of oxidant stress, anti-oxidant defences and resulting inflammation.

- For oxidant stress, the most popular approaches are to measure the thiobarbituric acid reactive species (TBARS) that are formed by the oxidation and degradation of polyunsaturated fatty acids in cell walls, or to determine F2 isoprostanes. Other potential markers include levels of protein carbonyls, homocysteine (which uncouples NO synthase, reduces circulating NO levels and encourages the production of free radicals), conjugated dienes (formed from peroxidation of polyunsaturated fatty acids), 4-hydroxyonenal and

DNA damage as diagnosed histologically by a cellular abnormality called comet tail formation.

- Markers of antioxidant defences include activity of the enzymes glutathione peroxidase, superoxide dismutase and catalase, levels of uric acid and reduced glutathione, and determinations of Vitamins A, C and E.
- Measures of inflammatory response include concentrations of c-reactive protein liberated during muscle injury and synthesized by the liver as a part of an acute-phase response, and levels of the pro-inflammatory cytokines IL-6 (liberated from liver, muscle and adipose tissue) and TNF-α; other possibilities are determinations of IL-12, and inflammatory chemokines (CXCL1,CXCL10).

What effects does exercise-induced oxidant stress have upon muscle?
Eccentric exercise causes oxidative damage to both proteins and lipids in the affected muscle fibres. Low levels of reactive oxygen species seem necessary for normal muscle function and force production, but in larger amounts they cause fatigue, muscular weakness and tissue damage [77].

How long do these effects persist?
The muscle soreness and biomechanical changes associated with eccentric exercise are usually reversed over a period of 1–3 days.

Several mechanisms increase the production and/or accumulation of *free radicals*. Inflammation is an important source of free radical production; it reflects an increased activity of the enzyme NADPH oxidase in phagocytic cells as they respond to tissue injury (for instance, in responding to injuries caused by excessive eccentric exercise). Inflammatory cells also produce *cytokines* such as tumor necrosis factor alpha (TNF-α), which can produce free radicals in the mitochondria. Vigorous exercise in itself is another significant factor.

The mitochondrial respiratory chain generates a continuous flux of free radicals as metabolism proceeds, with free radical production being proportional to the intensity and duration of activity. Several enzyme systems produce free radicals, using biochemical reactions such as xanthine oxidase and haeme oxygenase. Other potential adverse influences include nutritional deficits, mitochondrial pathology, and a low activity of tissue peroxidases.

On the other hand, the body has a system of antioxidant enzymes that serve to counter the accumulation of free radicals. *Superoxide dismutase* (SOD) is able to eliminate the superoxide radical. *Catalase* and *glutathione peroxidase* (GPx) are able to eliminate H_2O_2. Other enzymes such as glutathione transferase and thyrodoxine peroxidase also contribute to antioxidative defenses. Although the acute effect of exercise is to increase the production of oxidants, if the same exercise is practiced regularly, the individual develops a more than compensatory increase of antioxidant enzymes [16].

The quality of the diet has a major impact upon the activity of antioxidant enzymes. Vitamins, such as vitamin E, and beta-carotene, the precursor of vitamin A, trap and neutralize free radicals. Antioxidant status can thus be assessed by measuring the plasma, erythrocyte or leukocyte levels of such factors as vitamin E, vitamin C, vitamin A, zinc and selenium, as well as by measuring the activity of GPx activity and SOD.

Oxidative Stress during Exercise

The production of free radicals after intensive exercise has been assessed directly using a spectroscopic resonance technique [29], and it has been assessed indirectly by measuring increases in markers of oxidative stress (see Box 8.1). Three main mechanisms are involved in free radical production: (1) an increased overall consumption of oxygen; (2) the process of ischaemia and subsequent reperfusion of some tissues, both in the viscera (where blood flow is drastically reduced during vigorous exercise) and also in very vigorously contracting muscle, where perfusion may be limited because of the high intramuscular pressures [11,46]; and (3) reactions to muscular injury [24].

When the intensity of exercise is high, xanthine oxidase converts hypoxanthine to uric acid; the uric acid is an antioxidant, but also serves as a marker of protein breakdown. High-intensity exercise also induces microlesions in the active muscles [11,54,70], with the production of cytokines; the activation of monocytes, lymphocytes and macrophages; and in consequence the production of free radicals. Prolonged exercise is accompanied by an accumulation of neutrophils, and the macrophagic activity of these cells leads to the production of free radicals [57,67]. Plasma *malondialdehyde* (MDA) levels increase in proportion to the rise in intensity of exercise [25,62], and MDA is a popular marker of oxidant stress. Glycolytic muscle fibres, involved in anaerobic and prolonged exercise, generate more free radicals than oxidative muscle fibres [4,83]. Hypoxia plays probably a major role in the process of *lipoperoxidation*; even moderate exercise can cause substantial oxidative stress if it is performed under hypoxic conditions [10].

Eccentric contractions are more prone to cause muscular lesions than are concentric contractions [75]. The extent of muscular microlesions probably depends

---

BOX 8.1   Exercise and Oxidant Stress

Factors exacerbating stress during exercise:

- Muscle contraction at greater than 15% of maximal force
- Hypoxia and subsequent reperfusion of tissues
- Tissue injury

Factors minimizing oxidative stress:

- Avoidance of eccentric effort
- Dietary modification to increase the intake of anti-oxidants
- Aerobic training to increase the activity of oxidases

on the equilibrium that is struck between oxidative stress and antioxidative defenses. Increases in plasma concentrations of the enzymes creatine phospho-kinase, lactate dehydrogenase (LDH) and phosphofructokinase are seen after intensive eccentric exercise and prolonged endurance activity; Finsterer [38] has underlined the link between muscle fatigue, lipoperoxidation and plasma lev-els of these enzymes. MDA, LDH, catalase and superoxide dismutase were all increased after repeated sprints (6×35 m sprints with 10 seconds rest intervals [28]). Prolonged intensive exercise can also cause oxidative damage to both pro-teins and lipids in the contracting muscles, with changes in gene expression [78]. Arachidonic acid is released from the cellular membranes with the formation of prostaglandins, another marker of the severity of oxidant stress.

During the process of reperfusion of ischaemic tissue, xanthine dehydroge-nase is converted to xanthine oxidase, with the production of superoxide radicals ($O_2\cdot^-$). Furthermore, the oxidation of haemoglobin, myoglobin, cytochrome C and catecholamines can all lead to the production of free radicals [41,51].

Training and the Balance between Oxidative Stress and Antioxidant Defenses

Several studies have demonstrated that both aerobic and anaerobic training lead to decreases in oxidative stress and/or increases in antioxidant defenses [16,97]. For this reason, the initial status of a well-conditioned athlete is usually better than that of a sedentary individual. Margaritis et al. [66] observed positive correlations between training volume, maximal oxygen intake and glutathione levels, and in a cross-sectional comparison; ElAbed et al. [31] noted that judokas had a more effective antioxidant system than sedentary individuals. Bogdanis et al. [16] found lower levels of oxidative stress markers (thiobarbituric acid reactive spe-cies [TBARS], creatine kinase) and an upregulated activity of the antioxidant system in people who practised intensive interval training three times a week for as little as 3 weeks. Likewise, aerobic training reduced the concentrations of lipoperoxidation ·OH radicals in both plasma and muscle [58]. Trained individu-als also showed a greater activity of antioxidant enzymes (catalase, glutathione peroxidase, glutathione reductase and superoxide dismutase) in muscle samples after training [16,64]. Skrha [88] further noted increased gene expression of anti-oxidant enzymes. These enzymatic adaptations explain why well-trained individ-uals can undertake very vigorous physical activity without developing evidence of lipid peroxidation and oxidant stress.

Dietary Modifications and Oxidative Stress

Manipulation of the quality and/or quantity of dietary intake can have either a posi-tive or an adverse effect upon oxidative stress and immune function, depending upon a person's initial status. Modest dietary restriction is generally beneficial in sedentary individuals who are initially overweight or obese [19]. The production of free radicals, which occurs predominantly in the mitochondria, is decreased as food intake and daily energy expenditure is reduced. Micronutrient supplements have a beneficial effect upon oxidant status only if they are correcting a deficit related to fasting or a severely restricted food intake; there is little evidence that micronutrients have any effect upon oxidant levels in well-nourished individuals [15].

Muscle glycogen is depleted during prolonged fasting. This reduces the potential for aerobic activity, which could in turn increase oxidative stress. Glycogen stores can be spared by increased fat oxidation in a well-trained individual [17], but a greater reliance upon fat is likely to increase oxidative stress [27,48]. In addition, individuals who engage in fasting could lack the essential fats and micronutrients needed to support both exercise performance and antioxidant defense mechanisms [34]. Excessive training and/or a micronutrient deficiency may increase stress hormone levels, with adverse changes in several aspects of immunity such as neutrophil and lymphocyte counts, granulocyte oxidative capacity, and nasal and salivary immunoglobulin A levels; all of these changes predispose to an increased risk of acute infections [43,98]. An adequate intake of protein, carbohydrate, iron, zinc and B vitamins and an appropriate adjustment of the training/rest ratio are critical to reducing the risk of immunosuppression and acute infections during periods of intensive training [45].

Galassetti et al. [42] tested the effects of dietary restriction by exposing a half of their subjects to a 25% reduction of energy intake. They found a similar reduction in markers of lipid peroxidation (F-2 isoprostanes) and no difference of neutrophil-derived myeloperoxidases in both normal and low-energy intake subject groups after 7 days of exercise, despite a reduction of neutrophil counts in those whose diet was restricted; possibly, impairment of oxidant defenses might also have been seen with a longer period of dietary restriction. Adoption of a low-fat high-carbohydrate diet (15% fat, 65% CHO, 20% protein), such as might occur with Greek Orthodox fasting, can also increase proinflammatory and decrease anti-inflammatory immune factors, with depressed levels of antioxidants and negative effects upon blood lipoprotein ratios, at least in athletes [44]; however, increasing the total energy intake (+25%) to match energy expenditures and increasing the dietary fat intake to 32% appeared to reverse the negative effects reported when eating a much lower-fat diet [44]. In the same context, Meksawan et al. [71] found that decreasing fat intake to 19% of an energy-deficient diet caused higher plasma *TNF*-α levels than those seen with a 30% or 50% fat diet. Pendergast et al. [77] further found that if the fat intake was increased to provide 50% of energy needs while maintaining energy balance, this did not exacerbate proinflammatory responses relative to a 30% fat diet. However, others found that a very high-fat intake increased oxidant stress, with a resulting increase in the risk of atherosclerosis [39]. At least in athletes, it is likely that dietary fat can be increased to at least 50% of energy needs without compromising cardiovascular or immune function; presumably, in the active individual, much of the ingested fat is quickly used by the active muscles. Vogt et al. [99] found that muscle glycogen stores were well maintained after following a high-fat diet for 5 weeks, but at the same time, intramyocellular lipid stores were more than doubled. Endurance performance capacity was thus conserved at moderate to high-exercise intensities, with lipids making a significantly larger contribution to total energy turnover.

If glycogen and fat stores are reduced because of fasting or a combination of fasting and training processes, protein breakdown is increased, and the protein synthesis needed for muscle repair and hypertrophy is inhibited, so that a loss of muscle mass results [77].

Oxidative Stress and Ramadan Intermittent Fasting

The immune system may be adversely affected by Ramadan observance, due to dehydration, biochemical changes such as reduced plasma concentrations of iron, calcium and magnesium, and altered hormonal responses [69]. On the other hand, if the total energy intake is reduced during Ramadan, this could increase the capacity of the antioxidant system and thus improve immune function, particularly in an obese individual [80,88]. Findings differ substantially between sedentary individuals and athletes.

Sedentary people often use Ramadan fasting as an opportunity to reduce body mass, and as with other more prolonged periods of dietary restriction, the impact upon oxidant status is generally positive. Often, the weight loss is monitored by medical advisers, and care may be taken to provide adequate amounts of the micronutrients needed to sustain immune function and conserve antioxidant status. Antioxidants may be boosted by an increased intake of fresh fruit during the celebration of Ramadan [6]. In the majority of published studies of sedentary but otherwise healthy individuals, body mass has decreased, and oxidant status has improved with the observance of Ramadan and other forms of dieting (Table 8.1).

Athletes generally show no change of energy intake during Ramadan. A review of 15 studies found small decreases of dietary intake in 4 trials, but no significant change in the remaining 11 [93]. On the other hand, an increased intake of fat to allow ingestion of the required energy in two rather than three meals may have the effect of increasing oxidant stress [48]. Mele [72] pointed out that amino acids are a source of antioxidant activity, and an increased reliance on protein during fasting or dietary restriction could reduce this source of protection. Another variable that may affect the oxidant status of the athlete is the extent to which the normal training routine is sustained during dietary restriction; maintenance of normal training seems feasible during Ramadan [21], but it is not always achieved.

Empirical data on athletes show a varied oxidant status, depending in part on whether energy intake and training were maintained during dietary restriction (Table 8.2). Two reports found an enhanced oxidant status following an acute bout of exercise, in three studies, there was no change of resting status, and in two studies, the oxidant status worsened. Production of the cytokine IL-12 following completion of a Wingate test was less during Ramadan than during a control period

TABLE 8.1 Oxidant Stress in Sedentary but Otherwise Healthy Subjects during Ramadan and Other Forms of Dietary Restriction

Author	Subjects	Measures	Response
Ramadan Observance			
Akrami Mohajeri et al. [2]	58 healthy adults	Inflammatory chemokines (CXCL1, CXCL10)	Reduced oxidant stress, decrease of BMI during Ramadan
Aksungar et al. [3]	Healthy, non-obese young adults (20 M, 20 F) versus 28 matched volunteers	C-reactive protein, IL-6 and homocysteine	C-reactive protein, IL-6 and homocysteine reduced, increased HDL/total cholesterol ratio, no report on body mass
Al Hourani et al. [5]	57 healthy females	Uric acid	No change of uric acid, decrease of body mass
Asgary et al. [9]	50 healthy male adults	Malondialdehyde	Decreased, body mass not reported
El Ati et al. [32]	16 healthy young women	Uric acid	Increased, no change of energy intake or body mass
Faris et al. [35]	Healthy adults, 23 M, 27 F	Urinary 15 F_{2t} isoprostane	No significant change, decrease of body mass
Faris et al. [36]	Healthy adults, 23 M, 27 F	IL-1, IL-6, TNF-α	Proinflammatory cytokines greatly reduced, small decrease of body mass
Gumaa [49]	16 healthy males	Uric acid	Increased, body mass not reported
Ibrahim et al. [53]	Healthy adults, 9 M, 5 F	Serum malondialdehyde, aspartate aminotransferase, alanine aminotransferase, creatine kinase, red cell MDA, glutathione, glutathione peroxidase, catalase	Red cell MDA reduced on the 28th day of Ramadan, small decrease of body mass and lean body mass
Lahdimawan et al. [61]	30 healthy males	Complement C3, inducible nitric oxide synthase, superoxide dismutase, macrophage and TNF-α	Ramadan altered macrophage regulation and signalling, reducing macrophage oxidative stress. Body mass not reported
Sayedda et al. [84]	20 male medical students	Creatine phosphokinase	Reduction of CPK, decrease of body mass
Sülü et al. [91]	Healthy adults, 23 M, 22 F	Malondialdehyde, glutathione	Malondialdehyde increased (significant only in F), glutathione decreased in M and increased in F; no change of body mass

(*Continued*)

TABLE 8.1 (*Continued*) Oxidant Stress in Sedentary but Otherwise Healthy Subjects during Ramadan and Other Forms of Dietary Restriction

Author	Subjects	Measures	Response
Dietary Restriction			
Galassetti et al. [42]	Healthy male adults, 9 reduced energy intake, 10 control	F_2 isoprostanes, catalase, myeloperoxidase, IL-6	7-day study. No differences between 25% reduction and 10% increase of energy intake; decreased oxidative stress in both groups
Lee et al. [63]	52 healthy females	Urinary malondialdehyde, 8-isoprostaglandin F_{2a}(8-isoPGF), 8-hydroxdeoxyyguanosine, $1,n^6$-ethenodeoxyadenosine	Fasting 7 days, 7.5 and decrease of body mass. Decrease of malondialdehyde and 8-isoPGF
Velthuis-Te Wierik et al. [96]	24 non-obese M (16 experimental, 8 control)	Catalase, glutathione peroxidase, superoxide dismutase	20% reduction of energy intake for 10 weeks, 7.4 kg decrease of body mass. No change of oxidant status

[1], in association with a 2.5 kg decrease of body mass. In the study of Hammouda et al. [50], evening data obtained during Ramadan also showed increases in uric acid and total antioxidant status following performance of intermittent exercise (a Yo-Yo test); this group of investigators also observed a reduction of body mass during Ramadan. Of the two reports where oxidant status may have worsened, Chaouachi et al. [21] studied 15 elite male judoka, finding no change of energy intake or training during Ramadan; however, there was a 57% increase in levels of C-reactive protein and decreased levels of vitamin E. Chennaoui et al. [22] followed eight middle-distance runners. They saw no change of body mass during Ramadan, but IL-6 levels were increased. This could reflect a greater inflammatory response, but it is also possible that the IL-6 may have been playing a role in mobilizing glucose (Chapter 3), since levels of C-reactive protein were decreased during Ramadan.

Three studies examined the effects of 'making weight' in judoka who deliberately reduced their body mass in the week prior to competition (Table 8.2). Degoutte and associates [26] studied 20 national-level judoka, a half of whom decreased their food intake from 11 to 7 MJ/day with a 3.8 kg decrease of body mass. An increase of uric acid relative to the control group was attributed to increased protein catabolism, but it could also have indicated an enhanced oxidant status.

A second report looked at the lag phase before free radical–induced oxidation began, the maximum rate of oxidation, and maximum levels of conjugated dienes. No pre-competitive differences were seen between experimental and control groups [37].

A third study concerned 16 female judoka, a half of whom reduced their body mass by an average of 3.2 kg [92]. Both experimental (weight-loss) and control

TABLE 8.2 Oxidant Stress in Athletes during Ramadan Observance, when 'Making Weight', and during Deliberate Dieting

Author	Subjects	Measures	Response
Ramadan Observance			
Abedelmalek et al. [1]	9 young males	IL-12 production during exercise (Wingate test)	Reduced IL-12 production; 2.5 kg loss of body mass
Bouhlel et al. (unpublished data, [18])	10 young moderately trained male boxers	Malondialdehyde, total oxidants, catalase; C-reactive protein, IL-6, homocysteine	No effect on oxidant stress or inflammatory markers during Ramadan fasting, either before or after repeated sprinting; small decreases of body mass and lean mass
Chaouachi et al. [21]	15 elite male judoka	Blood vitamin A and E content, C-reactive protein, homocysteine	57% increase of C-reactive protein by end of Ramadan; increase of Vit. A, decrease of vitamin E; no change of energy intake or training
Chennaoui et al. [22]	8 male middle-distance runners	C-reactive protein IL-6	133% increase of IL-6 during Ramadan, but non-significant trend to decrease of C-reactive protein; no change of body mass
Hammouda et al. [50]	20 male adolescent soccer players	Total antioxidant status, uric acid, creatine phosphokinase following Yo-Yo intermittent exercise	CPK, TAS and uric acid higher in morning than in evening during Ramadan; evening shows significant decrease; decrease of body mass
Maughan et al. [68]	78 male adolescent soccer players, 48 observing Ramadan	C-reactive protein	Decrease of C-reactive protein in fasting and non-fasting subjects, but more persistent in those fasting; 0.7 kg decrease of body mass
Trabelsi et al. [94]	16 male recreational body builders, 8 fed normally during Ramadan	Uric acid, C-reactive protein	No change of C-reactive protein, but increase of uric acid; food intake unchanged
Athletes 'making weight'			
Degoutte et al. [26]	20 judoka, 10 lost 5% body mass	Uric acid	Greater increase with exercise in those losing 5% body mass in 1 week
Finaud et al. [37]	20 male judoka, 10 reducing body mass by 5% in week before competition	Conjugated diene accumulation	Competition causes similar change of oxidant stress in those losing 5% body mass and controls

(*Continued*)

TABLE 8.2 (*Continued*) Oxidant Stress in Athletes during Ramadan Observance, when 'Making Weight', and during Deliberate Dieting

Author	Subjects	Measures	Response
Suzuki et al. [92]	16 female judoka, 8 reducing body mass	Oxidative burst activity of neutrophils	Decrease of neutrophil phagocytic activity with 3.2 kg decrease of body mass
Deliberate Dieting			
Rankin et al. [80]	20 trained male cyclists	Glutathione, glutathione peroxidase	Glutathione antioxidant system enhanced with 4 days dieting (protein supplements, 2.7 kg decrease of body mass)

groups showed an increased oxidative burst activity in their neutrophils with competitive activity, but the weight loss group also showed a reduction of neutrophil phagocytic activity. One report looked at deliberately restricting 20 cyclists to an energy intake of 83 kJ/kg/day (with protein supplements) for 4 days [80]. A 2.7 kg decrease in body mass was accompanied by an increase in lymphocyte total glutathione and red cell glutathione peroxidase, but plasma lipid peroxidation was unchanged. Possibly, an initially high antioxidant capacity did not allow scope for improvement in oxidant status in this study.

Dietary Restriction in Patients with Clinical Conditions

Patients with clinical conditions have almost invariably shown an improvement of oxidant status during Ramadan and other forms of dietary restriction (Table 8.3).

Dietary Restrictions and Oxidant Stress in Laboratory Animals

Animal studies offer the potential of random assignment to severe dietary restriction, with or without vigorous exercise, and the assurance that the assigned regime will be maintained for several months. On the other hand, such requirements impose substantial stress upon the animals concerned, and often the treatment of the control group (sedentary life in a laboratory cage) is also far from normal. Whereas a short-term (72 hours) food deprivation of animals increased their oxidant stress [90], three studies where food intake was limited from an early age showed an enhanced oxidant status relative to control animals [14,20,59].

TABLE 8.3 Oxidant Status in Patients with Clinical Conditions during Dietary Restriction

Author	Subjects	Measures	Response
Ramadan Observance			
Al-Shafei [7]	40 hypertensive patients, 40 controls	Malondialdehyde, glutathione	Malondialdehyde decreased 25, 23%, glutathione increased 57, 53%; body mass not reported
Al-Shafei [6]	40 diabetic patients, 40 controls	Malondialdehyde, glutathione	Malondialdehyde decreased 47, 54$, glutathione increased 59. 53%; body mass not reported
El-Gendy et al. [33]	20 older diabetic patients, 20 controls	Malondialdehyde, glutathione	Malondialdehyde reduced 40, 58%, glutathione increased 241, 139%; no change of body mass
Khajafi et al. [56]	56 patients with stable cardiac disease (45 M, 11 F)	C-reactive protein	n.s. trend to decrease of C-reactive protein; no change of body mass
Nematy et al. [74]	38 M, 44 F with coronary or cerebrovascular disease or metabolic syndrome	C-reactive protein, homocysteine	Unchanged; no change of energy intake
Ozturk et al. [76]	Women in second trimester of pregnancy, 42 fasting, 30 non-fasting	Total antioxidant status, total oxidant status, oxidative stress index	Total antioxidant status higher in those observing Ramadan; no difference of weight gain
Radhakishun et al. [79]	25 ethnic obese adolescents	C-reactive protein	Decrease of C-reactive protein during Ramadan, no change of BMI
Shariatpanahi et al. [85]	65 adult M with metabolic syndrome	C-reactive protein	Decreased; decrease of BMI
Ünalacak et al. [95]	10 obese males, 10 males with normal BMI	IL-2, IL-8, TNF-α	Inflammatory cytokines and BMI reduced in both groups
Bastard et al. [13]	21 obese women, 8 controls	IL-6, TNF-α, C- reactive protein	Decrease of IL-6 but not TNF-α or C-reactive protein in obese women after 3 weeks of low-energy diet
Buchowski et al. [19]	Obese women (20 test, 20 control)	F_2-isoprostane, C-reactive protein	F_2 isoprostane fell within 5 days of 25% decrease in energy intake
Heilbronn et al. [52]	40 overweight adults	Protein carbonyls, DNA damage assessed by comet tail formation	No change of protein carbonyls but decrease of DNA damage with energy deficit $\pm$ exercise

(Continued)

TABLE 8.3 (*Continued*) Oxidant Status in Patients with Clinical Conditions during Dietary Restriction

Author	Subjects	Measures	Response
Sustained Dietary Restriction			
Johnson et al. [55]	10 obese subjects with asthma	8-isoprostane, nitrotyrosine, protein carbonyls, 4-hydroxynonenal, uric acid, TNF-α	All markers improved with 80% decrease of energy intake within alternate days for 8 weeks
Meydani et al. [73]	46 overweight adults	Glutathione peroxidase, superoxide dismutase, catalase, plasma protein carbonyls, 8-epi-prostaglandin F2α	Glutathione peroxidase increased, plasma protein carbonyls decreased with energy restriction of 30% over 6 months
Tchernof et al. [93]	25 obese post-menopausal women	C-reactive protein	32% decrease in CRP with 14.6 kg decrease of body mass over 14 months
Wycherley et al. [100]	29 obese diabetic adults (16 diet, 13 diet + exercise)	Malondialdehyde	Malondialdehyde reduced with 12 weeks 5 MJ/day ±exercise

Practical Implications for Athletes

The stress imposed by a combination of intensive exercise and/or training combined with dietary restrictions can have detrimental effects upon oxidative status, immune function, health and performance. It is thus important to begin a conditioning programme with low to moderate training loads and to increase the intensity and volume of training progressively, avoiding excessive training loads that could lead to chronic fatigue, illness or injury. Particularly if diet is restricted, a variety of forms of conditioning should be introduced to limit training monotony, with non-specific cross training to offset staleness, and adequate opportunities for rest and recovery should be ensured. Specific monitoring should be adopted to identify any signs of performance deterioration as conditioning continues.

A prolonged increase of oxidant stress and/or a proinflammatory reaction could predispose to diabetes mellitus and the metabolic syndrome [23,47,60,82], atherosclerosis [40,65,74], carcinogenesis [12] and accelerated aging [8,86,89]. However, the magnitude of the changes observed in athletes, and the relatively short-term nature of Ramadan observance make a long-term adverse health effect unlikely. The main effect of any change in oxidant status is upon the duration of muscle soreness, which is normally linked to increased serum creatine kinase activity and a proinflammatory reaction. This response may be a normal component of the body's reaction to resistance training, and changes in oxidant status could conceivably alter responses to muscular training. However, a study of recreational body builders found no reduction in gains of lean tissue among those who observed Ramadan [94].

During the intermittent fasting of Ramadan, the night-time food intake of athletes should be maximized so that their total energy intake matches energy expenditures, and carbohydrate and fat reserves are maintained. Some nutritional supplements such as quercetin, *Lactobacillus* probiotics, iron, zinc and vitamins A, D, E, B6 and B12 could be helpful to augment immune function and to reduce illness and injury rates if overall dietary intake is restricted, although benefit is unlikely if the diet contains adequate fruit and vegetables [101]; some supplements even reverse the normal exercise-induced increase of peroxidase activity [81].

Conclusions

Increases of oxidative stress depend on the intensity and duration of exercise in relation to the individual's physical fitness and dietary restrictions. Prolonged and/or intensive exercise increases free radical production, but on the other hand, a training programme progressively increases antioxidant defenses. The balance between oxidative and antioxidative processes is modulated by diet. In sedentary individuals, dietary restriction or fasting generally leads to a more favourable balance, but in athletes with a high-energy expenditure, a lack of micronutrients and other consequences of fasting can have negative consequences. Further studies of athletes should assess details of these relationships through accurate measurement of training loads, dietary intakes and physical performance.

Key Terms

Arachidonic acid: Arachidonic acid is a polyunsaturated omega-6 fatty acid; it is readily converted to prostaglandin with tissue breakdown.

Catalase: Catalase is an enzyme that can breakdown hydrogen peroxide.

Chemokines: Cytokines that induce chemotaxis (the attraction of specific cells to a given site).

Conjugated dienes: Conjugated dienes are carbohydrate chains that contain two double bonds.

Creatine kinase: Creatine kinase is an enzyme found in muscle tissue that transfers energy from adenosine triphosphate to creatine, forming the high-energy substance phosphocreatine.

Cytokines: Cytokines are chemical signals that affect the function of nearby cells and sometimes the function of the cells releasing them. They are an important component of the immune system.

Eccentric exercise: Eccentric exercise is performed when a muscle shortens as it contracts, as when running downhill.

Free radicals: A free radical is an atom or molecule that has an unpaired electron, and thus a dangling bond that can interact with other chemicals.

Glutathione peroxidase: Glutathione peroxidase is an enzyme that can break down hydrogen peroxide.

Homeostasis: Homeostasis implies a system that maintains conditions within narrow limits.

Hydrogen peroxide (H_2O_2): Hydrogen peroxide is the simplest form of peroxide and is a strong oxidizing agent.

Immunosuppression: A decreased function of the immune system that normally protects the body against infection.

Isoprostanes: Isoprostanes are used as measures of lipid peroxidation.

Lipoperoxidation: Lipoperoxidation is the oxidative degradation of lipids.

Malondialdehyde: MDA is an organic compound often used as a marker of oxidative stress.

Mitochondria: The mitochondrion is an organelle within a cell where many of the essential chemical reactions such as the generation of energy occur.

Nitric oxide (Nitrogen monoxide, NO˙): Nitric oxide functions as a free radical.

Oxidative stress: Oxidative stress reflects an imbalance between the accumulation of free radicals and the ability of the body to neutralize them.

Peroxidase: Peroxidase is an enzyme that can break down hydrogen peroxide.

Phagocytic cells: Phagocytes are cells that protect the body by ingesting bacteria, foreign particles, and dead or dying cells.

Reactive oxygen species: Reactive oxygen species are highly interactive molecules containing oxygen ions.

Redox potential: In terms of oxidation/reduction reactions, a substance that can accept electrons has a high redox potential, and a substance that liberates electrons has a low redox potential.

Superoxide ($O_2^{˙-}$ radical): Superoxide is a molecule of oxygen that carries an additional electron giving it a negative charge.

Superoxide dismutase: Superoxide dismutase is an enzyme that can breakdown the superoxide radical.

TBARS: TBARS are thiobarbituric reactive substances, formed as by-products of lipid peroxidation.

TNF-α: TNF-α is a cytokine that stimulates an inflammatory reaction.

Key Points

1. Intensive and/or prolonged exercise increases the generation of free radicals.
2. Training programmes enhance antioxidant mechanisms, generally with some reduction of free radicals levels in the individual concerned.
3. Short periods of fasting appear to enhance antioxidative mechanisms, at least in those who are initially overweight.
4. Some studies have shown enhanced antioxidative mechanisms in trained athletes during Ramadan, but often there is no improvement, and sometimes oxidant status is worsened.
5. Further studies are needed to examine the effects of combined fasting and training in promoting positive changes in antioxidative mechanisms.

Questions for Discussion

1. Which biomarker would you use to evaluate oxidant stress during fasting?
2. What factors might alter an athlete's resistance to oxidative stress during Ramadan observance and other forms of dietary restriction?
3. Are micronutrients helpful in enhancing resistance to oxidative stress when consuming a normal diet? Are recommended daily needs of micronutrients modified by dietary restriction?
4. What overall recommendations would you make to minimize oxidative stress in a high-performance athlete who is observing Ramadan?

References

1. Abedelmalek S, Souissi N, Takayuki A et al. Effect of acute maximal exercise on circulating levels of interleukin-12 during Ramadan fasting. *Asian J Sports Med* 2011; 2:154–160.
2. Akrami Mohajeri F, Ahmadi Z, Hassanshahi G et al. Does Ramadan fasting affect inflammatory responses: Evidence for modulatory roles of this unique nutritional status via chemokine network. *Iran J Basic Med Sci* 2013;16:1217–1222.
3. Aksungar FB, Topkaya AE, Akyildiz M. Interleukin-6, C-reactive protein and biochemical parameters during prolonged intermittent fasting. *Ann Nutr Metab* 2007;51:88–95.
4. Alessio HM. Exercise-induced oxidative stress. *Med Sci Sports Exerc* 1993;25(2):218–222.
5. Al Hourani HM, Atoum MF, Akel S et al. Effects of Ramadan fasting on some haematological and biochemical parameters. *Jordan J Biol Sci* 2009;2:103–108.
6. Al-Shafei AI. Ramadan fasting ameliorates oxidative stress and improves glycemic control and lipid profile in diabetic patients. *Eur J Nutr* 2014;53(7):1475–1481.
7. Al-Shafei AI. Ramadan fasting ameliorates arterial pulse pressure and lipid profile, and alleviates oxidative stress in hypertensive patients. *Blood Pressure* 2014;23:160–167.
8. Ames BN, Shigenaga MK. Oxidants are a major contributor to aging. *Ann NY Acad Sci* 1992;663:85–96.
9. Asgary S, Aghaeı A, Naderı GA et al. Effects of Ramadan fasting on lipid peroxidation, serum lipoproteins and fasting blood sugar. *Med J Islamic Acad Sci* 2000;13:35–38.
10. Askew EW. Work at high altitude and oxidative stress: Antioxidant nutrients. *Toxicology* 2002 Nov 15;180(2):107–119.
11. Banerjee AK, Mandal A, Chanda D, Chakraborti S. Oxidant, antioxidant and physical exercise. *Mol Cell Biochem* 2003 Nov;253(1–2):307–132.
12. Barocas DA, Motley S, Cookson MS et al. Oxidative stress measured by urine F2-isoprostane level is associated with prostate cancer. *J Urol* 2011;185:2102–2107.
13. Bastard J-P, Jardel C, Briuckert E et al. Elevated levels of interleukin 6 are reduced in serum and subcutaneous adipose tissue of obese women after weight loss. *J Clin Endocrinol Metab* 2000;86:3338–3342.
14. Bevilacqua L, Ramsdey JJ, Hagopian K et al. Effects of short- and medium-term calorie restriction on muscle mitochondrial proton leak and reactive oxygen species production. *Am J Physiol* 2004;86:E852–E861.
15. Bishop NC, Blannin AK, Walsh NP et al. Nutritional aspects of immunosuppression in athletes. *Sports Med* 1999 Sep;28(3):151–76.
16. Bogdanis GC, Stavrinou P, Fatouros IG et al. Short-term high-intensity interval exercise training attenuates oxidative stress responses and improves antioxidant status in healthy humans. *Food Chem Toxicol* 2013;61:171–177.

17. Bouhlel E, Salhi Z, Bouhlel H et al. Effect of Ramadan fasting on fuel oxidation during exercise in trained male rugby players. *Diabetes Metab* 2006;32:617–624.

18. Bouhlel H, Bogdanis GC, Hamila A et al. Effects of Ramadan observance on repeated cycle ergometer sprinting and associated inflammatory and oxidative stress responses in trained young men. "Still under review".

19. Buchowski MS, Hongu N, Acra S et al. Effect of modest caloric restriction on oxidative stress in women, a randomized trial. *PLoS ONE* 2012;7:e47079.

20. Castello L, Froio T, Maina M et al. Alternate-day fasting protects the rat heart against age-induced inflammation and fibrosis by inhibiting oxidative damage and NF-kB activation. *Free Radic Biol Med* 2009;48:47–64.

21. Chaouachi A, Leiper JB, Souissi N et al. Effects of Ramadan intermittent fasting on sports performance and training: A review. *Int J Sports Physiol Perform* 2009;4:419–434.

22. Chennaoui M, Desgorces F, Drogou C et al. Effects of Ramadan fasting on physical performance and metabolic, hormonal, and inflammatory parameters in middle-distance runners. *Appl Physiol Nutr Metab* 2009 Aug;34(4):587–594.

23. Chung S-W, Kang S-G, Rho J-S et al. The associations between oxidative stress and metabolic syndrome in adults. *Korean J Fam Med* 2013;34:420–428.

24. Closa D, Folch-Puy E. Oxygen free radicals and the systemic inflammatory response. *IUBMB Life* 2004;56:185–191.

25. Córdova Martínez A, Martorell Pons M, Sureda Gomila A et al. Changes in circulating cytokines and markers of muscle damage in elite cyclists during a multi-stage competition. *Clin Physiol Funct Imaging* 2014 May 26.

26. Degoutte F, Jouanel P, Bègue RJ et al. Food restriction, performance, biochemical, psychological and endocrine changes in judo athletes. *Int J Sports Med* 2006;27:9–18.

27. Dembach AR, Sherman WM, Simonsen JC et al. No evidence of oxidant stress during high intensity rowing. *J Appl Physiol* 1993;74:2140–2145.

28. Deminice R, Rosa FT, Franco GS et al. Effects of creatine supplementation on oxidative stress and inflammatory markers after repeated-sprint exercise in humans. *Nutrition* 2013 Sep;29(9):1127–1132.

29. Dikalov SI1, Dikalova AE, Mason RP et al. Noninvasive diagnostic tool for inflammation-induced oxidative stress using electron spin resonance spectroscopy and an extracellular cyclic hydroxylamine. *Arch Biochem Biophys* 2002;402(2):218–226.

30. Donoshow JH. Glutathione peroxidase and oxidative stress. *Toxicol Lett* 1995; 82–83:395–398.

31. ElAbed K, Rebai H, Bloomer RJ et al. Antioxidant status and oxidative stress at rest and in response to acute exercise in judokas and sedentary men. *J Strength Cond Res* 2011 Sep;25(9):2400–2409.

32. El Ati J, Bell C, Danguir J. Increased fat oxidation during Ramadan fasting in healthy women: An adaptive mechanism for body-weight maintenance. *Am J Clin Nutr* 1995;62:302–307.

33. El-Gendy OA, Roikaya M, El-Batae HE et al. Ramadan fasting improves kidney functions and ameliorates oxidative stress in diabetic patients. *World J Sports Sci* 2012;7:38–48.

34. Evans P, Halliwell B. Micronutrients: Oxidant/antioxidant status. *Br J Nutr* 2001:85 (Suppl. 2):S67–S74.

35. Faris MAE, Husein RN, Al-Kurd RA et al. Impact of Ramadan intermittent fasting on oxidative stress as measured by urinary 15-F21-isoprostane. *J Nutr Metab* 2012;ID802924:1–9.

36. Faris MA, Kacimi S, AlKurd RA et al. Intermittent fasting during Ramadan attenuates proinflammatory cytokines and immune cells in healthy subjects. *Nutr Res* 2012 Dec;32(12):947–955.

37. Finaud J, Degoutte F, Scislowski V et al. Competition and food restriction effects on oxidative stress in judo. *Int J Sports Med* 2006;27:834–841.

38. Finsterer J. Biomarkers of peripheral muscle fatigue during exercise. *BMC Musculoskelet Disord* 2012;8;13:218.
39. Folmer V, Soares CM, Gabriel D et al. A high fat diet inhibits D-aminolevulinate dehydratase and increases lipid peroxidation in mice. *J Nutr* 2003;133:2165–2170.
40. Fontana L, Meyer TE, Klein S et al. Long-term calorie restriction is highly effective in reducing the risk for atherosclerosis in humans. *Proc Natl Acad Sci USA*. 2004;101:6659–6663.
41. Fridovich I. Superoxide dismutases: Regularities and irregularities. *Harvey Lect* 1983–1984;79:51–75.
42. Galassetti PR, Nemet D, Pescatello A et al. Exercise, caloric restriction, and systemic oxidative stress. *J Investig Med* 2006 Mar;54(2):67–75.
43. Gleeson M, Bishop NC. Elite athlete immunology: Importance of nutrition. *Int J Sports Med* 2000 May;21(Suppl. 1):S44–S50.
44. Gleeson M, Lancaster GI, Bishop NC. Nutritional strategies to minimise exercise-induced immunosuppression in athletes. *Can J Appl Physiol* 2001;26(Suppl.):S23–S35.
45. Gleeson M, Niman DC, Pedersen BK. Exercise, nutrition and immune function. *J Sports Sci* 2004 Jan;22(1):115–125.
46. Gonzalez-Fleche B, Reides C, Cutrin JC et al. Oxidative stress produced by suprahepatic occlusion and reperfusion. *Hepatology* 1993;18:881–889.
47. Goodwill AG, Frisbee JC. Oxidant stress and skeletal muscle microvasculopathy in the metabolic syndrome. *Vasc Pharmacol* 2012;57:150–159.
48. Gregersen S, Samnocha-Bonet D, Heilbronn LK et al. Inflammatory and oxidative stress responses to high carbohydrate and high-fat meals in healthy humans. *J Nutr Metab* 2012;(ID 238056).
49. Gumaa KA, Mustafa KY, Mahmoud NA et al. The effects of Ramadan fasting: 1. Serum uric acid and lipid concentrations. *Br J Nutr* 1978;40:573–581.
50. Hammouda O, Chtourou H, Aloui A et al. Does Ramadan fasting affect the diurnal variations in metabolic responses and total antioxidant capacity during exercise in young soccer players? *Sport Sci Health* 2014;10:97–104.
51. Hassan HM, Fridovich I. Chemistry and biochemistry of superoxide dismutases. *Eur J Rheumatol Inflamm* 1981;4(2):160–172.
52. Heilbronn LK, de Jonge L, Frisard MI et al. Effect of 6-month calorie restriction on biomarkers of longevity, metabolic adaptation, and oxidative stress in overweight individuals. A randomized controlled trial. *JAMA* 2006;295:1539–1548.
53. Ibrahim WH, Habib HM, Jarrar AH et al. Effect of Ramadan fasting on markers of oxidative stress and serum biochemical markers of cellular damage in healthy subjects. *Ann Nutr Metab* 2008;53:175–181.
54. Ji LL. Antioxidants and oxidative stress in exercise. *Proc Soc Exp Biol Med* 1999 Dec;222(3):283–292.
55. Johnson JB, Summer W, Cutler RG et al. Alternate day calorie restriction improves clinical findings and reduces markers of oxidative stress and inflammation in overweight adults with moderate asthma. *Free Radic Biol Med* 2007 Mar 1;42(5):665–674.
56. Khajafi HARH, Bener A, Osman M et al. The impact of diurnal fasting during Ramadan on the lipid profile, hs-CRP, and serum leptin in stable cardiac patients. *Vasc Health Risk Manag* 2012;8:7–14.
57. Knez WL, Jenkins DG, Coombes JS. Oxidative stress in half and full Ironman triathletes. *Med Sci Sports Exerc* 2007 Feb;39(2):283–288.
58. Kretzschmar M, Müller D. Aging, training and exercise. A review of effects on plasma glutathione and lipid peroxides. *Sports Med* 1993 Mar;15(3):196–209.
59. Koizumi A, Weindruch R, Walford RL. Influences of dietary restriction and age on liver enzyme activities and lipid peroxidation in mice. *J Nutr Health Aging* 1987; 117:361–367.

60. Kotani K, Yamada T. Oxidative stress and metabolic syndrome in a Japanese female population. *Australas J Ageing* 2012;31:124–127.
61. Lahdimawan A, Handono K, Indra MR et al. Effect of Ramadan fasting on classically activated, oxidative stress and inflammation of macrophage. *OSR J Pharmacy* 2013;3:14–22.
62. Leaf DA, Kleinman MT, Hamilton M, Barstow TJ. The effect of exercise intensity on lipid peroxidation. *Med Sci Sports Exerc* 1997 Aug;29(8):1036–1039.
63. Lee K-H, Bartsch H, Nair JY et al. Effect of short-term fasting on urinary excretion of primary lipid peroxidation products and on markers of oxidative DNA damage in healthy women. *Carcinogenesis* 2006;27:1398–1403.
64. Leonardo-Mendonça RC, Concepción-Huertas M, Guerra-Hernández E et al. Redox status and antioxidant response in professional cyclists during training. *Eur J Sport Sci* 2014;14(8):830–838.
65. Magliano DJ, Liew D, Ashton EL et al. Novel biomedical risk markers for cardiovascular disease. *J Cardiovasc Risk* 2003;10:41–55.
66. Margaritis I, Tessier F, Richard MJ, Marconnet P. No evidence of oxidative stress after a triathlon race in highly trained competitors. *Int J Sports Med* 1997;18:186–190.
67. Marzatico F, Pansarasa O, Bertorelli L et al. Blood free radical antioxidant enzymes and lipid peroxides following long-distance and lactacidemic performances in highly trained aerobic and sprint athletes. *J Sports Med Phys Fitness* 1997 Dec;37(4):235–239.
68. Maughan RJ, Leiper JB, Bartagi Z et al. Effect of Ramadan fasting on some biochemical and haematological parameters in Tunisian youth soccer players undertaking their usual training and competition schedule. *J Sports Sci* 2008;26(Suppl. 3):539–546.
69. Meckel Y, Ismaeel A, Eliakim A. The effect of Ramadan fast on physical performance and dietary habits in adolescent soccer players. *Eur J Appl Physiol Occup Physiol* 2008;102:651–657.
70. Meckel Y, Eliakim A, Seraev M et al. The effect of a brief sprint interval exercise on growth factors and inflammatory mediators. *J Strength Cond Res* 2009;23(1):225–230.
71. Meksawan K, Venkatraman JT, Awad AB, Pendergast DR. Effect of dietary fat intake and exercise on inflammatory mediators of the immune system in sedentary men and women. *J Am Coll Nutr* 2004 Aug;23(4):331–340.
72. Mele MC. Amino acids and plasma antioxidant activity. *Amino Acids* 1997;12:373–377.
73. Meydani M, Evans WJ, Handelman G et al. Protective effect of vitamin E on exercise-induced oxidative damage in young and older adults. *Am J Physiol* 1993 May;264(5 Pt 2): R992–R998.
74. Nematy M, Alinnezhad-Namaghi M, Rashed MM et al. Effects of Ramadan fasting on cardiovascular risk factors: A prospective observational study. *Nutr J* 2012;11:69–75.
75. Nosaka K, Clarkson PM. Effect of eccentric exercise on plasma enzyme activities previously elevated by eccentric exercise. *Eur J Appl Physiol Occup Physiol* 1994;69(6):492–497.
76. Ozturk E, Balat O, Ugur MG et al. Effect of Ramadan fasting on maternal oxidative stress during the second trimester: A preliminary study. *J Obstet Gynaecol Res* 2011 Jul;37(7):729–733.
77. Pendergast DR, Horvath PJ, Leddy JJ, Venkatraman JT. The role of dietary fat on performance, metabolism, and health. *Am J Sports Med* 1996;24(6 Suppl.):S53–S58.
78. Powers SK, Jackson MJ. Exercise-induced oxidative stress: Cellular mechanisms and impact on muscle force production. *Physiol Rev* 2008;1243–1276.
79. Radhakishun N, Blokhuis C, van Vliet M et al. Intermittent fasting during Ramadan causes a transient increase in total, LDL, and HDL cholesterols and hs-CRP in ethnic obese adolescents. *Eur J Pediatr* 2014;173:1103–1106.
80. Rankin JW, Shute M, Heffron SP, Saker KE. Energy restriction but not protein source affects antioxidant capacity in athletes. *Free Radic Biol Med* 2006 Sep 15;41(6):1001–1009.

81. Ristow M, Zarse K, Oberbach A et al. Antioxidants prevent health-promoting effects of physical exercise in humans. *Proc Natl Acad Sci USA* 2009;106:8665–8670.
82. Roberts CK, Sindhu KK. Oxidative stress and metabolic syndrome. *Life Sci* 2009; 84:705–709.
83. Sachdev S, Davies KJ. Production, detection, and adaptive responses to free radicals in exercise. *Free Radic Biol Med* 2008 Jan 15;44(2):215–223.
84. Sayedda K, Kamal S, Ahmed QS. Effect of Ramadan fasting on anthropometric parameters, blood pressure, creatine phosphokinase activity, serum calcium and phosphorus in healthy students of Shri Ram Murti Smarak Institute of Medical Sciences, Bareilly-UP. *Nat J Physiol Pharm Pharmacol* 2013;3:48–52.
85. Shariatpanahi MV, Shariatpanahi ZV, Shahbazi S et al. Effect of fasting with two meals on BMI and inflammatory markers of metabolic syndrome. *Pak J Biol Sci* 2012;15:255–258.
86. Shephard RJ. *Aging, Physical Activity and Health.* Human Kinetics, Champaign, IL, 1997.
87. Shephard RJ, Shek PN. Immune responses to inflammation and trauma: A physical training model. *Can J Physiol Pharm* 1998;76:469–472.
88. Skrha J. Effect of caloric restriction on oxidative markers. *Adv Clin Chem* 2009; 47:224–247.
89. Sohal RS, Weindruch R. Oxidative stress, caloric restriction, and aging. *Science* 1996;273:59–63.
90. Sorensen M, Sanz A, Gómez G et al. Effects of fasting on oxidative stress in rat liver mitochondria. *Free Rad Res* 2006;40:339–347.
91. Sülü B, Öztürk B, Güven A et al. The effect of long-term controlled fasting (the Ramadan model) on body mass index, blood biochemistry and oxidative stress factors. *Turk Klin J Med Sci* 2010;30:855–863.
92. Suzuki M, Nakaji S, Umeda T et al. Effects of weight reduction on neutrophil phagocytic activity and oxidative burst activity in female judoists. *Luminescence* 2003;18:214–217.
93. Tchernof A, Nolan A, Sites CK et al. Weight loss reduces C-reactive protein levels in obese postmenopausal women. *Circulation* 2002 Feb 5;105(5):564–569.
94. Trabelsi K, Chaker A, Ghlisssi Z et al. Physical activity during Ramadan fasting: Effects on body composition, hematological and biochemical parameters. *IOSR J Pharm* 2012;2:33–41.
95. Ünalacak M, Kara IH, Baltaci D et al. Effects of Ramadan fasting on biochemical and haematological parameters and cytokines in healthy and obese individuals. *Metab Syndr Relat Disord* 2011;9:157–161.
96. Velthuis-Te Wierik EJ, van Leeuwen RE, Hendricks JF et al. Short-term moderate energy restriction does not affect indicators of oxidative stress and genotoxicity in humans. *J Nutr Health Aging* 1995;125:2631–2639.
97. Venditti P, Di Meo S. Effect of training on antioxidant capacity, tissue damage and endurance of adult male rats. *Int J Sports Med* 1997;18:497–502.
98. Venkatraman JT, Pendergast DR. Effect of dietary intake on immune function in athletes. *Sports Med* 2002;32(5):323–337.
99. Vogt M, Puntschart A, Howald H et al. Effects of dietary fat on muscle substrates, metabolism, and performance in athletes. *Med Sci Sports Exerc* 2003 Jun;35(6):952–960.
100. Wycherley TP, Brinkworth GD, Noakes M et al. Effect of caloric restriction with and without exercise training on oxidative stress and endothelial function in obese subjects with type 2 diabetes. *Diabetes Obes Metab* 2008 Nov;10(11):1062–1073.
101. Yavari A, Javadi M, Mirmiran P et al. Exercise-induced oxidative stress and dietary antioxidants. *Asian J Sports Med* 2015 March;6(1):e24898.

Further Reading

Alessio HM, Hagerman AE. *Oxidative Stress, Exercise and Aging*. Imperial College Press, London, U.K., 2006.

Reznick AZ. *Oxidative Stress in Skeletal Muscle*. Birkhauser Verlag, Basel, Switzerland, 1998.

Walsh NP, Gleeson M, Shephard RJ et al. Position statement. Part one: Immune function and exercise. *Exerc Immunol Rev* 2011;17:6–63.

Walsh NP, Gleeson M, Pyne DB, Nieman DC, Dhabhar FS, Shephard RJ, Oliver SJ, Bermon S, Kajeniene A. Position statement. Part two: Maintaining immune health. *Exerc Immunol Rev* 2011;17:64–103.

9

Effects of Dietary and Fluid Restrictions upon Physical Performance, Cognition and Vigilance

Ezdine Bouhlel and Roy J Shephard

Learning Objectives

1. To understand the effects of Ramadan observance upon high-intensity exercise performance and the mechanisms underlying observed changes, including both inherent factors such as a diminution of energy stores and/or a reduction in body fluids, and extraneous factors such as alterations in training regimen, the duration or quality of sleep, and circadian rhythms
2. To explore the effects of Ramadan observance upon exercise of moderate and low intensity, in relation to changes in muscle glycogen stores, body fluid reserves, altered sleeping patterns, and/or modification of training loads
3. To know the effects of Ramadan observance upon aerobic and anaerobic metabolism and the development of muscular force and to explore the determinants of the observed changes
4. To gain insight into the effects of Ramadan observance upon the various components of cerebral function and to explain the main mechanisms involved

Introduction

Prolonged fasting almost inevitably leads to a reduction of both physical and psychomotor performance. A progressive decrease of blood glucose and glycogen reserves limits the possibility of undertaking the anaerobic component of near-maximal exercise and hampers isometric muscular contraction; it also impairs many components of cerebral function, since glucose is the primary metabolite of the brain. In a longer-term perspective, the depletion of lean tissue mass weakens the muscles, reducing their maximal contractile force. These changes are exacerbated by a reduction of motivation (which is an important determinant of most laboratory tests of physical performance), and in athletes there is also likely to be a relaxation of training schedules. On the positive side, the decrease in body mass as fat and lean tissue are metabolized reduces the energy cost of activities that involve the displacement of body mass. However, a substantial dehydration reduces blood volume and maximal cardiac output, thus impairing peak aerobic performance, and an alteration of sodium ion concentrations at the muscle membrane impairs muscle contraction. Although many of the impediments to performance have a physiological cause, the psychological element is also important, and for this reason, effects are usually greater in human studies than in animal research.

The relatively brief and intermittent periods of fasting required by Ramadan observance are likely to have little adverse effect upon blood glucose levels or fluid balance in sedentary individuals, and any loss of performance seen in such subjects reflects a combination of deliberate dieting and diminished motivation. Ramadan observance almost inevitably has a greater impact upon the all-out physical performance of top athletes than upon sedentary individuals. In athletes, there is a progressive reduction of muscle and hepatic glycogen over each day of fasting, and this could have a negative impact upon endurance and ultraendurance performance, particularly if competitions are scheduled during the afternoon or early evening. Nevertheless, the magnitude of such changes will depend on the extent of pre-fast preparation (endurance training and carbohydrate loading), the care taken to maximize night-time food and fluid intake during Ramadan, the extent of any relaxation of training and the motivation to maximal effort while fasting.

Classification of Physical Work

Scherrer and Monod [67] distinguished three categories of muscular exercise: local, regional and general, involving, respectively, less than a third, between 1/3 and 2/3, and most of the body's muscle mass. Local exercise is limited primarily by the muscles that are immediately involved, but exercise using a larger fraction of the total muscle mass is increasingly influenced by any changes in cardiac and respiratory function, thermoregulation and overall nutrition.

During the early 1960s–1970s, physiologists such as Lange Andersen [1] and Rudolfo Margaria [48] classified maximal exercise into three main categories: activities requiring anaerobic power, anaerobic capacity and aerobic power. This distinction was based upon the primary source of energy that was exploited.

- **Anaerobic power.** Anaerobic power exploits local tissue reserves of oxygen and the high-energy phosphate molecules (ATP and creatine phosphate) stored in the active muscles. This energy store is only available for very brief sprints and is depleted during 2–4 s of all-out effort.
- **Anaerobic capacity.** Anaerobic capacity is based upon muscle energy stores such as glucose and glycogen, in the absence of a matching supply of oxygen. Maximal anaerobic effort is halted within about 45 s by the intramuscular accumulation of lactate; this is painful and inhibits the metabolic process of energy release.
- **Aerobic power.** Aerobic power depends upon the ability of the circulation to deliver oxygen to the working tissues, and it progressively assumes responsibility for ongoing exercise as anaerobic power and anaerobic capacity are exhausted.

Andersen and Margaria both viewed the three processes as proceeding sequentially, although more recent research has emphasized that exploitation of the aerobic supply of energy begins within a few seconds of commencing an activity.

A further refinement to this schema is the definition of an aerobic capacity. This reflects the oxygen consumption that can be sustained over a prolonged (1–2 h) period of physical activity. It is determined by a progressive build-up of lactate as the aerobic power is approached. An ordinary person can sustain only about 75% of their aerobic power over a long period of exercise, but endurance athletes such as marathon runners may be able to maintain 85%–90% of maximal oxygen intake through much of an event.

Findings are affected by the latitude and season of the year when Ramadan is observed and by ambient conditions; fluid loss will occur much more quickly if an athlete must exercise in hot and humid weather. Finally, the alteration of meal and sleep times during Ramadan can displace circadian rhythms of performance (Chapter 7), influencing the physiological and psychomotor data obtained with a fixed time of evaluation. Although the impact of observing Ramadan for a single day is often small, if a competitor engages repeatedly in heavy exercise, there could be a cumulative loss of fat, lean tissue and protein over the 29 days of fasting, with final effects similar to those seen with a continuous fast. Changes of circadian rhythm associated with Ramadan observance (Chapter 7) could also have a negative impact upon some activities, particularly those requiring rapid reactions, careful thought, and cooperation between team members.

The impact of total fasting and/or dehydration upon body mass and energy balance has been detailed in Chapter 2. We will now examine the large volume of empirical data relating to the effect of Ramadan observance upon physical and cognitive performances in both sedentary and physically active subjects, remembering that many of the reports lack critical information on preparations for Ramadan, the duration of the daily fasts, evidence of test motivation and allowance for possible circadian shifts in peak performance.

Anaerobic Performance

Anaerobic performance has two components: anaerobic power (mainly the breakdown of phosphagen molecules) and anaerobic capacity (anaerobic metabolism, with a build-up of lactate). The relative contribution of these two processes depends upon the duration of activity [1,48]. Much of the available data seems to have been collected during autumn or winter celebrations of Ramadan, when periods of fasting were relatively short. Several studies where athletes were living under well-controlled conditions with little disruption of sleep or training patterns have shown little effect, but other investigators have seen changes, particularly when the living conditions of athletes were less well regulated, tests were conducted in the late afternoon or evening, and repeated brief efforts were required either by competition or by the test measurements.

Anaerobic Power

An athlete exploits anaerobic power in single, all-out efforts, such as a high jump or a javelin throw. Performance is tested in the laboratory through such measures as the height of a standing jump, the sprint performance on a track or the peak power generated in a Wingate or a Vandewalle cycle ergometer test [72]. Ramadan fasting generally has little effect on measures of this type [11] (Table 9.1); 7 of 12 studies reported no change. However, it is interesting that one group of investigators found a greater effect under free-living conditions than under controlled living conditions [74,75]; loss of function could conceivably occur if sleep disturbance impaired the coordination of all-out effort or if dehydration was sufficient to impair maximal muscular contraction.

Although glycogen reserves may remain adequate for a single sprint during Ramadan, problems can arise if the activity is repeated (e.g., if a contestant must participate in several heats). Thus, Bouhlel et al. [11], using a Vandewalle force–velocity test, found that early during Ramadan there were decreases in the ability to exert peak anaerobic power repeatedly, whether using the arms or the legs. Likewise, Meckel et al. [52] found a decrease of performance in repeated sprints, which they attributed to a decrease in glycolytic capacity and a slower replenishment of muscle creatine phosphate stores between sprints. However, physiological or behavioural adaptations may occur over the 29 days of intermittent fasting, and Bouhlel et al. [11] saw a recovery of performance toward the end of Ramadan.

The time of day when observations are made is obviously critical to data interpretation. Thus, Souissi et al. [69] found that during Ramadan, peak anaerobic

TABLE 9.1 Effects of Ramadan Observance on Anaerobic Power of Athletes

Sample	Effect of Ramadan	Author
12 trained men	Decrease of the maximal anaerobic power of the arms and legs during the first week of Ramadan, with a partial return to initial values at the end of fasting. Vertical jump height unchanged	Bouhlel et al. [11]
15 young national-level judokas	No change of 5, 10 or 30 m sprint performance	Chaouachi et al. [18,20]
10 soccer players	Decrease of peak power on Wingate test	Chtourou et al. [24]
10 assorted power athletes	No change of anaerobic power on Wingate test	Karli et al. [39]
Information not available	Decrease in 100 m race performance and in sprint tests on cycle ergometer	Khedder et al. [40]
53 junior soccer players	No change of speed on *fastest* 10 or 30 m run, but improvement in 10 m sprint average time	Kirkendall et al. [41]
Adolescent soccer players	No change of morning sprint speed, but increased fatigue over 6 sprints	Meckel et al. [52]
14 male collegiate wrestlers	No effect on anaerobic power or strength	Mirzaei et al. [55]
12 physical education students	Less than normal afternoon increase of peak power on Wingate test, increased fatigue	Souissi et al. [69]
8 male karatekas	Time to exhaustion at 75% of voluntary contraction unchanged	Zarrouk et al. [73]
55 free-living soccer players	Decrease of sprint speed during Ramadan	Zerguini et al. [74]
64 soccer players living in a controlled environment	Sprint speed unchanged during Ramadan	Zerguini et al. [75]

power, mean power and fatigue index were unaffected in the morning (when blood glucose levels would presumably have been close to normal), but values were impaired in the evening (when blood glucose levels and muscle glycogen levels would likely have been decreased). Motivation is also an issue, with two studies reporting greater fatigue during Ramadan [23,41].

Anaerobic Capacity

A common method of assessing anaerobic capacity is to undertake an all-out effort for 30 seconds on a cycle ergometer (the Wingate anaerobic capacity test, [8]). With this test, it is possible to examine not only the total work performed during 30 seconds (the mean power, or anaerobic capacity), but also the decrease of effort over the 30 seconds (the fatigue index). Another approach to the evaluation of anaerobic capacity is to measure sprint performance on a track.

Five of seven studies reported increased fatigue and/or a decrease of anaerobic capacity during Ramadan (Table 9.2). However, Karli et al. [39] found no change

TABLE 9.2 Effects of Ramadan Observance on Anaerobic Capacity of Athletes

Sample	Effect of Ramadan	Author
9 trained athletes	Decrease of the total work completed during six Wingate test bouts during Ramadan	Aziz et al. [3]
10 healthy young male	Unchanged total work performed during four Wingate bouts	Aziz et al. [4]
12 junior level soccer players	Increased fatigue index on ergometer sprint test	Chtourou et al. [23]
10 soccer players	Increased fatigue index on Wingate test	Chtourou et al. [24]
Ten 200 and 400 m runners	Poorer times over 200 and 400 m track events	Faye et al. [30]
10 assorted power athletes	No change of anaerobic capacity on Wingate test	Karli et al. [39]
Adolescent soccer players	Increased fatigue over six sprints	Meckel et al. [52]
12 physical education students	Increased fatigue on Wingate test during Ramadan	Souissi et al. [69]
55 free-living soccer players	Decrease of sprint speed during Ramadan, particularly in events of >15 seconds duration	Zerguini et al. [74]
64 soccer players living in controlled environment	Sprint speed unchanged during Ramadan	Zerguini et al. [75]

of anaerobic capacity in a group of athletes who controlled their lifestyle carefully during Ramadan observance.

Likewise, Chaouachi et al. [18] found that Ramadan fasting had little effect on 30 m sprint performance in elite Judokas, particularly if training load and food intake were well controlled. Nevertheless, this group of athletes showed a reduction in the average power during a 30-second repeated jump test when values from the end of Ramadan were compared with control data, and this impairment was associated with an increase in total fatigue scores. Zerguini et al. [74] observed decreases in speed, agility and dribbling speed during Ramadan in young soccer players. They concluded that the phase shift associated with Ramadan observance had a larger impact upon anaerobic capacity test scores than upon anaerobic power, and they saw associated increases in ratings of perceived exertion and fatigue with the intermittent fasting. As in the studies of Karli et al. [39] and Chaouachi et al. [18], these decrements of performance were not seen in a second group of soccer players who observed Ramadan while living in a well-controlled environment. Scores on the Wingate test are susceptible to circadian rhythms of muscular performance, and Chtourou et al. [24] suggested that in an uncontrolled environment, the sleep disturbances associated with Ramadan might have modified the circadian rhythm and thus affected muscle power and fatigue scores.

Repetition of testing seems particularly likely to bring out the adverse effects of Ramadan. Thus, Meckel et al. [52] found a reduction of running speed during Ramadan when young soccer players repeated 40 m sprints six times. Aziz et al. [2] also found a poorer response during repeated sprinting efforts.

In terms of anaerobic performance on the sports field, Faye et al. [30] showed reductions in the 200 and 400 m run performances during Ramadan. They attributed this to poor glycolytic function and recommended countering the loss of performance by adopting a high-carbohydrate diet during the hours of darkness.

Aerobic Performance

Aerobic Power

Maximal aerobic power is the largest oxygen intake that the body can develop during an effort of a few minutes duration, and it is important to performance in events such as a 1.5 or 5 km run. It reflects mainly the maximal pumping ability of the heart and is particularly vulnerable to changes of circulating blood volume and thus dehydration, whether this develops over a single day or cumulatively over the month of Ramadan observance. Maximal aerobic power can be expressed in absolute units, measured in L/min, but it is often expressed in mL/(kg·min); in the latter case, the reported value is influenced not only by cardiac function but also by any loss of body mass caused by fasting or dehydration. Laboratory measurements of maximal aerobic power or the corresponding running velocity are usually based on some 10 minutes of maximal exercise on a cycle ergometer or a treadmill, and scores are thus susceptible to any reduction of motivation that may occur during Ramadan. Unfortunately, not all investigators have indicated their criteria for determination of a plateauing of oxygen consumption, nor have they provided measures of the quality of maximal effort elicited, such as peak heart rate, peak respiratory gas-exchange ratio and blood lactate levels.

Eight of sixteen studies found no deterioration in the directly measured or estimated maximal oxygen intake during Ramadan (Table 9.3), and in one other report [29], a decrease of maximal heart rate suggested that there had been a decrease in motivation to all-out effort. Two other studies found an initial decrease of maximal aerobic power, but recovery as Ramadan continued [70,74]; it is unclear whether this reflected a physiological adaptation [70], a reduction of resting oxygen consumption, or a better organization of lifestyle as the intermittent fasting continued. One report noted the absence of the usual circadian increase of aerobic power during the afternoons of Ramadan [34], but morning values remained unchanged, emphasizing the importance of the timing of observations.

Maximal Oxygen Intake

The maximal oxygen intake is a standard laboratory measure of aerobic performance. It depends on a person's ability to transport oxygen from the atmosphere to the working tissues. Values (expressed per unit of body mass) can vary from 90 mL/(kg·minutes) in a very fit cross-country skier to 30 mL/(kg·minutes) in a sedentary older adult. In a moderately fit person, the maximal oxygen intake is limited by the pumping ability of the heart; values are reduced by administering a beta-blocking drug, which limits the maximal heart rate and thus the maximal cardiac output. In very fit athletes, the respiratory system may also impose some limitation; in such individuals, haemoglobin does not become fully oxygenated as the red cells pass through the lungs. Possibly, a reduction in sensitivity of arterial chemoreceptors leads to an inadequate compensatory increase in ventilation at peak effort [26], and/or the rapid speed of blood flow through the lungs may allow insufficient time for oxygen to diffuse from the lungs into the blood stream. In sedentary individuals, muscle weakness may become a dominant factor, and in this situation, the maximal oxygen intake is unaffected by the administration of beta-blocking drugs.

Brisswalter et al. [16] observed a 5% decrease in 3000 m track performance at the end of Ramadan, although they saw no change in either the maximal oxygen intake or maximal aerobic velocity of 18 middle-distance runners. In one of the other studies with an adverse effect [21], there were substantial decreases of sleep times and energy intake, and increased fatigue scores, and it seems possible that performance could have been maintained if there had been a better regulation of personal lifestyle; the authors of this report recommended daytime napping or a reduction of training loads during Ramadan.

Aerobic Capacity

A person's aerobic capacity reflects the ability to sustain an oxygen transport close to the individual's maximal oxygen intake over a long period, as in a marathon run or in the repeated runs of a typical team game. This can be assessed quite easily as the distance run or cycled in 60 or 90 minutes and is a variable vulnerable to both a low initial muscle glycogen and decreased motivation. Another measure of the tolerance of near-maximal effort is the individual's anaerobic threshold.

Among empirical observations (Table 9.3), Zerguini et al. [74] found that the endurance capacity and agility of 55 free-living Algerian professional soccer players were significantly reduced by the end of Ramadan; most of these players reported reductions in sleep quality and a sensation of poorer physical performance. The authors concluded that disturbances of mood and motivation were likely responsible for at least part of the reduction in physical performance that was seen. In contrast, Kirkendall et al. [41] found unchanged speed, power, agility, endurance, passing and dribbling skills in a group of 45 soccer players. Likewise, two studies of sedentary subjects reported no adverse effect of Ramadan observance upon submaximal aerobic performance [59,60].

Bouhlel et al. [12] noted that whereas the first ventilatory threshold (V_{T1}) was unchanged during Ramadan, the second ventilatory threshold (V_{T2}) occurred at a lower than normal intensity of effort. This suggests that anaerobic processes may have made a larger contribution to the energy supply during fasting, as would be

TABLE 9.3 Effects of Ramadan Observance upon Aerobic Power and Capacity

Subjects	Performance Change	Authors
Aerobic Power		
10 healthy subjects	Unchanged maximal oxygen intake	Aziz et al. [4]
9 well-trained middle-distance runners, 9 controls	No change on maximal oxygen intake or running efficiency on treadmill; 5% increase of 5000 m run times	Brisswalter et al. [16]
9 trained karatekas	No change in maximal oxygen intake or maximal power output on cycle ergometer	Bouhlel et al. [12,14]
Review article; fasts of varying length, mainly involving non-athletes, but also 15 judokas	Little change of multistage shuttle-run score	Chaouachi et al. [19]
8 middle-distance athletes	Decrease of maximal aerobic velocity at days 7 and 21 of Ramadan observance	Chennaoui et al. [21]
30 junior soccer players	No change of Léger shuttle run score or endurance at 85% of maximal oxygen intake during Ramadan	Chiha [22]
12 junior level soccer players	Decrease of aerobic performance during the Yo-Yo intermittent running test	Chtourou et al. [23]
12 young trained men	Decrease of maximal aerobic power and maximal heart rate during Ramadan	Fall et al. [29]
16 male soccer players	Peak velocity, distance and time in shuttle run unchanged	Güvenç [34]
10 junior soccer players	Decrease of performance of Yo-Yo intermittent shuttle running test during Ramadan	Hamouda et al. [35]
53 junior soccer players	No effect on multistage shuttle run performance during Ramadan	Kirkendall et al. [41]
19 junior soccer players	0.9% increase of time over 3000 m run	Meckel et al. [52]
10 male distance runners	No change of maximal oxygen intake, small increase of endurance effort during Ramadan	Mehdioui et al. [54]
14 male collegiate wrestlers	Decrease of maximal aerobic power in the fourth week of Ramadan	Mirzaei et al. [55]
14–16-year-old soccer players	Decrease of maximal oxygen intake in the first week of Ramadan, but subsequent recovery	Sweileh et al. [70]
48 professional soccer players	16% decrease in distance run during 12 minutes at start of Ramadan, partial recovery after 2 weeks	Zerguini et al. [74]

(*Continued*)

TABLE 9.3 (*Continued*) Effects of Ramadan Observance upon Aerobic Power and Capacity

Subjects	Performance Change	Authors
Aerobic Capacity		
10 moderately trained runners	60 minutes of endurance running: shorter distance covered during Ramadan, with slowing mainly in later phases of run	Aziz et al. [2]
9 karatekas	Second ventilatory threshold at lower intensity of exercise	Bouhlel et al. [12]
53 junior soccer players	No deterioration of speed, power, agility, endurance, passing and dribbling skills	Kirkendall et al. [41]
6 active, 7 sedentary men	No significant change	Ramadan [59]
18 sedentary men	No significant change	Ramadan and Barac-Nieto [60]
15 endurance runners	Small decrease of endurance in 90 minutes test	Shaygun Asl [66]
411 male, 323 female junior athletes	24% of subjects perceived decrease of sports performance across all types of sport	Singh et al. [68]
55 free-living professional soccer Players	Reduction of endurance capacity and agility despite unchanged explosive power of leg muscles	Zerguini et al. [75]

anticipated if the maximal cardiac output and thus muscle oxygen supply had been reduced by dehydration. A more rapid buildup of lactate could impair prolonged aerobic effort during Ramadan observance. Gutierrez et al. [33] hypothesized that a longer period of fasting (3 days) also modified fibre recruitment patterns during high-intensity exercise; such a change would cause an earlier glycogen depletion of type I (slow twitch) muscle fibres, an earlier recruitment of type II (fast twitch) fibres, and in consequence a greater activation of anaerobic processes during exercise.

Muscular Strength and Endurance

Muscular strength can be estimated either from simple field tests such as jump height (where the performance of a fasting person could show an apparent improvement due to a decrease in body mass) or in the laboratory, using such devices as dynamometers and force platforms. Strength could be impaired during Ramadan because of poor motivation, less effective coordination of motor units, changes in fibre recruitment patterns [33] and dehydration. As intermittent fasting continues, additional effects could arise from a progressive loss of lean tissue and a reduction in training loads. Repeated muscular efforts and sustained contractions are also compromised because of a low initial store of glycogen.

Other potential influences are changes in meal times and food habits, hormonal changes associated with dehydration [50,60], and disturbed sleep patterns and circadian rhythms [52].

Muscle Strength

If hydration and training are maintained during Ramadan, changes in muscle strength seem relatively small (Table 9.4). The extent of change observed seems to depend on the duration of exercise and the muscle mass involved [11,18,52].

Bigard et al. [9] saw a 10%–12% reduction of maximal voluntary force in the elbow flexor muscles of fighter pilots during Ramadan observance. Brisswalter et al. [16] found smaller decrease in the maximal voluntary contraction (MVC) of middle-distance runners (3.2%), associated with a 5% decrease in their 3000 m

TABLE 9.4 Effects of Ramadan Observance on Muscular Strength, Endurance, and Agility

Sample	Effect of Ramadan	Authors
Muscle Strength		
11 male fighter pilots	Maximum isometric force of elbow flexors reduced 10%–12%	Bigard et al. [9]
10 trained men	No effect on handgrip force. Initial decrease of vertical jump height and 5 jump test, but recovery over course of Ramadan	Bouhlel et al. [11]
9 well-trained middle-distance runners, 9 controls	3.2% decrease of maximal voluntary contraction force of knee extensors	Brisswalter et al. [16]
15 young national-level judokas	No change of standing jump or counter-movement jump, but slight (4%) decrease of power during 30 seconds repeated jump test	Chaouachi et al. [18]
53 junior soccer players	Decrease of vertical jump, especially in the afternoon	Kirkendall et al. [41]
34 elite athletes (volleyball, karate, taekwondo and soccer)	No change of explosive strength	Kordi et al. [42]
19 junior soccer players	1.8% decrease of vertical jump performance	Meckel et al. [52]
12 female athletes	No change of vertical jump or balance	Memari et al. [53]
Muscle Endurance		
11 male fighter pilots	Maximum isometric force of elbow flexors reduced 10%–12%	Bigard et al. [9]
Agility		
53 junior soccer players	Dribbling and passing skills unaffected	Kirkendall et al. [41]
34 elite athletes	No effect on agility	Kordi et al. [42]
19 junior soccer players	No effect on agility	Meckel et al. [52]
12 female athletes	No change of balance but decrease of agility	Memari et al. [53]

run performance. The latter authors suggested that decreased motivation might account for the strength impairments that they saw. Maximal handgrip force was unaffected either during Ramadan observance [11] or in longer periods of fasting [33]. In terms of jump height, some authors have found no change [18,42,53], but others have reported decreases [41,52].

Muscular Strength

Gains of muscular strength achieved by a power athlete reflect two main types of adaptation: morphological and neural. There are two main mechanisms of morphological adaptation: hypertrophy and hyperplasia. Hypertrophy is due to an increase in the diameter of existing muscle fibres (with an increase in their content of contractile proteins). Hyperplasia is a proliferation of fibres through activation of 'satellite cells'; this increases the number of myofibrillar units within a given muscle [31]. The extent of hyperplasia remains a somewhat controversial topic, although this mechanism of hypertrophy has been observed in adults [7,38]. Strength training also induces modifications in the structure of the heavy myosin chain, and there are changes in muscle fibre type (particularly increases in fast twitch IIa fibres and decreases in intermediate type IIx fibres [17,36]). These changes are associated with increases of tendon stiffness [44], reducing the electromechanical delay between the nerve impulse and contraction, and in consequence increasing force production. As the number of fibres increases, there are also increases of the pennation angle (the angle of insertion of fibres into the muscle tendon) and the cross-sectional area of the muscle, further contributing to the increase in strength [5,62].

Neural adaptations (more effective muscle coordination and recruitment patterns) also play a major role in increasing muscle force production following a period of strength training. Optimal force production requires not only an increased activation of the muscle directly involved (the agonist), but also a parallel decrease in activation of its antagonists [43,57,61].

Mechanisms that could explain decreases of force production during Ramadan observance remain unclear. The duration of a given effort and the need to repeat it may play critical roles, but participant motivation is also likely to be important. Muscle fatigue is usually specific to the activity that has been performed. The relative importance of central versus peripheral mechanisms remains to be clarified.

Muscular Endurance

The only examination of muscular endurance during Ramadan seems that of Bigard et al. [9]; they found a lesser ability to sustain contractions at both 35% and 70% of maximal voluntary force, with endurance reduced by 28% and 22%, respectively, at the end of Ramadan.

Agility

Three studies found no change of agility during Ramadan [41,42,52]. A group of female athletes (Memari et al. [53]) also showed no change of balance, but there was a decrease of agility in this sample.

In general, it seems that during Ramadan observance, muscle force and power are maintained for short efforts, but performance is impaired if a prolonged or repeated contraction is required.

Psychomotor Performance

Cognitive function plays a major role in sports. It enables the athlete to minimize learning times, develop skills, interact appropriately with other team members and avoid physical injuries. The results of psychomotor tests depend on many factors. The delivery of oxygen and metabolites to the brain can be compromised by reductions of cardiac output and blood glucose. But there can also be adverse effects from loss of sleep, shifts of circadian rhythm and impaired motivation, particularly in tasks requiring vigilance and rapid reactions. Dehydration can also affect cognitive function through (1) alterations of cerebral neurotransmission due to hyperosmolarity and electrolyte shifts; (2) changes in blood–brain barrier permeability; (3) alterations in the activity of nitric oxide synthase, a key enzyme facilitating learning and memory; (4) changes in central dopaminergic and noradrenergic pathways; (5) reductions in activity of the reticular activating system and the autonomic nervous system; and (6) alteration of the cortical and/or subcortical structures responsible for memory and perception [49].

Glucose is the most important substrate for brain metabolism, and glucose consumption is increased during cognitive tasks. Any deterioration of cognitive function could thus be related to the reduction of blood glucose observed at the end of a day of fasting. In keeping with this hypothesis, the adverse effects of Ramadan upon psychomotor performance are greater during afternoons than mornings [71]. In the study just cited, afternoon capillary glucose readings dropped to an average of 4.6 mmol/L (as compared with 5.4 mmol/L at the same time of day before Ramadan). However, sleep patterns were also disturbed; night-time sleep was shortened from 7.0 to 5.3 hours, and subjects took a compensatory 3 hours daytime nap.

It remains puzzling why the effects of Ramadan seem to depend on the task that is performed. Time (attention and information processing) and spatially-dependent tasks (non-verbal recognition, memory, problem solving, verbal naming and visual–spatial skills) seem particularly prone to deteriorate during Ramadan observance.

Empirical studies of changes in psychomotor function during Ramadan are relatively few (Table 9.4). In reviewing these findings, it is important to remember that laboratory test scores do not necessarily reflect the psychomotor performance that will be achieved during training or competition.

Cognition and Reaction Times

In general, cognition and reaction times have remained unchanged during the mornings of Ramadan, but impairments have been seen during the afternoons. Tian et al. [71] found a temporal and functional variability in the deterioration of memory, with a reduction in verbal learning and memory at 16 hours, but no change in visual learning and working memory at this time of day. Cognitive tests requiring sustained (Table 9.5) rapid responses were performed better in the morning than in the late afternoon, whereas performance of measures that were not speed dependent remained unchanged. Hakkou et al. [37] also noted a deterioration of memory during Ramadan, and others reported slowed reaction times [13,14,26,47,63].

Lofti et al. [47] reported no change of physical performance in a group of resistance athletes during Ramadan. They did see deterioration in both recognition and total reaction times, but motor performance time was unchanged, particularly during the first week of fasting. In this study, the subjects had napped for much of the morning, and tests were performed after about 8 hours of fasting.

Gutierrez et al. [33] found no fasting-related changes in perception–reaction time following a longer (3 day) fast, despite a significant decrease in the serum glucose concentrations in their group of 8 male athletes.

Vigilance

Almost all reports have noted increased sleepiness, with a decreased alertness and concentration and (with one exception, Lofti et al. [47]) a decreased flicker fusion frequency during Ramadan observance. However, it remains unclear how far these changes were due to fasting and how far they reflected disturbances of sleep patterns that were an incidental consequence of Ramadan.

Mood State

The mood state of athletes has commonly been assessed using a simple questionnaire known as the profile of mood states. Most studies except that of Aziz et al. [3] have reported a change in one of the indices derived from this questionnaire, usually an increase in the fatigue score [18,21,23], during Ramadan. A deterioration of mood state plainly could have an adverse effect upon other areas of cognitive function.

Several investigators have used a simple 6–20 rating of perceived effort [10] to assess possible changes in an athlete's perception of the intensity of exercise during Ramadan. Most studies have found unchanged ratings of effort [3,46,75].

Cognitive Function during Exercise

Exercise in itself modifies cognitive function. There have been few assessments of how cerebral function during and immediately following fasting is altered by a bout of exercise [47], but this is an interesting question. Performance may be maintained,

TABLE 9.5 Effects of Ramadan Observance on Cognition, Vigilance and Mood State

Sample	Effect of Ramadan	Author
Cognition and Reaction Times		
10 karatekas	Impairment of simple reaction time at rest and after maximal exercise during Ramadan. No effect of Ramadan observance upon choice reaction time	Bouhlel et al. [13]
Information not available	Slowed reaction time to auditory stimulus	Dolu et al. [27]
Information not available	Impaired memory	Hakkou et al. [37]
9 healthy males	No change of memory between before and after exercise values during Ramadan. Slowing of recognition and total reaction time	Lofti et al. [47]
10 healthy young subjects	Increase of movement reaction times at the beginning of Ramadan	Roky et al. [63]
18 male athletes	Decreased learning and verbal memory in afternoon	Tian et al. [71]
Vigilance		
20 men and 20 women	Decrease of perceptual sensitivity; decreased flicker fusion frequency	Ali and Amir [6]
18 soccer players	Decrease of alertness and concentration	Aziz et al. [3]
Information not available	Decrease of both reaction amplitude and continuous attention	Dolu et al. [27]
Information not available	Decreased functional attention	El Moutawakil et al. [28]
9 healthy males	No change of flicker fusion frequency	Lofti et al. [47]
10 healthy young subjects	Decreased subjective alertness during Ramadan. Decreased flicker fusion frequency	Roky et al. [63]
8 healthy young males	Decrease in daytime alertness at 12:00 at the beginning of Ramadan, but no change by the end of Ramadan	Roky et al. [64]
Review	Decrease of daytime alertness and psychomotor performance	Roky et al. [65]
Mood State and Perception of Exertion		
18 soccer players (fasting group = 10, non-fasting group = 8)	No change of mood profile or perception of exertion	Aziz et al. [3]
15 judokas	Increase of fatigue score on profile of mood states	Chaouachi et al. [18]
8 middle-distance athletes	Increase of fatigue score as estimated by the profile of mood states questionnaire at the end of Ramadan	Chennaoui et al. [21]

(*Continued*)

TABLE 9.5 (*Continued*) Effects of Ramadan Observance on Cognition, Vigilance and Mood State

Sample	Effect of Ramadan	Author
12 junior male soccer players	Increases of rating of perceived exertion (RPE) scores and fatigue score estimated by the profile of mood state questionnaire during Ramadan	Chtourou et al. [23]
87 soccer players (54 fasting players, 33 non-fasting)	No change in perceived effort during training in the group observing Ramadan	Leiper et al. [46]
10 healthy young subjects	Impairment of mood state	Roky et al. [63]
8 healthy young males	Impairment of subjective mood state at 16:00 h, both at the beginning and the end of Ramadan	Roky et al. [64]
734 (411 male and 323 female) Malaysian junior-level Muslim athletes (mean age 16.3 ± 2.6 year)	24% of the athletes perceived that there was an adverse effect of Ramadan observance upon sport performance	Singh et al. [68]
64 soccer players living in a controlled environment	No change in perception of exertion	Zerguini et al. [75]

enhanced or impaired, depending on the duration of fasting, the environmental conditions (particularly temperature and humidity), the time when performance is measured, the intensity and/or the duration of the exercise [15], the physical fitness level of the participant [56], the type of cognitive task that is selected, and the type of exercise that is performed [45]. If poor psychomotor function is due to a loss of sleep, then it may be helped by the arousing effect of physical activity. On the other hand, if it reflects a low blood glucose and/or dehydration and an impaired cerebral blood flow, this is likely to be made worse by physical activity.

Reaction times tend to be maintained following exercise, probably because of concomitant increases in blood catecholamine levels [25,32]. The hormonal response to exercise could play a pivotal role in countering the adverse effects of fasting upon cognitive function. Pivik and Dykman [58] also hypothesized a neuronal influence, involving the activity of occipital cortex, although they did not observe any change of alpha frequency in the occipital cortex, which is the primary area of the brain associated with the visual processing and integration involved in a choice reaction time test. Maughan and Shirreffs [51] underlined the importance of hydration to cognitive performance. They argued that a 1%–2% decrease in body mass could indicate sufficient fluid loss to impair cerebral function. It is uncertain how often such dehydration arises over the day during Ramadan; such fluid deficits seem probable in athletes who are undertaking prolonged bouts of exercise (greater than 1 hour) under hot and humid conditions, or who are engaging in repeated exercise (whether in competition or in training sessions).

Bouhlel et al. [13] found that a short bout of maximal cycle ergometer exercise in itself had no effect on simple reaction time (SRT) or choice reaction time (CRT). However, Ramadan observance slowed SRT both at rest and after exercise. Surprisingly, they saw no significant effects of Ramadan observance on a choice reaction time task that involved identification of four white squares and one black square, located at differing positions on a computer screen, and making an appropriate decision (pressing an appropriate key to indicate the location of the black square).

Areas Requiring Further Research

Any effects of Ramadan observance upon physical performance are quite slight, and the precision of many laboratory measurements is insufficient to detect changes that nevertheless could make the difference between a gold medal and an unplaced performance. There is a need for more epidemiological research, particularly a careful comparison of competitive performance between athletes who are observing Ramadan and those who are not. It may be possible to make these comparisons both during Ramadan and at other times of the year. It is also far from clear in those cases where performance appears to have deteriorated, if training was well maintained, and whether all permissible remedies to minimize disturbances of sleep, blood glucose levels and hydration were followed. Finally, there is need to include the issues of altered motivation and displaced circadian rhythms as covariates in future research. If indeed a measurable decrease in performance during Ramadan is confirmed, then the main causes need to be pinpointed through detailed studies of fluid balance and muscle glycogen stores, and further practical measures must be developed to minimize such changes.

Practical Applications

Current scientific evidence suggests that not only sustained fasting and/or major dehydration, but also the brief intermittent fasting of Ramadan can lead to decrements in both physical and psychomotor performance. The changes are relatively small in both absolute and percentage terms and, sometimes are at the limit of detection with the tools available to the exercise scientist. Nevertheless, they are sufficient in magnitude to cause a considerable deterioration of placing in athletic competitions. Often, decrements of performance seem at least in part an incidental consequence of Ramadan observance, due to a reduction in training, disruption of timing of meals and sleep, and impaired motivation, and it is possible to find examples of athletes whose performance has remained unchanged in most types of competition. This should encourage other athletes to emulate such achievements by maintaining motivation and training and adopting all permitted adaptations of lifestyle to accommodate the constraints inherent in Ramadan.

Conclusions

Ramadan observance seems to lead to small decrements in both physical and psychomotor performance, more marked with sustained or repeated effort using a large muscle mass that challenges glycogen and fluid reserves than with brief activities that involve smaller muscle groups. There are many potential extraneous causes of impairment—a decrease in training schedules, disturbances of sleep, displacement of circadian rhythms, and above all a depression of mood and a loss of motivation. There remains a need for further research to distinguish extraneous influences from the unavoidable consequences of Ramadan observance. Nevertheless, the fact that the effects of the intermittent fast are more marked in the afternoon than in the morning tend to point to cumulative effects of glycogen depletion and/or dehydration. Athletes and their coaches should thus undertake all possible measures to avoid disruption of lifestyle and maximize night-time intake of foodstuffs and fluids. A few studies where normal performance has been maintained suggest that with appropriate planning, competitors can overcome both the effects of food and fluid restrictions and the incidental disturbances associated with the celebration of Ramadan by maintaining a normal training regimen and maximizing personal fitness level.

Key Terms

Anaerobic power: The peak anaerobic power is usually defined as the peak power output observed during performance of an all-out test (typically seen during the first 5 seconds of a force–velocity test or an all-out Wingate cycle ergometer test). The mean anaerobic power or anaerobic capacity is the average of the power output maintained over the 30 seconds of an all-out Wingate test. The fatigue index is the difference between the peak power and the minimum power observed during the Wingate test.

Alertness: Alertness in the context of this text is the fully attentive state for a given task, the ability to perceive and to act as quickly as possible.

Arousal: Arousal is a state of cerebral activation with rapid perception, a high level of cognition, and treatment of information with an adequate and rapid motor response.

Cognition: Cognition involves the mental processes related to the acquisition, storage and use of knowledge, including the functions of memory, attention, perception, information treatment and decision making.

Dehydration: Dehydration reflects a sufficient loss of body water to have an adverse effect upon metabolic reactions and performance, probably at least 1–2 L.

Force–velocity test: The force–velocity test was developed by Henry Vandewalle et al. [72]. During this test, the subject completes six to eight short (about 7 seconds) all-out sprints on a cycle ergometer, using braking forces that are selected relative to the individual's body mass.

Each repetition is separated by 5 minutes of passive recovery. The instantaneous peak velocity is used to calculate the maximal power output at each of the selected braking forces. Maximal anaerobic power is defined as the highest power calculated for the different braking forces.

Handgrip strength: The handgrip strength is assessed using a small dynamometer that the subject grips as strongly as possible after being allowed several practice attempts to master technique.

Maximal aerobic power or maximal oxygen intake: This represents the peak oxygen consumption of an individual. It is usually measured by a cycle ergometer or treadmill test of progressively increasing intensity, carried out over a period of 8–12 minutes, until a plateau of oxygen consumption is reached. This plateau is arbitrarily defined as an increase in oxygen consumption of less than 2 mL/(kg minutes) with a further increase in the individual's rate of working. Other evidence of a well-motivated effort include a heart rate close to the age-related maximum value, a respiratory gas exchange ratio >1.1, and an arterial blood lactate >10 mmol/L.

Maximum voluntary contraction: The MVC is the peak force developed by an individual during the isometric contraction of a specific muscle group.

Mechanical efficiency: The mechanical efficiency is the ratio of power output to energy consumed during a task such as riding a cycle ergometer. It may be expressed as a gross efficiency or a net efficiency (the latter taking account of the individual's resting energy expenditure).

Memory: Memory reflects the mental ability to retain or to recall past experience, for example verbal memory.

Mood: Mood refers to the emotional state of a subject; it is commonly measured by the profile of mood states questionnaire, which evaluates the individual's experience over the immediately preceding 7 days.

Muscular endurance: Muscular endurance is the ability to sustain the contraction of a given muscle or group of muscles at a specified fraction of maximal force.

Reaction time: The reaction time is the time taken by a subject to react to a given stimulus. In the case of a physical response, it includes response time (the interval needed to initiate a movement) and the movement time (the time to complete the movement).

Sleeping: Sleeping is associated with a general relaxation of the body and a reduction of energy expenditures. A full analysis of sleep includes not only its duration but also its latency, quality and depth.

Ventilatory thresholds: The first ventilatory threshold (VT_1) is the point during a progressive exercise test where the ventilation begins to increase in a non-linear fashion relative to oxygen consumption, but still bears a consistent relationship to carbon dioxide output. The second ventilatory threshold (VT_2) is the point at which there is also an excessive increase in carbon dioxide output relative to ventilatory minute volume.

Wingate test: The Wingate test is an all-out cycle ergometer test of 30 seconds duration. It permits the estimation of anaerobic power and capacity.

Yo-yo intermittent run test: This test is a progressive shuttle run that incorporates a brief recovery period after each of a series of 40 m runs (2 × 20 m). The subject runs at a progressively increasing speed, as imposed by a beep. The test is halted when the subject is unable to follow the imposed rhythm. The test assesses the maximal aerobic velocity and permits an approximate estimation of the individual's maximal oxygen intake.

Key Points

1. Ramadan observance has little or no effect on brief, anaerobic performance, such as jumping, handgrip force or dribbling a ball, but some reduction in maximal anaerobic capacity is commonly seen, particularly if the test measurement is repeated.
2. Ramadan observance also has very little impact on maximal aerobic power. The detrimental effect of fasting is observed mainly if high rates of oxygen consumption are sustained over very prolonged or repeated bouts of exercise.
3. Ramadan observance has only small effects on the MVC force of the muscles, although the ability to sustain a vigorous submaximal contraction may be reduced.
4. Ramadan fasting commonly has some negative effects on cognitive function, vigilance, reaction times, mood state and perceptions of effort, although the response varies, depending upon the type of cognitive function that is examined.
5. Vigorous exercise can combat some of the negative effects of Ramadan observance upon cognitive function, probably by increasing blood levels of catecholamine and having a general arousing effect.
6. At least a part of the adverse effect upon other aspects of performance can be countered by appropriate pre-fast training, maintenance of a normal conditioning programme, and an optimization of lifestyle during Ramadan.

Questions for Discussion

1. What factors are likely to cause a decrease of aerobic capacity during Ramadan?
2. What mechanisms may impair cognitive performance during Ramadan?
3. What suggestions do you have for countering the adverse effects of Ramadan observance upon physical and cognitive performance?

References

1. Andersen LK. Energy cost of swimming. *Acta Chir Scand* 1960 Suppl 253:1–169.
2. Aziz AR, Wahid MF, Png W et al. Effects of Ramadan fasting on 60 min of endurance running performance in moderately trained men. *Br J Sports Med* 2010;44:516–521.
3. Aziz AR, Chia M, Singh R, Wahid MF. Effects of Ramadan fasting on perceived exercise intensity during high-intensity interval training sessions in elite youth soccer players. *Int J Sports Sci Coach* 2011;6:87–98.
4. Aziz AR, Slater GJ, Chiac MY et al. Effects of Ramadan fasting on training induced adaptations to a seven-week high-intensity interval exercise programme (Effets du jeûne du Ramadan sur les adaptations induites par un programme de sept semaines d'entraînement à haute intensité par intervalles). *Sci Sports* 2012;27:31–38.
5. Aagaard P, Andersen JL, Dyhre-Poulsen P et al. A mechanism for increased contractile strength of human pennate muscle in response to strength training: Changes in muscle architecture. *J Physiol* 2001 Jul 15;534(Pt. 2):613–623.
6. Ali MR, Amir T. Effects of fasting on visual flicker fusion. *Perceptual Motor Skills* 1989;69:627–631.
7. Appell HJ. Muscular atrophy following immobilization. A review. *Sports Med* 1990; 10:42–58.
8. Bar-Or O. The Wingate anaerobic test. An update on methodology, reliability and validity. *Sports Med* 1987 November–Dec;4(6):381–394.
9. Bigard AX, Boussif M, Chalabi H, Guezennec CY. Alterations in muscular performance and orthostatic tolerance during Ramadan. *Aviat Space Environ Med* 1998;69:341–346.
10. Borg G. The perception of physical performance. In: Shephard RJ (ed.), *Frontiers of Fitness*. C.C. Thomas, Springfield, IL, 1971, pp. 280–294.
11. Bouhlel H, Shephard RJ, Gmada N et al. Effect of Ramadan observance on maximal muscular performance of trained men. *Clin J Sport Med* 2013;23(3):222–227.
12. Bouhlel H, Shephard RJ, Adela H et al. Ramadan observance and aerobic exercise in male Karetakas. *Health Fitness J Can* 2013;6(4):99–107.
13. Bouhlel H, Latiri I, Zarrouk N et al. Effet du jeûne du Ramadan et de l'exercice maximal sur le temps de réaction simple et de choix chez des sujets entraînés (Effect of Ramadan observance and maximal exercise on simple and choice reaction times in trained men). *Sci Sports* 2014;39(3):131–137.
14. Bouhlel H. *Effet du jeûne du Ramadan sur le métabolisme et la performance physique chez le sujet entraîné*. 2014, Thèse de Doctorat en Biologie, mention physiologie de l'exercice musculaire. Faculté des Sciences de Bizerte, Université de Carthage.
15. Brisswalter J, Collardeau M, René A. Effects of acute physical exercise characteristics on cognitive performance. *Sports Med* 2002;32(9):555–566.
16. Brisswalter J, Bouhlel E, Falola JM, Abbiss CR, Vallier JM, Hauswirth C. Effects of Ramadan intermittent fasting on middle-distance running performance in well-trained runners. *Clin J Sport Med* 2011;21:422–427.
17. Campos GE, Luecke TJ, Wendeln HK et al. Muscular adaptations in response to three different resistance-training regimens: Specificity of repetition maximum training zones. *Eur J Appl Physiol* 2002 Nov;88(1–2):50–60.
18. Chaouachi A, Coutts AJ, Chamari K et al. Effect of Ramadan intermittent fasting on aerobic and anaerobic performance and perception of fatigue in male elite judo athletes. *J Strength Cond Res* 2009;23(9):2702–2709.
19. Chaouachi A, Leiper JB, Souissi N et al. Effects of Ramadan intermittent fasting on sports performance and training: A review. *Int J Sports Physiol Perform* 2009;4:419–434.
20. Chaouachi A, Leiper JB, Chtourou H et al. The effects of Ramadan intermittent fasting on athletic performance: Recommendations for the maintenance of physical fitness. *J Sports Sci* 2012;30(Suppl. 1):S53–S73.

21. Chennaoui M, Desgorces F, Drogou C et al. Effects of Ramadan fasting on physical performance and metabolic, hormonal, and inflammatory parameters in middle-distance runners. *Appl Physiol Nutr Metab* 2009;34:587–594.

22. Chiha F. Changes in metabolism and the energetics of exercise in footballers during Ramadan fasting (in French). Thesis of the University of Constantine, 2008.

23. Chtourou H, Hammouda O, Souissi H et al. The effect of Ramadan fasting on physical performances, mood state and perceived exertion in young footballers. *Asian J Sports Med* 2011;2:177–185.

24. Chtourou H, Hammouda O, Chaouachi A et al. The effect of time of day and Ramadan fasting on anaerobic performances. *Int J Sports Med* 2012;33:142–147.

25. Chmura J, Nazar K, Kaciuba-Uściłko H. Choice reaction time during graded exercise in relation to blood lactate and plasma catecholamine thresholds. *Int J Sports Med* 1994;15(4):172–176.

26. Dempsey JA. JB. Wolffe memorial lecture. Is the lung built for exercise? *Med Sci Sports Exerc* 1986 Apr;18(2):143–155.

27. Dolu N, Yüksek A, Sizer A, Alay M. Arousal and continuous attention during Ramadan intermittent fasting. *J Basic Clin Physiol Pharmacol* 2007;18(4):315–322.

28. El Moutawakil B, Hassounr S, Sibai M et al. Effect of Ramadan fasting upon functions of attention (in French). *Rev Neurol* 2007;163(Suppl. 4):60.

29. Fall A, Sarr M, Mandengue S-H et al. Effets d'une restriction hydrique et alimentaire prolongée (Ramadan) sur la performance et les réponses cardiovasculaires au cours d'in exercice incrémental en milieu tropical chaud. *Sci Sports* 2007;22:50–53.

30. Faye J, Fall A, Badji L et al. Effets du jeûne du ramadan sur le poids, la performance et de la glycémie lors de l'entraînement à la résistance (Effects of Ramadan fasting on weight, performance and glycemia during training for resistance). *Dakar Med* 2005; 50:146–151.

31. Folland JP, Williams AG. The adaptations to strength training: Morphological and neurological contributions to increased strength. *Sports Med* 2007;37(2):145–168.

32. Grego F, Vallier J-M, Collardeau M et al. Effects of long duration exercise on cognitive function, blood glucose, and counterregulatory hormones in male cyclists. *Neurosci Lett* 2004;364:76–80.

33. Gutierrez A, Gonzalez-Gross M, Delgado M, Castillo MJ. Three days fast in sportsmen decreases physical work capacity but not strength or perception-reaction time. *Int J Sport Nutr Exerc Metab* 2001;11(4):420–429.

34. Güvenç A. Effects of Ramadan fasting on body composition, aerobic performance and lactate, heart rate and perceptual responses in young soccer players. *J Hum Kinet* 2011;29:79–91.

35. Hamouda O, Chtourou, H, Farjallah MA et al. The effect of Ramadan fasting on the diurnal variations in aerobic and anaerobic performances in Tunisian youth soccer players. *Biol Rhythm Res* 2011;1:1–15.

36. Häkkinen K, Newton RU, Gordon SE et al. Changes in muscle morphology, electromyographic activity, and force production characteristics during progressive strength training in young and older men. *J Gerontol A Biol Sci Med Sci* 1998 Nov;53(6):B415–B423.

37. Hakkou F, Wast D, Jaouan C. Does Ramadan impair vigilance and memory? *Psychopharmacology* 1988;96:213.

38. Kadi F, Thornell LE. Concomitant increases in myonuclear and satellite cell content in female trapezius muscle following strength training. *Histochem Cell Biol* 2000 Feb;113(2):99–103.

39. Karli U, Guvenc A, Aslan A et al. Influence of Ramadan fasting on anaerobic performance and recovery following short time high intensity exercise. *J Sports Sci Med* 2007;6:490–497.

40. Khedder A, Achour N, Abou-Messad N et al. Comparative study of the adaptation of the body to cycle ergometry during and after Ramadan (in French). *Tunisie Med* 1983;57:16–17.

41. Kirkendall DT, Leiper JB, Bartagi Z et al. The influence of Ramadan on physical performance measures in young Muslim footballers. *J Sports Sci* 2008 Dec;26(Suppl. 3): S15–S27.
42. Kordi R, Abdullahi M, Memari M-H, Najafabadi MG. Investigating two different training time frames during Ramadan. *Asian J Sports Med* 2011;2:205–210.
43. Kraemer WJ, Fry AC, Frykman PN et al. Resistance training and Youth. *Pediatr Exerc Sci* 1989;1:336–350.
44. Kubo K, Kanehisa H, Fukunaga T. Effects of different duration isometric contractions on tendon elasticity in human quadriceps muscles. *J Physiol* 2001 Oct 15;536(Pt 2): 649–655.
45. Lambourne K, Tomporowski P. The effect of exercise-induced arousal on cognitive task performance: A meta-regression analysis. *Brain Res* 2010;23(1341):12–24.
46. Leiper JB, Watson P, Evans G, Dvorak J. Intensity of a training session during Ramadan in fasting and non-fasting Tunisian youth football players. *J Sports Sci* 2008;26:571–579.
47. Lofti S, Madani M, Abassi A et al. CNS activation, reaction time, blood pressure and heart rate variation during Ramadan intermittent fasting and exercise. *World J Sports Sci* 2010;3:37–43.
48. Margaria R. The sources of muscular energy. *Sci Am* 1972;226(3):84–91.
49. Maughan R. Physiology of sport. *Br J Hosp Med (Lond)* 2007 Jul;68(7):376–379.
50. Maughan RJ, Fallah J, Coyle EF. The effects of fasting on metabolism and performance. *Br J Sport Med* 2010;44:490–494.
51. Maughan RJ, Shirreffs SM. Hydration and performance during Ramadan. *J Sports Sci* 2012;30(Suppl. 1):S33–S41.
52. Meckel Y, Ismaeel A, Eliakim A. The effect of Ramadan fast on physical performance and dietary habits in adolescent soccer players. *Eur J Appl Physiol* 2008;102:651–657.
53. Memari A-H, Kordh R, Panahl N et al. Effect of Ramadan fasting on body composition and physical performance in female athletes. *Asian J of Sports Med* 2011;2:161–166.
54. Mehdioui H, Aberkane A, Bouroubi O et al. Influence de la pratique du jeûne Ramadan sur l'endurance maximale aérobie des coureurs de fond (Influence of Ramadan fasting on the maximal aerobic endurance of distance runners). *J Algér Méd* 1996;6(1).
55. Mirzaei B, Rahmani-Nia F, Moghadam MG et al. The effect of Ramadan fasting on biochemical and performance parameters in collegiate wrestlers. *Iran J Basic Med Sci* 2012 November;15(6):1215–1220. Spriet (1990).
56. Mouelhi-Guizani S, Bouzaouach I, Tenenbaum G et al. Simple and choice reaction times under varying levels of physical load in high skilled fencers. *J Sports Med Phys Fitness* 2006;46(2):344–351.
57. Ozmun JC, Mikesky AE, Surburg PR. Neuromuscular adaptations following prepubescent strength training. *Med Sci Sports Exerc* 1994 Apr;26(4):510–514.
58. Pivik RT, Dykman RA. Event-related variations in alpha band activity during an attentional task in preadolescents: Effects of morning nutrition. *Clin Neurophysiol* 2007 March;118(3):615–632.
59. Ramadan J. Medical principles and practice: Does fasting during Ramadan alter body composition, blood constituents and physical performance? *Int J Kuwait Univ Health Sci Centre* 2002;11(Suppl. 2):41–46.
60. Ramadan JM, Barac-Nieto M. Cardio-respiratory responses to moderately heavy aerobic exercise during the Ramadan fasts. *Saudi Med J* 2000;21:238–244.
61. Ramsay JA, Blimkie CJ, Smith K et al. Strength training effects in prepubescent boys. *Med Sci Sports Exerc* 1990 Oct;22(5):605–614.
62. Reeves ND, Narici MV, Maganaris CN. Effect of resistance training on skeletal muscle-specific force in elderly humans. *J Appl Physiol* (1985). 2004 Mar;96(3):885–892.
63. Roky R, Iraki L, HajKhlifa R et al. Daytime alertness, mood, psychomotor performances, and oral temperature during Ramadan intermittent fasting. *Ann Nutr Metab* 2000;44(3):101–107.

64. Roky R, Chapotot F, Benchekroun MT et al. Daytime sleepiness during Ramadan intermittent fasting: Polysomnographic and quantitative waking EEG study. *J Sleep Res* 2003 June;12(2):95–101.
65. Roky R, Houti I, Moussamih S et al. Physiological and chronobiological changes during Ramadan intermittent fasting. *Ann Nutr Metab* 2004;48(4):296–303.
66. Shaygan Asl N. The effects of Ramadan fasting on endurance running performance in male athletes. *Int J Sport Studies* 2011;1:18–22.
67. Scherrer J, Monod H. Local muscle work and fatigue. *J Physiol* (Paris) 1960;52:419–501.
68. Singh R, Hwa OC, Roy J et al. Subjective perceptions of sports performance, training, sleep and dietary patterns of Malaysian junior Muslim athletes during Ramadan intermittent fasting. *Asian J Sports Med* 2011;2:167–176.
69. Souissi N, Souissi H, Sahli S et al. Effect of Ramadan on the diurnal variation in short-term high power output. *Chronobiol Int* 2007;24:991–1007.
70. Sweileh N, Schnitzler A, Hunter GR, Davis B. Body composition and energy metabolism in resting and exercising Muslims during Ramadan fast. *J Sports Med Phys Fitness* 1992;32:156–163.
71. Tian HH, Aziz AR, Png W et al. Effects of fasting during Ramadan month on cognitive function in Muslim athletes. *Asian J Sports Med* 2011;2(3):145–153.
72. Vandewalle H, Pérès G, Monod H. Standard anaerobic exercise tests. *Sports Med* 1987 July–August;4(4):268–289.
73. Zarrouk N, Hug F, Hammouda O et al. Effect of Ramadan intermittent fasting on body composition and neuromuscular performance in young athletes: A pilot study. *Biol Rhytm Res* 2013;44:697–709.
74. Zerguini Y, Kirkendall D, Junge A, Dvorak J. Impact of Ramadan on physical performance in professional soccer players. *Br J Sports Med* 2007;41:398–400.
75. Zerguini Y, Dvorak J, Maughan RJ et al. Influence of Ramadan fasting on physiological and performance variables in football players: Summary of the F-MARC 2006 Ramadan fasting study. *J Sports Sci* 2008;26(Suppl. 3):S3–S6.

Further Reading

Aziz AR, Png W. Ramadan fasting and sports performance. In: Lanham-New S, Stear S, Shirrefs S, Collins A (eds.), *Sport and Exercise Nutrition*. Wiley-Blackwell, Chichester, U.K., 2011.
Jeukendrup A, Gleeson M. Dehydration and its effects on performance. In: *Sport Nutrition*, 2nd edn. Human Kinetics, Champaign, IL, 2010.
Shephard RJ. Anaerobic metabolism and endurance performance. In: Shephard RJ, Åstrand P-O (eds.), *Endurance in Sport.* Blackwell Science, Oxford, U.K., 2000, pp. 311–327.
Shephard RJ. The impact of Ramadan performance upon athletic performance. *Nutrients* 2012;4:491–505.
Shephard RJ. Ramadan and sport: Minimizing effects upon the observant athlete. *Sports Med* 2012;43:1217–1241.

10

Nutritional Recommendations for Dietary Restriction

Roy J Shephard and Ezdine Bouhlel

Learning Objectives

1. To consider tactics to restore and/or maintain carbohydrate reserves during recovery from prolonged exercise and/or fasting in trained athletes
2. To review strategies for enhancing carbohydrate before and during competition in long-distance athletes
3. To determine practical implications for athletes, coaches and trainers when regulating the percentage of lipid intake
4. To assess the minimum protein needs of strength athletes during dietary restriction
5. To develop tactics to maintain hydration during periods of fluid restriction
6. To consider the merits of antioxidant supplementation during dietary restriction and fasting

Introduction

Nutritional recommendations are required equally by the sedentary person who is seeking to reduce body fat, by the athlete who is dieting or undergoing deliberate dehydration in an attempt to make a specific weight category, and by the competitor who wishes to maintain health and physical performance in the face of a partial or complete fast because of religious beliefs. The needs of the sedentary person can be summarized quite briefly, but in the case of the athlete, we will examine carbohydrate, fat, protein and fluid needs in more detail, with specific reference to the intermittent fasting of Ramadan.

Athletes adopt various dietary tactics during Ramadan, either on their own initiative or with the advice of a coach. Some opt to eat a very large breakfast, others take a large evening meal and some supplement this with a midnight snack. A common choice is a high-carbohydrate, low-fat diet with or without nutritional supplements [56]. Fluids are often ingested late into the night and sometimes regularly throughout the night, although this has the disadvantage of disrupting normal sleep patterns [34,56], with an impairment of vigilance. One danger is that taking a heavy meal together with copious fluids late at night may cause a feeling of bloating that impedes sleeping [73].

Dieting and the Sedentary Person

The sedentary person who wishes to reduce body fat content by a few kilos should opt to create a negative energy balance of around 4 MJ/day. If such a loss can be developed and sustained, this should reduce body fat content at a rate of about 137 g/day or a loss of 13.8 kg over 100 days. Attempts to develop a larger negative energy balance will have negative effects upon mood state that will make it difficult to sustain the diet and may also lead to a substantial metabolism of lean tissue.

The negative energy balance can be created simply by almost halving the daily intake of food, but it is better to combine a 2 MJ/day reduction of food intake with a 2 MJ/day increase of energy expenditure. The added physical activity carries a wide panoply of health benefits [7], and in the specific context of dieting, an active regimen reduces the tendency to metabolize lean tissue; often, a person who augments their daily activity can reduce body fat with a simultaneous gain of lean tissue and little overall change in body mass. Dieters often look for a large and immediate change of readings on their bathroom scales, and they should be warned that losses are likely to be slow, and that loss of fat without change of body mass is an excellent outcome of their efforts.

The main factor reducing the efficacy of either dieting or dieting plus exercise is that the negative energy balance tends to induce a compensatory reduction of resting metabolism. This is in part a hormonal adjustment and in part a consequence of a decreased tissue mass and a lesser energy cost of displacing a lighter body. The decrease can be as large as 1 MJ/day, a quarter of the intended energy deficit. However, it seems that the reduction of resting metabolism is smaller and may not even occur if the dieter at the same time engages in a systematic exercise programme [16].

Controversy continues concerning the relative merits of a carbohydrate- or a fat-centred diet when attempting to reduce body fat content. Either approach can be effective, provided that the person achieves a negative energy balance. The advantage of a high-carbohydrate diet is that muscle glycogen stores are maintained; this may avoid feelings of weakness and thus encourage a greater daily total level of physical activity [4]. The disadvantage of a carbohydrate emphasis is that the ingestion of carbohydrates, particularly refined sugar, triggers an increased secretion of insulin with a resulting increase of appetite that all except a very strong-willed individual may find hard to resist. A high-fat diet is less likely to stimulate appetite, and by remaining longer in the stomach than carbohydrate, a fat-based meal sustains a feeling of satiety. However, one potential danger of a high-fat diet is an increase of oxidant stress (Chapter 8), and if the diet is continued for a long period, it could contribute to the development of various chronic conditions such as metabolic syndrome, atherosclerosis, cancer and accelerated aging.

The current consensus of sedentary dieters seems slightly in favour of the high-fat diet, but whether the focus is upon fat or carbohydrate, it is essential to ensure an adequate intake of protein and micronutrients. The sedentary individual's daily consumption of first-class protein, providing a full range of essential amino acids, should be at least 0.7 to 1.0 g/kg of body mass; this level of protein intake should be sufficient to maintain nitrogen balance and avoid a loss of lean tissue during the dieting process.

Carbohydrate Requirements and Dietary Restriction

Carbohydrate intake is important in terms of maintaining glycogen reserves in the muscles and the liver, and because of the associated molecules of hydration, it provides a reserve of two or more litres of water that can be exploited during sustained endurance exercise. A minimum intake of carbohydrate is required to maintain plasma glucose levels. If adequate carbohydrate is not available, glucose is synthesized in the liver, mainly from amino acids derived from the body musculature.

CHO and Recovery Processes

The rate of depletion of glycogen stores caused by endurance activity, dietary restriction or fasting is minimized by maintenance of training, since the well-trained person metabolizes a larger fraction of fats. The immediate depletion of carbohydrate reserves during a sustained bout of exercise and/or fasting stimulates the process of glycogen resynthesis, particularly if there is subsequent access to a high-carbohydrate diet, and often glycogen stores are boosted above their initial values as replenishment proceeds [12].

Studies assessing glycogen store kinetics in response to several days of exercise have shown that if an athlete ingests a mixed diet that provides only 200–300 g of carbohydrate per day, there is a progressive reduction of glycogen stores. However, if the carbohydrate intake is increased to 400–600 g/day, muscle glycogen resynthesis is enhanced during recovery periods [12,29] with a progressive enhancement of glycogen stores and consequently an improved aerobic performance.

The capacity for glycogen resynthesis is influenced by the type of carbohydrate that is ingested. Glycogen resynthesis is greater with glucose than with an equivalent amount of fructose [48]; indeed, Png et al. [49] found that ingesting a pre-dawn meal with a low glycaemic index did not enhance either metabolic or physical performance in athletes who were performing an endurance run during Ramadan. Carbohydrates with a high glycaemic index are recommended to restore carbohydrate stores rapidly, although complex carbohydrates with a low glycemic index can also enhance the performance of physical activity and the overall recovery process [19].

The optimal proportions of water and sugar in an athletic drink depend upon ambient conditions. In a hot environment, there is a substantial need for water, and a glucose concentration of 20 g/L should permit ready absorption and increase carbohydrate stores, but under cold conditions (5°C–10°C), the need for water is less, and the glucose concentration can be increased to 30–60 g/L. Drinks should be taken in relatively small volumes in order to facilitate gastric emptying and efficient subsequent intestinal absorption [14].

Some nutritionists have recommended taking drinks where carbohydrates are mixed with proteins during and/or following exercise [54,60,65]. The added protein or amino acid may help to reduce muscle fatigue and microinjuries and maintain peak performance [60]. A mixed carbohydrate and protein drink is also reported to enhance muscle glycogen resynthesis (although not necessarily performance) relative to a drink of glucose alone with an equivalent energy content [6,41]. Beelen et al. [5] argued that consuming CHO and protein during the early phases of recovery positively affected subsequent exercise performance for athletes who were involved in multiple training or competitive sessions on the same or consecutive days. The underlying mechanisms have yet to be clarified. Possibly, the addition of small amounts of protein to a drink stimulates the endogenous secretion of insulin and thus enhances glycogen storage.

Plasma glucose is well maintained even if exercise is performed after 23 hours of fasting [15], probably through increased gluconeogenesis. Oliver et al. [45] imposed 2 days of dietary restriction (1.2 MJ/day) with or without fluid restriction (<200 mL/day); dietary restriction reduced the subsequent 30 minutes treadmill performance by 10%, but dehydration alone did not affect subsequent performance, at least under temperate conditions. A helpful tactic with the intermittent fasting of Ramadan is to engage in carbohydrate overloading after sundown [56]. A high-carbohydrate intake during recovery periods immediately after training and a day of fasting should boost muscle and hepatic glycogen levels and maximize physical performance in endurance events.

Carbohydrate Intake before Competition

A short-term (3 day) pre-event increase of carbohydrate intake to 75% of energy needs can double muscle glycogen stores. However, the classic Scandinavian carbohydrate boosting regimen is of 6 days duration; a competitor depletes glycogen stores by avoiding carbohydrates for 3 days and follows this by a high-carbohydrate diet for the final 3 days before an event. Glycogen stores are boosted, with an increase of endurance performance. However, this type of regimen has some practical disadvantages. Greater fatigue is perceived during the period without carbohydrate, and this predisposes to a reduction of training and an increase of injuries. Moreover, 3 days of carbohydrate overloading in itself seems sufficient to boost glycogen stores and to increase endurance capacity, without the initial 3-day period of glycogen depletion. Supplements of B group vitamins should be added to a high-carbohydrate diet in order to sustain biochemical reactions (glucose transporters, enzymatic activities) and thus aerobic performance.

Carbohydrate Intake on the Day before and on the Day of Competition

The athlete's aim is for glycogen levels to peak as competition approaches. Meals based on spaghetti and rice are typically chosen by athletes to provide a high-carbohydrate intake and thus to augment muscle glycogen levels. Care should be taken in the choice of carbohydrates immediately before an event. The ingestion of large amounts of simple carbohydrate with a high glycaemic index is likely to stimulate insulin secretion and may thus exacerbate hypoglycaemia during an event. In addition, high concentrations of monosaccharides such as glucose can slow gastric emptying and reduce blood volumes by drawing water into the intestines. Complex carbohydrates with a low glycaemic index are thus the best choice immediately before competition. Cereals (400–500 kJ) can be ingested up to 1 hour before competition. Such nutritional tactics offer high levels of carbohydrate, optimal hydration and a minimum of digestive discomfort.

Carbohydrate Intake during Competition

The ingestion of carbohydrate during an event can enhance aerobic performance, especially in activities that continue for more than 90 minutes and thus deplete muscle glycogen stores [21]. During competition, the volume of fluid ingested must be small enough to avoid problems of gastric emptying; a maximum of 600 mL/h is suggested, depending upon environmental conditions. Several studies have shown improvements of performance with a carbohydrate intake of 30–60 g/h (5%–10%, if the fluid volume is 600 mL/h). Increases in gastric osmolarity (glucose concentrations >8%), slow gastric emptying and complaints of abdominal distension are a common reason for abandoning an endurance event [47]. Although an excessive secretion of insulin is less likely with fructose than with glucose, gastric discomfort is more common with fructose ingestion. The ingestion of a mixed fructose/glucose solution (30–40 g/h) is perhaps the optimum choice. Sanchez et al. [58] pointed out that some abdominal complaints reflect a dehydration-related decrease of mesenteric blood flow rather than gastric distension. At the other end of the nutritional spectrum, symptomatic hyponatraemia is another serious but largely preventable problem, arising when competitors ingest excessive volumes of water under cool conditions. Hew et al. [25] argued that an excessive fluid intake could induce both vomiting and hyponatraemia.

For the athlete who is observing Ramadan, although there are advantages in maximizing carbohydrate intake at the post-sundown meal, the delayed emptying of a high-fat intake may offer an advantage for the pre-dawn meal.

Lipid Requirements and Dietary Restriction

The daily lipid intake can vary within a wide range, although there is a minimal requirement of two essential fatty acids that the body is unable to synthesize (linoleic and alpha-linoleic acid), and a very high-lipid diet increases the risk of oxidative stress (Chapter 8). In terms of dietary quality, it is also important to avoid synthetic trans fats.

Lipids play an important energetic role, particularly in the fasting state and during prolonged exercise of mild-to-moderate intensities, as carbohydrate reserves become depleted [37]. Average individuals take 30%–35% of their total daily energy requirement in the form of fat. In athletes who are boosting their glycogen stores, this could decrease to 20%–25%, but on the other hand because the energy content per gram is greater for fat than carbohydrate, they may elect a high-fat diet when undertaking an event that requires a very high-energy expenditure for many days (e.g., the 'Tour de France', or a cross-Canada run).

A minimum lipid intake of 1–1.2 g/kg/day is recommended to ensure an adequate supply of liposoluble vitamins. Monounsaturated fatty acids such as oleic acid (found in olive, arachnid and avocado oils) and polyunsaturated fatty acids such as *linoleic acid*, *alpha-linolenic acid* and *arachidonic acid* (found mainly in vegetables and fat fish) should (comprising 65% and 20% of total fats, respectively). The minimum requirements of linoleic and alpha-linolenic acids are 7–10 and 1–2 g/day, respectively. The intake of saturated fatty acids (butter, palm oil, coconut oil, fat meats and whole milk) should be limited, in order to reduce the risk of developing cardiovascular and metabolic diseases.

Dietary manipulation aimed at increasing fat oxidation could reduce the risk of developing metabolic diseases such as obesity, type 2 diabetes and fatty liver [1,62]. The rate of fat oxidation is influenced by many factors, including exercise intensity and duration, mode of exercise, training status and diet.

Exercise Intensity and Duration

Exercise intensity and duration are important factors influencing the rate of fat oxidation. The proportional utilization of fat increases with intensity, peaking at moderate intensities of effort, and decreasing at high intensities (when muscle oxygen supply may not be adequate to allow aerobic metabolism, Chapter 4). The peaking of fat oxidation rates occurs at higher relative intensities of effort in trained than in sedentary subjects (59%–64% vs. 47%–52% of $\dot{V}O_{2\,max}$, Achten and Jeukendrup [1]). During moderate aerobic exercise, the metabolism of fat is greater in trained than in untrained individuals, but during intensive exercise athletes develop an enhanced circulation and are thus able to metabolize fat to a high fraction of maximal effort [9,17].

Type of Exercise

The type of exercise also influences the extent of fat metabolism. Fat oxidation is generally greater during running than when cycling, because when running, activity is distributed over a larger fraction of the body muscles, and anaerobic metabolism does not commence until the person is closer to maximal effort [1].

Endurance Training

Endurance training induces a multitude of adaptations that increase the potential for fat oxidation [1], with an increased oxidation of fatty acids derived from tissue fat depots [27].

Fasting or Dietary Restriction

Fasting or dietary restriction generally increases fat metabolism. Ingestion of carbohydrate in the hours immediately preceding a bout of exercise reduces fat oxidation relative to fasting conditions, whereas fasting for longer than 6 hours maximizes fat oxidation [1].

During a period of fasting, fat oxidation is enhanced both at rest and during exercise demanding up to 60% of $\dot{V}O_{2\,max}$ [8,64]. The increased reliance upon fat as a source of energy should theoretically conserve existing glycogen reserves during prolonged effort, although Aziz et al. [3] found no difference in the relative usage of fat and carbohydrate during Ramadan when subjects ran on a treadmill for 30 minutes at 65% of $\dot{V}O_{2\,max}$.

Most studies have seen no major impact of high-fat-intake diets upon aerobic performance [24,59], although Muoio et al. [43] found that with a diet where 38% of total energy intake was attributable to fat, there was an increase in fat oxidation, with an increase of $\dot{V}O_{2\,max}$ and running endurance on a treadmill.

High-Lipid Diets

The rate of fat oxidation during exercise is determined by the availability of fatty acids and the rate of carbohydrate utilization [26,43]. Turcotte [69] noted that a high-carbohydrate diet increased plasma glucose levels, with a decrease of lipolysis in adipose tissues and a decrease of fat metabolism. On the other hand, a high-fat/low-carbohydrate diet increases the relative contribution of fat to oxidative metabolism and increases the sympathoadrenal response to exercise, with reduced plasma insulin concentrations [30,36].

Fat utilization of endurance-trained subjects during submaximal exercise (60% of O_{2peak}) was increased after ingesting a high-fat (60%–70% of energy intake) low-CHO (15%–20% of energy intake) diet for 7–10 days [22,23]. Zderic et al. [75] also reported an increased oxidation of fats when trained cyclists exercised after only 2 days on a high-fat diet (60% fat of total energy intake). Rowlands and Hopkins [55] again found that a high-fat intake (66% ± 10% of total energy intake) for 2 weeks induced greater lipolysis and free fatty acid availability in cyclists: lower plasma insulin concentrations before and during exercise, higher plasma glucose concentrations, higher plasma glycerol levels, and two- to three-fold increases in the peak fat oxidation rate were also noted. In their study,

100 km cycling performance was enhanced relative to high-carbohydrate ingestion. Pendergast et al. [46] maintained that high-fat diets (42%–55%) when combined with an adequate carbohydrate intake enhanced endurance relative to low-fat diets (10%–15%). Vogt et al. [71] noted that muscle glycogen stores were still well maintained after 5 weeks on a high-fat diet, but that the intramyocellular lipid content was more than doubled. They also reported larger contribution of lipids to total energy turnover when following this regimen.

The acute ingestion of exogenous substrates, usually carbohydrates, during a bout of exercise has little effect upon rates of muscle glycogenolysis [74]. However, short-term (<1–2 weeks) dietary manipulations can increase endogenous muscle stores of both glycogen and lipids. One recently adopted tactic is 'fat adaptation', where well-trained endurance athletes continue their normal training regimen but consume a high-fat, low-carbohydrate diet for 2 weeks; they then switch to a high-carbohydrate diet with a tapering of training for 1–3 days before competition. This regimen appears to optimize fatty acid availability and rates of fat oxidation and attenuates glycogen utilization during submaximal exercise at 60%–70% of $\dot{V}O_{2\,max}$ [74].

Another dietary tactic proposed by Burke and Hawley [10] involved a 5–6-day period ingesting a high-fat diet (60%–70% of energy intake), followed by 1–2 days of a high-carbohydrate intake (70%–80% of energy intake). Again, it was claimed that athletes showed higher rates of fat oxidation and concomitant muscle glycogen sparing during submaximal exercise [10]. The higher rates of fat oxidation seem to persist even if a high-carbohydrate meal is provided shortly before exercise and/or glucose solutions are ingested during exercise [10]. However, the increased fat utilization does not necessarily enhance the performance of prolonged endurance exercise [10]. Burke and Hawley [10] concluded that 'there is insufficient scientific evidence to recommend that athletes either ingest fat, in the form of medium-chain triglyceride, during exercise, or "fat adapt" in the weeks prior to a major endurance event to improve athletic performance'.

The ingestion of small quantities of medium-chain triglycerides (8–10 carbon chains) has no major effects on either fat metabolism or exercise performance [22]. However, if such triglycerides are combined with carbohydrate, there is a sparing of muscle glycogen stores during 2 hours of submaximal cycling exercise at 70% of O_{2peak}, and improved 40 km time-trial performance [35]. The medium-chain triacylglycerols are fatty acids found in butter and coconut. They have a high solubility; they are absorbed rapidly by the small intestine and transported to the liver, where they can be metabolized, thus sparing glycogen reserves. Nevertheless, any benefit from ingesting long-chain or medium-chain triacylglycerols during exercise has yet to be confirmed [27]. Indeed, most studies to date have seen no gains in aerobic performance [2,18,22,32]. Angus et al. [2] reported that carbohydrate ingestion during exercise improved 100 km times, but the addition of medium-chain triacylglycerols to an athlete's drink did not further enhance performance in endurance-trained men. Furthermore, some studies have suggested that the ingestion of medium-chain triacylglycerols can exacerbate gastrointestinal symptoms [18,31].

Low-Lipid Diets

Low-lipid diets are encountered by those practising the fasts required by the Greek Orthodox Church. Classically, other endurance athletes have also reduced their fat intake substantially in order to permit a high-carbohydrate intake. Coyle et al. [13] showed that very low-fat (2% of energy) and high-CHO diet reduced body lipolysis, total fat oxidation and non-plasma fatty acids oxidation during exercise in the fasted state. In addition, decreases of intramuscular triglyceride levels were seen in endurance-trained cyclists.

Consuming low levels of fat may lead to a vitamin E deficiency and, in consequence, an increase of oxidative stress [57]. Venkatraman et al. [70] reported that a low-fat high-carbohydrate diet (15% fat, 65% CHO) increased inflammatory and decreased anti-inflammatory immune factors, with depressed levels of antioxidants, and negative effects upon blood lipoprotein ratios. A low-fat intake may also compromise zinc intake, leading to a decrease of body mass, fatigue, decreased endurance performance and a risk of osteoporosis [40]. Pogliaghi and Veicsteinas [50] found unchanged $\dot{V}O_{2\,max}$ and endurance times in sedentary subjects who were submitted to 4 weeks of several different diets (a spontaneous diet, 30% fat, 15% fat, 55% fat). However, Horvath et al. [28] found that a low-fat diet (16% fat) decreased treadmill endurance times in runners.

Protein Needs of the Athlete during Ramadan

The body has a daily minimum requirement of protein that varies with habitual activity and the need for hypertrophy and/or tissue repair. The quality of the protein must also be appropriate; there are nine amino acids that humans are unable to synthesize (phenylalanine, valine, threonine, tryptophan, methionine, leucine, isoleucine, lysine and histidine), and these must be provided in the diet, preferably all in the same meal. Meats generally contain all of the necessary amino acids, but if a vegetable-based diet has been adopted for religious or philosophical reasons, the constituents of each meal must be carefully balanced. Additional protein may be required to compensate for the catabolism of lean tissue during the gluconeogenesis induced by any form of dieting, including the intermittent fasting of Ramadan; the tendency for protein-based gluconeogenesis is greatest among athletes who are participating in endurance and ultraendurance events, and unfortunately, there has been little study of such individuals during Ramadan. If competitive events are held in the afternoon or early evening, glycogen reserves are likely to be depleted, with a corresponding increase in the likelihood of protein-based gluconeogenesis. Studies to date suggest that if efforts are made to maximize the intake of nutrients during the hours of darkness, there is no cumulative decrease of lean tissue mass over the month of intermittent fasting. Nevertheless, it is prudent to adopt nutritional tactics that maximize daytime blood glucose levels within the limits imposed by the fast, ensuring a sufficient intake of good quality protein each evening to maintain a positive nitrogen balance, and maintaining normal training-induced anabolism throughout Ramadan. If estimating dietary requirements, it is important to remember that the minimum protein needs of the athlete, particularly the strength athlete, are substantially larger than those of a sedentary person. When the overall energy intake is restricted, the protein intake should be in the range 1.7–2.0 g/kg, perhaps as high as 20% of total energy intake.

The matching of training sessions to the time when protein is ingested seems a substantive issue for those observing Ramadan (Chapter 11). Vigorous muscular exercise (particularly eccentric exercise) increases the permeability of the muscle fibre membranes, allowing proteins such as troponin and enzymes such as creatine kinase to escape into the blood stream. Nevertheless, this increase of membrane permeability also facilitates entry into the muscle fibre of the amino acids needed in muscle hypertrophy. It is thus important to match the timing of peak plasma levels of amino acids with this training-induced increase of permeability. Ramadan does not allow great flexibility in the scheduling of meals, but it is usually possible for the athlete to align training sessions with the time when plasma amino acids are presumed to be at their peak.

Moore et al. [42] reported that protein synthesis was encouraged by the ingestion of 20 g of high-quality protein immediately following a bout of resistance exercise. This suggests that the best time to ingest protein may be immediately following a training session [20,67]. However, some authors have noted benefit if appropriate proteins or amino acids are ingested either immediately before or as late as 3 hours after a training session [53,73].

Issues of Hydration

With most forms of dieting, people tend to increase their intake of fluids as a means of minimizing the pangs of hunger. However, this is not the case for athletes who are observing Ramadan or are attempting to make a specific weight category.

Empirical data suggest that problems in maintaining a normal level of body hydration during Ramadan are commonest during the first few days of fasting [52,64,66]. Somewhat surprisingly, a cumulative dehydration over the 29 days is more commonly observed in sedentary individuals than in athletes [52]. Presumably, experienced competitors have been taught or learned and have the self-discipline to follow simple tactics that maximize their nighttime ingestion of fluids and minimize their daytime fluid losses. Any effects upon the hydration of the athlete seem acute rather than cumulative, reaching their maximum immediately before sunset each day. If possible, the times of both training sessions and competition should thus be postponed until the late evening, giving the athletes time to rehydrate before exercising.

In terms of fluid ingestion, a useful recommendation for the athlete is to drink 600 mL/hours of fluid (corresponding to the normal gastric emptying rate) from breaking of the fast at sundown until bedtime and to take at least an additional 1 L at breakfast. The aim should be to leave 500–600 mL of unabsorbed water in the stomach at the moment the fast is resumed. It may also be useful to boost intra-muscular glycogen stores. The metabolism of glycogen and release of its associ-ated water molecules normally contributes up to 2 L to the body's daily fluid requirements, and this reserve could theoretically be as much as doubled if adop-tion of a high-carbohydrate diet maximized pre-competition glycogen stores [61]. If a competitor deliberately maximizes fluid intake at night, the total daily water intake may show little change during Ramadan [38], and there may be little change in either haemoglobin or haematocrit values as the month proceeds [39]. Nevertheless, observant Muslims usually show some increase of serum electrolyte concentrations over the course of the day, even if they have not been physically active, and there is an associated increase in the specific gravity of their urine [68].

Maughan et al. [38] noted that in one group of observant soccer players, the salt intake was substantially reduced during Ramadan (from 5.4 to 4.3 g/day). The reason for this change is unclear, but it would seem an inappropriate tactic; in fact, a small increase of salt consumption might be helpful in maximizing fluid ingestion and retention. Another potential method of expanding plasma volume would be to take a mixture of glycerol and creatine. This tactic would help to expand the intracellular water volume [33,51], but unfortunately, athletes are now prohibited from adopting such an approach under rules of the World Anti-Doping Association.

The main source of fluid loss over the day is sweating. In order to minimize sweating, athletes should if possible remain in a cool room away from sun-light and avoid unnecessary physical activity until immediately before com-petition. Sweating during an event can be reduced by pre-cooling of the body. The most effective method of pre-cooling is internal, through the ingestion of cold water or ice cream [63], but this is not an option for those who are observ-ing Ramadan. External cooling by immersion of the body in cold water is an alternative, but athletes must use this approach judiciously; it eliminates the benefits associated with a 'warm-up', slowing metabolic processes, competitive speed and power [44]. Nevertheless, competitors could consider wetting their clothing immediately before an event, so that body cooling is derived from the evaporation of this water rather than from sweating. In some types of competi-tion such as a soccer match, it might even be possible to rewet the clothing at half-time.

Che Muhamed et al. [11] recently found improvements of 10 km run times when athletes who were observing Ramadan and exercising in a hot and humid cham-ber rinsed their mouths with a carbohydrate solution. Mouth rinsing also reduced the perception of effort during Ramadan. However, this tactic is not permitted under Muslim law. Further studies are needed to examine the effect of mouth rinsing water on fasting athletes under thermally neutral ambient conditions.

Antioxidant Supplementation during Fasting

Periods of prolonged and intensive exercise increase the production of free radicals. There is thus a danger that dietary restriction or fasting may reduce the body's store of antioxidants. Some authors have advocated the use of nutritional supplements, including flavonoids such as quercetin and *Lactobacillus* probiotics to cover the postulated deficiency, enhance immune function, and reduce the risk of acute infections in athletes [72]. However, there is no strong evidence for the effectiveness of this tactic in those observing Ramadan.

Conclusions

Carbohydrates and lipids are normally the two major energy sources during the performance of aerobic exercise. Glycogen is plainly depleted during prolonged fasting, and even during Ramadan, the cumulative effects of the intermittent fast and heavy training can lead to a cumulative glycogen depletion that compromises aerobic performance. In such situations, pre-fast carbohydrate boosting is helpful in maintaining adequate glycogen reserves. Nutrients with a high glycaemic index are recommended at the beginning of recovery from training or the breaking of the fast; they speed up the recovery process. However, nutrients with a low glycaemic index are advisable immediately prior to competition, in order to avoid an insulin surge and resulting hypoglycaemia. There is as yet little overall evidence to commend prolonged ingestion of a high-lipid diet, although a fatty pre-dawn meal may give athletes a longer period of satiety when they are observing Ramadan. Medium-chained triacylglycerols supplements do not seem to enhance performance. The choice of a very low-fat diet may induce mineral and vitamin deficits, decrease antioxidants, and increase in inflammatory and oxidative responses to exercise.

Minimum protein requirements of strength athletes are quite high, and care should be taken to maintain a nitrogen balance during any form of dietary restriction, in order to avoid the breakdown of lean tissue; during Ramadan, it is helpful to match peak plasma amino acid levels with the timing of training sessions in order to maximize the anabolic response.

Athletes should prepare themselves for fasting by maximizing training and eating a well-balanced diet with a focus upon carbohydrate boosting. The amounts of carbohydrate, proteins and fat needed during refeeding will depend upon individual requirements, guided by sensations of fatigue. Micronutrient supplements of vitamins and minerals may help to reduce oxidative stress during some forms of dieting, but there is no evidence that they enhance muscular performance.

Key Terms

Alpha linolenic acid: Alpha linoleic acid is a polyunsaturated omega-3 fatty acid that is an essential constituent of the human diet. It is found in vegetable oils and plays a major role in reducing the risk of cardiovascular disease.

Carnitine: Carnitine is a molecule that plays a major role in the transport of fatty acids from the cytosol to the mitochondria during lipid catabolism.

Complex carbohydrates: Simple carbohydrates are built from one or two sugar molecules, but complex carbohydrates such as starch contain many sugar molecules; these must be broken down during digestion, slowing the rise of blood sugar and thus the rise of insulin secretion.

Essential amino acids: Essential amino acids are needed for good health, but cannot be synthesized within the body. Meats usually provide all essential amino acids, but a vegetarian diet must be planned carefully to ensure that its elements provide all nine essential amino acids.

Essential fatty acids: Essential fatty acids are needed for good health, but cannot be synthesized in the body; in humans, the two essential fatty acids are linoleic and alpha-linoleic acid.

First-class protein: First-class proteins provide a good balance of essential amino acids.

Fructose: Fructose is a monosaccharide fruit sugar that provides palatability to many prepared foods.

Gastric emptying: The emptying of the stomach takes between 2 and 3 hours in normal subjects. The emptying rate is slowed during exercise and in patients with diabetes mellitus, gastric ulcer and other digestive troubles.

Gastric osmolarity: Gastric osmolarity defines the molar concentration of the stomach contents.

Glycaemic index: The glycaemic index provides a measure of the increase in plasma glucose seen following the ingestion of a carbohydrate.

Intestinal absorption: Intestinal absorption is the process by which nutrients pass from the intestines into the blood stream.

Linoleic acid: Linoleic acid is a polyunsaturated omega-6 fatty acid found in the lipids of membrane cells and hormones. It is abundant in many vegetable oils, poppy seed, safflower, sunflower and corn oils.

Metabolic diseases: Metabolic diseases are any diseases or disorders that disrupt normal metabolism. Perhaps the best known is diabetes mellitus, where there is a lack of the hormone insulin that regulates blood glucose.

Micronutrients: Micronutrients are substances required in small quantities (less than 100 mg/day) to ensure good health. They include traces of elements such as iron, cobalt, chromium, copper, iodine, manganese, selenium, zinc and molybdenum and various vitamins.

Molecules of hydration: Each molecule of glycogen is associated with three water molecules of hydration. The water is liberated into the body fluid pool as the glycogen is metabolized.

Monosaccharides: Monosaccharides are the simplest, 6-carbon forms of sugar such as glucose, fructose and galactose.

Monounsaturated fatty acids: Fatty acids that have one double bond in their carbon chain.

Nitrogen balance: A situation where the intake of nitrogen in the form of proteins and amino acids matches the excretion of nitrogen as ammonia, urea and uric acid. It provides a measure of the adequacy of daily protein intake.

Polyunsaturated fatty acids: Fatty acids that have multiple double bonds in their carbon chain.

Trans fats: Trans fats are uncommon in nature but, until recently, were a major component of synthetic fats, for example, saturated fats produced by the hydrogenation of vegetable oils. In trans fats, the fatty acid chains are arranged at 180° to each other (the *trans* formation), whereas in natural fat they are parallel (the *cis* formation). Trans fats have an adverse effect upon blood lipids and increase the risk of cardiovascular disease.

Vegan diet: A vegan diet avoids the consumption of animal products. It may be imposed at some times of the year by religious fasting.

Vitamins: Vitamins are essential dietary constituents that are important to the body's metabolism. They are classified as fat soluble (vitamins A, D, E and K) or water soluble (vitamins B and C).

Key Points

1. Carbohydrates and fats are normally the main energy sources during exercise.
2. If trained athletes must compete or continue vigorous conditioning during a period of fasting, they are likely to develop a progressive depletion of glycogen stores, with associated fatigue and reductions in their exercise performance.
3. Maximizing training and carbohydrate boosting are recommended as preparations for fasting, in order to maximize glycogen stores, boost fat oxidation, and enhance aerobic performance.
4. A drink containing a mixture of carbohydrate and protein may facilitate recovery periods during the intermittent fasting of Ramadan.
5. There is no evidence that the sustained adoption of a high-fat regime will enhance the aerobic performance of athletes, although greater feelings of satiety may help both the sedentary dieter and the athlete immediately before he or she begins the daily fast of Ramadan.
6. During Ramadan observance, training sessions must be matched to times of the day when plasma levels of amino acids are high in order to maximize anabolism.
7. A progressive dehydration is likely to challenge endurance athletes who must compete late in the day while observing Ramadan. Helpful tactics in minimizing dehydration are to maximize glycogen stores, to keep in a cool place between events, to wet the clothing when moving into the sun, and to rinse the mouth with a sugar solution.

Questions for Discussion

1. Which form of carbohydrate would you recommend to an athlete who was breaking a fast?
2. What changes in glycogen stores would you anticipate in an athlete during Ramadan observance?
3. Which micronutrients are necessary to safeguard health and aerobic performance during dietary restriction and fasting?
4. What nutritional preparations would you recommend to minimize the effects of Ramadan observance upon the aerobic and anaerobic performances of elite athletes?
5. How can the challenges of dehydration be minimized in athletes observing Ramadan?

References

1. Achten J, Jeukendrup AE. Optimizing fat oxidation through exercise and diet. *Nutrition* 2004 Jul–Aug;20(7–8):716–727.
2. Angus DJ, Hargreaves M, Dancey J, Febbraio MA. Effect of carbohydrate or carbohydrate plus medium-chain triglyceride ingestion on cycling time trial performance. *J Appl Physiol* 2000 Jan;88(1):113–119.
3. Aziz AR, Che Muhamed AM, Chong E, Singh R. Effects of Ramadan fasting on substrate utilization, physiological and perceptual responses during submaximal intensity running in active men. *Sport Sci Health* 2014;10(1):1–10.
4. Bandini LG, Schoeller DA, Dietz WH. Metabolic differences in response to a high-fat vs. a high carbohydrate diet. *Obes Res* 1994;2(4):348–354.
5. Beelen M, Burke LM, Gibala MJ, van Loon LJC. Nutritional strategies to promote postexercise recovery. *Int J Sport Nutr Exerc Metab* 2010 Dec;20(6):515–532.
6. Berardi JM, Price TB, Noreen EE, Lemon PW. Postexercise muscle glycogen recovery enhanced with a carbohydrate-protein supplement. *Med Sci Sports Exerc* 2006 Jun;38(6):1106–1113.
7. Bouchard C, Shephard RJ, Stephens T. *Physical Activity, Fitness and Health*. Human Kinetics, Champaign, IL, 1994.
8. Bouhlel E, Salhi Z, Bouhlel H et al. Effect of Ramadan fasting on fuel oxidation during exercise in trained male rugby players. *Diabetes Metab* 2006 Dec;32(6):617–624.
9. Brooks GA, Mercier J. Balance of carbohydrate and lipid utilization during exercise: The "crossover" concept. *J Appl Physiol* 1985, 1994 Jun;76(6):2253–2261.
10. Burke LM, Hawley JA. Effects of short-term fat adaptation on metabolism and performance of prolonged exercise. *Med Sci Sports Exerc* 2002 Sep;34(9):1492–1498.
11. Che Muhamed AM, Mohamed NG, Ismail N et al. Mouth rinsing improves cycling endurance performance during Ramadan fasting in a hot humid environment. *Appl Physiol Nutr Metab* 2014 Apr;39(4):458–464.
12. Costill DL. Carbohydrates for exercise: Dietary demands for optimal performance. *Int J Sports Med* 1988 Feb;9(1):1–18.
13. Coyle EF, Jeukendrup AE, Oseto MC et al. Low-fat diet alters intramuscular substrates and reduces lipolysis and fat oxidation during exercise. *Am J Physiol Endocrinol Metab* 2001 Mar;280(3):E391–E398.
14. Coyle EF. Fluid and fuel intake during exercise. *J Sports Sci* 2004 Jan;22(1):39–55.
15. Dohm GL, Beeker RT, Israel RG, Tapscott EB. Metabolic responses to exercise after fasting. *J Appl Physiol* 1985, 1986 Oct;61(4):1363–1368.

16. Frey-Hewitt B, Vranizan KM, Dreon DM, Wood PD. The effect of weight loss by dieting or exercise on resting metabolic rate in overweight men. *Int J Obes* 1990;14(4):327–334.

17. Gleeson M, Greenhaff PL, Maughan RJ. Influence of a 24 h fast on high intensity cycle exercise performance in man. *Eur J Appl Physiol Occup Physiol* 1988;57(6):653–659.

18. Goedecke JH, Clark VR, Noakes TD, Lambert EV. The effects of medium-chain triacyl-glycerol and carbohydrate ingestion on ultra-endurance exercise performance. *Int J Sport Nutr Exerc Metab* 2005 Feb;15(1):15–27.

19. Guezennec CY. Oxidation rates, complex carbohydrates and exercise. Practical recommendations. *Sports Med* 1995 Jun;19(6):365–372.

20. Hartman JW, Tang JE, Wilkinson SB et al. Consumption of fat-free milk after resistance exercise promotes greater lean mass accretion than does consumption of soy or carbohydrate in young, novice, male weightlifters. *Am J Clin Nutr* 2007;86:373–381.

21. Hawley JA, Schabort EJ, Noakes TD, Dennis SC. Carbohydrate-loading and exercise performance. An update. *Sports Med* 1997 Aug;24(2):73–81.

22. Hawley JA, Brouns F, Jeukendrup A. Strategies to enhance fat utilisation during exercise. *Sports Med* 1998 Apr;25(4):241–257.

23. Hawley JA. Fat adaptation science: Low-carbohydrate, high- fat diets to alter fuel utilization and promote training adaptation. *Nestle Nutr Inst Workshop Ser* 2011;69:59–71.

24. Helge JW, Richter EA, Kiens B. Interaction of training and diet on metabolism and endurance during exercise in man. *J Physiol* 1996 Apr 1;492(Pt 1):293–306.

25. Hew TD, Chorley JN, Cianca JC, Divine JG. The incidence, risk factors, and clinical manifestations of hyponatremia in marathon runners. *Clin J Sport Med* 2003 Jan;13(1):41–47.

26. Holloszy JO, Kohrt WM, Hansen PA. The regulation of carbohydrate and fat metabolism during and after exercise. *Front Biosci* 1998 Sep 15;3:D1011–D1027.

27. Horowitz JF, Klein S. Lipid metabolism during endurance exercise. *Am J Clin Nutr* 2000 Aug;72(2 Suppl.):558S–563S.

28. Horvath PJ, Eagen CK, Fisher NM et al. The effects of varying dietary fat on performance and metabolism in trained male and female runners. *J Am Coll Nutr* 2000 Feb;19(1):52–60.

29. Hultman E. Liver as a glucose supplying source during rest and exercise with special reference to diet. In Parizkova J. Rogozkin VA, *Nutrition, Physical Fitness and Health.* University Park Press, Baltimore, MD, 1978, pp. 9–30.

30. Jansson E, Hjemdahl P, Kaijser L. Diet induced changes in sympatho-adrenal activity during submaximal exercise in relation to substrate utilization in man. *Acta Physiol Scand* 1982 Feb;114(2):171–178.

31. Jeukendrup AE, Thielen JJ, Wagenmakers AJ et al. Effect of medium-chain triacylglyc-erol and carbohydrate ingestion during exercise on substrate utilization and subsequent cycling performance. *Am J Clin Nutr* 1998 Mar;67(3):397–404.

32. Jeukendrup AE, Raben A, Gijsen A et al. Glucose kinetics during prolonged exercise in highly trained human subjects: Effect of glucose ingestion. *J Physiol* 1999 Mar 1;515(Pt 2):579–589.

33. Kilduff LP, Georgiades E, James N et al. The effects of creatine supplementation on cardiovascular, metabolic, and thermoregulatory responses during exercise in the heat in endurance-trained humans. *Int J Sport Nutr Exerc Metab* 2004;14:443–460.

34. Kirkendall DT, Chaouachi A, Aziz A-R, Chamari BK. Strategies for maintaining fitness and performance during Ramadan. *J Sports Sci* 2012;30(Suppl. 1):S103–S108.

35. Lambert EV, Hawley JA, Goedecke J et al. Nutritional strategies for promoting fat utilization and delaying the onset of fatigue during prolonged exercise. *J Sports Sci* 1997 Jun;15(3):315–324.

36. Langfort J, Pilis W, Zarzeczny R et al. Effect of low-carbohydrate-ketogenic diet on metabolic and hormonal responses to graded exercise in men. *J Physiol Pharmacol* 1996 Jun;47(2):361–371.

37. Martin WH 3rd. Effects of acute and chronic exercise on fat metabolism. *Exerc Sport Sci Rev* 1996;24:203–231.

38. Maughan RJ, Bartagi Z, Dvorak J, Zerguini Y. Dietary intake and body composition of football players during the holy month of Ramadan. *J Sports Sci* 2008;26(Suppl. 3): S20–S38.

39. Maughan RJ, Leiper JB, Bartagi Z et al. Effect of Ramadan fasting on some biochemical and haematological parameters in Tunisian youth soccer players undertaking their usual training and competition schedule. *J Sports Sci* 2008;26(Suppl. 3):539–546.

40. Micheletti A, Rossi R, Rufini S. Zinc status in athletes: Relation to diet and exercise. *Sports Med* 2001;31(8):577–582.

41. Millard-Stafford M, Childers WL, Conger SA, Kampfer AJ, Rahnert JA. Recovery nutrition: Timing and composition after endurance exercise. *Curr Sports Med Rep* 2008 Jul–Aug;7(4):193–201.

42. Moore DR, Robinson MJ, Fry JL et al. Ingested protein dose response of muscle and albumin protein synthesis after resistance exercise in young men. *Am J Clin Nutr* 2009;89:161–168.

43. Muoio DM, Leddy JJ, Horvath PJ et al. Effect of dietary fat on metabolic adjustments to maximal VO$_2$ and endurance in runners. *Med Sci Sports Exerc* 1994 Jan;26(1):81–88.

44. Nybo L. Hyperthermia and fatigue. *J Appl Physiol* 2008;104:871–878.

45. Oliver SJ, Laing SJ, Wilson S et al. Endurance running performance after 48 h of restricted fluid and/or energy intake. *Med Sci Sports Exerc* 2007 Feb;39(2):316–322.

46. Pendergast DR, Leddy JJ, Venkatraman JT. A perspective on fat intake in athletes. *J Am Coll Nutr* 2000 June;19(3):345–350.

47. Pfeiffer B, Stellingwerff T, Hodgson AB et al. Nutritional intake and gastrointestinal problems during competitive endurance events. *Med Sci Sports Exerc* 2012 Feb;44(2): 344–351.

48. Plowman SA, Smith D. *Exercise Physiology for Health, Fitness and Performance*. Wolters Kluwer, Philadelphia, PA, 2013.

49. Png W, Bhaskaran K, Sinclair AJ, Aziz AR. Effects of ingesting low glycemic index carbohydrate food for the sahur meal on subjective, metabolic and physiological responses, and endurance performance in Ramadan fasted men. *Int J Food Sci Nutr* 2014;65(5):629–636.

50. Pogliaghi S, Veicsteinas A. Influence of low and high dietary fat on physical performance in untrained males. *Med Sci Sports Exerc* 1999 Jan;31(1):149–155.

51. Polyviou TP, Easton C, Beis L et al. Effects of glycerol and creatine hyperhydration and doping-relevant blood parameters. *Nutrients* 2012;4:1171–1186.

52. Ramadan J, Telahoun G, Al-Zaid NS, Barac-Nieto M. Responses to exercise, fluid, and energy balances during Ramadan in sedentary and active males. *Nutrition* 1999;15:735–739.

53. Rasmussen BB, Tipton KD, Miller SL et al. An oral essential amino acid-carbohydrate supplement enhances muscle protein anabolism after resistance exercise. *J Appl Physiol* 2000;88:386–392.

54. Romano-Ely BC, Todd MK, Saunders MJ, Laurent TS. Effect of an isocaloric carbohydrate-protein-antioxidant drink on cycling performance. *Med Sci Sports Exerc* 2006 Sep;38(9):1608–1616.

55. Rowlands DS, Hopkins WG. Effects of high-fat and high-carbohydrate diets on metabolism and performance in cycling. *Metabolism* 2002 Jun;51(6):678–690.

56. Roy J, Hwa OC, Singh R, Aziz A-R, Jin CW. Self-generated coping strategies among Muslim athletes during Ramadan fasting. *J Sports Sci Med* 2011;10:137–144.

57. Sacheck JM, Decker EA, Clarkson PM. The effect of diet on vitamin E intake and oxidative stress in response to acute exercise in female athletes. *Eur J Appl Physiol* 2000 Sep;83(1):40–46.

58. Sanchez LD, Corwell B, Berkoff D. Medical problems of marathon runners. *Am J Emerg Med* 2006 Sep;24(5):608–615.

59. Satabin P, Portero P, Defer G et al. Metabolic and hormonal responses to lipid and carbohydrate diets during exercise in man. *Med Sci Sports Exerc* 1987 Jun;19(3):218–223.

60. Skillen RA, Testa M, Applegate EA et al. Effects of an amino acid carbohydrate drink on exercise performance after consecutive-day exercise bouts. *Int J Sport Nutr Exerc Metab* 2008 Oct;18(5):473–492.

61. Shephard RJ. *Physiology & Biochemistry of Exercise*. Praeger Publications, New York, 1982.

62. Shephard RJ, Johnson N. Physical activity and the liver. *Eur J Appl Physiol* 2014;Jan;115(1):1–46.

63. Siegel R, Laursen PB. Keeping your cool. Possible mechanisms for enhanced exercise performance in the heat with internal cooling methods. *Sports Med* 2012;42:89–98.

64. Stannard SR, Thompson MW. The effect of participation in Ramadan on substrate selection during submaximal cycling exercise. *J Sci Med Sport* 2008;11:510–517.

65. Stearns RL, Emmanuel H, Volek JS, Casa DJ. Effects of ingesting protein in combination with carbohydrate during exercise on endurance performance: A systematic review with meta-analysis. *J Strength Cond Res* 2010 Aug;24(8):2192–2202.

66. Sweileh N, Schnitzler A, Hunter GR, Davis B. Body composition and energy metabolism in resting and exercising Muslims during Ramadan fast. *J Sports Med Phys Fitness* 1992;32:156–163.

67. Tipton KD, Elliot TA, Cree MG et al. Stimulation of net muscle protein synthesis by whey protein ingestion before and after exercise. *Am J Physiol* 2007;292:E71–E76.

68. Trabelsi K, el-Abed K, Trepanowski JF et al. Effects of Ramadan fasting on biochemical and anthropometric parameters in physically active men. *Asian J Sports Med* 2011;2:134–144.

69. Turcotte LP. Role of fats in exercise. Types and quality. *Clin Sports Med* 1999 Jul; 18(3):485–498.

70. Venkatraman JT, Leddy J, Pendergast D. Dietary fats and immune status in athletes: clinical implications. *Med Sci Sports Exerc* 2000 Jul;32(7 Suppl.):S389–S395.

71. Vogt M, Puntschart A, Howald H et al. Effects of dietary fat on muscle substrates, metabolism, and performance in athletes. *Med Sci Sports Exerc* 2003 Jun;35(6):952–960.

72. Walsh NP, Gleeson M, Shephard RJ et al. Position statement. Part one: Immune function and exercise. *Exerc Immunol Rev* 2011;17:6–63.

73. Waterhouse J. Effects of Ramadan on physical performance: Chronobiological considerations. *Br J Sports Med* 2010;44:509–515.

74. Yeo WK, Carey AL, Burke L et al. Fat adaptation in well-trained athletes: Effects on cell metabolism. *Appl Physiol Nutr Metab* 2011 Feb;36(1):12–22.

75. Zderic TW, Davidson CJ, Schenk S et al. High-fat diet elevates resting intramuscular triglyceride concentration and whole body lipolysis during exercise. *Am J Physiol Endocrinol Metab* 2004 Feb;286(2):E217–E225.

Further Reading

Aziz AR, Png W. Ramadan fasting and sports performance. In: Lanham-New S, Stear S, Shirrefs S, Collins A (eds.), *Sports and Exercise Nutrition*. Wiley-Blackwell, Chichester, U.K., 2011.

Graham TE. The importance of carbohydrate, fat and protein for the endurance athlete. In: *Endurance in Sport*. Shephard RJ, Åstrand P-O (eds.), Blackwell Scientific, Oxford, U.K., 2000.

Lowman SA, Smith DL. *Exercise Physiology for Health Fitness and Performance*, 4th edn. Wolters Kluwer, Lippincott Williams & Wilkins, Philadelphia, PA, 2013.

Shephard, RJ. The impact of Ramadan performance upon athletic performance. *Nutrients* 2012;4:491–505.

11

Tactics to Sustain Training and Competitive Performance during Fasting

Ezdine Bouhlel and Roy J Shephard

Learning Objectives

1. To examine the role of physical activity in fat loss for the obese
2. To review some concepts underlying current training techniques
3. To consider what changes in training patterns are required during fasting or dietary restriction
4. To learn tactics appropriate to a continuation of training during Ramadan observance
5. To understand practical implications for athletes, coaches and trainers

Concepts Underlying Modern Training Techniques

Athletic training essentially involves a sequence of bouts of exhausting exercise, followed by adequate recovery periods, leading to a progressive increase in the individual's competitive performance. The task-specific capacity of the athlete passes through three phases:

1. A phase of fatigue immediately following the training stimulus
2. A recovery (compensation) period that allows the restoration of initial physical abilities
3. A phase of overcompensation, when the physical capacity exceeds the initial level

Performance is not optimized unless the recovery period is adequate. Too rigorous training or a lack of adequate recovery particularly if it is coupled with fasting or dietary restriction, can lead to overreaching or even overtraining, with a marked deterioration in performance [38,42,55]. Training seeks to develop many body functions [1], including the alactic anaerobic, lactic anaerobic and aerobic systems, muscle strength, and coordination. Aerobic training enhances a competitor's endurance and reduces fatigue during prolonged submaximal exercise. It is marked by increased glycogen stores, an enhanced activity of oxidative enzymes and a greater contribution of fat to submaximal metabolism. Anaerobic training is based on repeated bouts of high-intensity exercise. It is marked by increases of anaerobic power and capacity, with an increased activity of anaerobic enzymes, and the development of muscle mass with an increased proportion of fast-twitch fibres.

Laboratory assessments of training include measurements of maximal oxygen intake, anaerobic thresholds (lactic thresholds, LT1 or LT2 and/or ventilatory thresholds, VT1 and VT2), time to exhaustion on a treadmill or cycle ergometer, the critical velocity that can be sustained on a treadmill or cycle ergometer, the fast and slow components of oxygen kinetics, anaerobic capacity and power, heart rate recovery curves, and muscle strength and endurance.

There are many possible patterns of training, often specific to an athlete's type of sport. Sprint interval training (SIT) is one relatively new approach recommended by many scientists and coaches [15,57]; this technique is claimed to enhance both aerobic and anaerobic metabolism.

Changes in Patterns of Training during Fasting or Dietary Restriction

The need for athletes to modify their pattern of training during fasting or dietary restriction depends on both the duration of the fast and the nature of the physical task to be performed. It may be necessary to modify both the volume and the timing of training sessions. There are usually no difficulties in undertaking the normal conditioning programme if the duration of fasting is short and/or the energy cost of the activity is only moderate. However, if the combination of fast duration and exercise volume is enough to deplete muscle glycogen reserves, a fall of blood glucose may cause feelings of weakness, reduce motivation and predispose to muscular injury. Increased catabolic activity may also militate against the normal process of tissue hypertrophy.

Sedentary Individuals

Sedentary individuals who wish to reduce body fat should combine moderate exercise with a moderate restriction of food intake to create a negative energy balance of around 4 MJ/day, at the same time ensuring an increased intake of protein and an adequate minimum ingestion of micronutrients. The cumulative negative energy balance must be sufficient to deplete a person's glycogen reserves, and progressively deplete fat stores, while at the same time it must not be so large as to reduce fat-free body mass. A moderate rather than a high intensity of exercise encourages the metabolism of excess fat rather than carbohydrate and protein. The big issue for those operating fat-loss programmes is usually maintaining programme compliance in terms of adherence to exercise and dietary restrictions over what is necessarily a long process. In some studies, more than a half of those initially enrolled are no longer compliant 6 months after beginning a programme; many have already regained the fat that they initially lost [27].

Programme adherence is helped if details of both the training programme and the dietary restriction are individualized, taking due account of a person's initial physical fitness, their personality and mood state, and the environmental conditions in which they live. A combined programme of exercise and dietary restriction may achieve better adherence than dieting alone, in part because the exercise sessions have a mood-elevating effect. The planning of interventions is helped by the development of sophisticated attitude–behavioural models [30], but to date, there have been few applications of this technique to reductions in body fat. Many obese people have a low initial level of fitness, and they may also be embarrassed by their physical appearance in a gymnasium; walking or swimming programmes may be the best option for attaining and maintaining the required energy expenditures in such individuals.

Some people are naturally gregarious and welcome the support of other dieters in a group programme, but if attendance at a central facility is required several times per week, there may be a discouraging ratio of exercise to travel times, particularly in large city. One practical option is to meet once a week as a group, but to provide a detailed home prescription and exercise log for the remainder of the week. More introverted individuals may be deterred by the enforced bonhomie that seems characteristic of many gymnasia, and they will appreciate suggestions for solitary exercise such as active transportation to and from their place of employment. Extremes of hot and cold weather can hamper maintenance of the required exercise volume. Particularly if physical activity is combined with a restricted fluid intake, attempts to exercise under hot ambient conditions can cause dehydration and a variety of medical problems ranging from muscle cramps to cardiovascular collapse and renal failure. The main issue with very cold weather is the danger of slipping on icy surfaces; fasting may also reduce the ability to maintain body temperature by shivering, although this problem is easily overcome by adjustments of clothing.

The simplest remedy at times of either heat or cold weather is to move the required daily bout of physical activity into an air-conditioned environment; for example, a person could walk briskly for a substantial distance around an air-conditioned shopping mall.

If the fasting is intermittent, as when observing Ramadan, exercise could be performed just before eating the post-sunset meal or some 3 hours later; the latter tactic avoids the weakness associated with carbohydrate and fluid depletion, but has the disadvantage of disturbing sleep patterns.

Athletes

Athletes restrict their energy intake for two main reasons: the making of a specific body mass in weight-categorized sports and when attempting to enhance their appearance in activities such as gymnastics and figure skating. Such dietary restrictions could induce metabolic changes and health disorders, particularly a reduced secretion of testosterone and oestrogen, which could impair their response to strength training [48,64].

From the viewpoint of the sports physician, neither of these two reasons for dietary restriction are to be commended. But if an athlete is determined to follow such a plan, it is important to maintain training while dieting. The main item to cut from the diet is lipids. Carbohydrate intake should be maintained to avoid fatigue, and protein intake should be increased to avoid a loss of lean tissue. It may also be wise to vary the pattern of training and to make an allowance for longer recovery times following a training session. The adoption of SIT [14,15,57] may be a useful tactic, allowing a decrease in total training time, while continuing to develop both aerobic and anaerobic performance. The intensive exercise required by such a regimen stimulates the quasi-totality of muscle fibres, inducing favourable enzymatic and biochemical changes in both slow- and fast-twitch fibres. It may also be possible to reduce the total volume of conditioning by focusing on the quality of training (coordination, technical skills, and tactics) and incorporating the fasting period into a final pre-competitive tapering of exercise intensity [33].

Changes in Volume and Time of Training during Ramadan Observance

Given disturbances of sleep, acute disturbances of blood sugar and fluid balance, and fears of impaired performance, it is not surprising that some athletes report increased perceptions of effort when exercising during Ramadan [2,39,68]. There is a risk that because of such perceptions, athletes may lighten the duration [66] or volume [20,21] of training, in an attempt to reduce sensations of fatigue and to compensate for the absence of energy and fluid intake during daylight hours [47] (Table 11.1). Ramadan observance can have an adverse impact upon both training and competitive performance [52], although a brief daytime fast of perhaps 12 hours duration should have only minor physiological effects [36]. Low- to moderate-intensity exercise can be well tolerated by athletes during Ramadan [49,50,54,58], and some competitors have succeeded in maintaining their normal conditioning regimen, apparently without any significant disadvantage to either health or performance.

One investigation noted that during Ramadan, the intensity of training continued unchanged at 62% of the players' heart rate reserve [40]. Another report found no significant decrease in the daily training load, as measured in training impulse (TRIMPS) units, despite a shortening of training sessions [66]. National-level rugby players [10,11] continued to undertake their customary five 2 h training sessions per week, although since much of their training involved sport practice, intensity

TABLE 11.1 Changes in the Pattern of Athletic Training during Ramadan Observance

Authors	Subjects	Training Regimen	Response
Aziz et al. [4]	20 adolescent males, half fasting	High-intensity cycle ergometer interval training	Training maintained with intermittent fasting, equivalent training response
Bouhlel et al. [10,11]	9 rugby players	Five 2-hour sessions per week, mainly practice games	No change in frequency or duration of training; intensity not reported
Bouhlel et al. [12]	6 throwers, 4 sprinters	Training 30 h/week	No change in frequency or duration of training; intensity not reported
Bouhlel et al. [13]	10 karatekas	Five 2-hour sessions/ week	No change in frequency or duration of training; intensity not reported
Burke [16], Burke and King [17]	Review articles	Athletes cautioned not to exceed their capacity during fast	3 options for training: after sunrise, 3 hours after fast at night, or just before breaking fast
Chaouachi et al. [19–21]	15 judoka	Training 6 days/week	Training maintained; no details given
Chennaoui et al. [23]	8 middle-distance runners	Training 8.8 h/week	Training maintained; no details given
Chtourou et al. [24]	10 junior soccer players	Training 2 h/day, 4 days/week	No change in training; details not reported
Damit et al. [26]	Review article		Training response unaltered if sufficient training intensity maintained
Karli et al. [34]	11 elite power athletes	Training 2 h/day, 6 days/week	No change in frequency, duration or intensity of training
Kirkendall et al. [35]	53 junior soccer players	No details	No change in training; details not recorded
Kirkendall et al. [36]	Review article		Training commonly reduced
Kordi et al. [37]	34 athletes (volleyball, karate, taekwondo and soccer)	No details	Subjects able to maintain normal training 1 hour before or 3 hours after Iftar
Leiper et al. [39]	48 junior soccer players	No details	No change in training heart rate, training duration, load or TRIMPS
Maughan et al. [43]	Review article		Elite athletes maintain training, close to sunset best time
Meckel et al. [44]	Adolescent soccer players	Training 6.4 h/week	Training dropped from 6.4 to 4.5 h/week, physical education classes cancelled

(*Continued*)

TABLE 11.1 (*Continued*) Changes in the Pattern of Athletic Training during Ramadan Observance

Authors	Subjects	Training Regimen	Response
Mujika et al. [47]	Review article		Decreased training in many athletes, maintained in elite
Roy et al. [54]	65 national elite athletes		Training frequently modified as coping tactic; training early morning or late evening
Sweileh et al. [60]	14- to 16-year-old soccer players	Normally training 6.4 h/week	Training decreased from 6.4 to 5.2 h/week
Waterhouse [65]	Review article		Nighttime training recommended
Wilson et al. [66]	20 professional soccer players	Details not given	Training shortened, but no change of TRIMPS; nighttime training
Zerguini et al. [67]	55 professional soccer players	Details not given	70% of players thought training was impaired
Zerguini et al. [68]	64 young soccer players	Details not given	Heart rates show no change during training sessions

could conceivably have been reduced. Likewise, throwers and sprinters at a regional sports school continued 18 h/week of training during Ramadan [12]. Leiper et al. [40] found that the intensity of training was similar in fasted and non-fasted young soccer players, whether their regimen was quantified in terms of TRIMPS [7], training loads [28] or ratings of perceived exertion [9]. Performances improvements were also similar in fasted and non-fasted subjects, although heart rate increases were larger in the fasted individuals. In contrast, less experienced 14–16-year-old soccer players allowed their duration of training to decrease from 6.4 to 5.2 h/week during Ramadan [61], and in a second study a decrease of training from 6.4 to 4.5 h/week was exacerbated by cancelling of their physical education classes [44].

Mujika et al. [47] and Chaouachi et al. [22] argued that experienced elite Muslim athletes could maintain a normal training programme during Ramadan, with at most only minor adverse effects upon their physical performance. Maughan et al. [43] agreed that high-level athletes who observed Ramadan could maintain their performance if physical training, food and fluid intake, and sleep were all well controlled. An individualized regulation of the daily training load was recommended, using ratings of perceived exertion, heart rate measurements and questionnaires to prevent fatigue, overreaching or overtraining with their associated risks of illness and injury [18]. Aziz et al. [4] found unchanged aerobic and anaerobic training responses during Ramadan fasting. Damit et al. [26] also maintained that the training response was unchanged during Ramadan, provided that the training programme was adequate and dietary intake was optimized. Further, Eirale et al. [29] found no significant change in the incidence of total, match, or training injuries between Ramadan and non-Ramadan periods in top-level soccer players, suggesting that with good planning, adequate adjustments of lifestyle could be organized to avoid the danger of overtraining.

A number of authors have offered practical advice to athletes who are training and competing during the month of Ramadan [41,47,54]. Their suggestions include potential modifications to the frequency, intensity, timing and type of training [41]. Meckel et al. [44] proposed reducing the frequency, intensity and/or duration of training, although admitting that this could have the disadvantage of allowing some detraining to occur [44,56]. Even if an athlete lacks the motivation to undertake all-out training when fasting, continued sport practice is helpful in maintaining skill levels. Possibly, as during pre-competition tapering, training during Ramadan could focus upon the development of technical skills and the quality of training [47], with an emphasis upon high-intensity activities such as repeated sprints [14,15]. Burgomaster et al. [15] found that 2 weeks of SIT induced changes in aerobic and anaerobic potential that matched those obtained with 8 weeks of traditional aerobic training.

Methods of Controlling Training Load

Three simple methods of controlling the training load have been proposed by Banister, Edwards and Borg.

(1) Banister's method: Eric Banister [7] suggested measuring the TRIMPS in units that he called TRIMPS. The calculation was

$$\text{TRIMPS} = \text{Duration (min)} \times \text{Intensity (\% max)}$$
$$\times \text{Correction factor K (dimensionless)}$$

$$\text{Intensity} = (Fc_{exercise} - Fc_{rest})/(Fc_{max} - Fc_{rest})$$

Example: 100 min of training at a heart rate of 150 beats/min in an athlete with resting and maximal heart rates of 50 and 200 beats/min, respectively.

$$\text{Intensity} = (150 - 50)/(200 - 50) = 0.66$$

$$K = 0.64e^{1.92 \times \text{intensity}} = 0.64e^{1.92 \times 0.66} = 2.3$$

$$\text{TRIMPS} = 100 \times 0.66 \times 2.3 = 152$$

The recommended daily training load is 125 TRIMPS for a regional-level runner aged 30–40 years and 250 TRIMPS for young adult elite athletes.

(2) Edwards et al. [28]

$$\text{Training load} = \Sigma \, (\text{Duration (min)} \times (\mathbf{1}: 50\%-60\%; \mathbf{2}: 60\%-70\%;$$
$$\mathbf{3}: 70\%-80\%; \mathbf{4}: 80\%-90\% \text{ and } \mathbf{5}: 90\%-100\% \, Fc_{max})$$

(3) Borg [9]

$$\text{TRIMPS} = \text{RPE} \times \text{Training duration (min)}$$

Changes in Training Time

Training is normally thought to be most effective if it coincides in timing with the daily peak of body temperature, although there may also be some tactical advantage in practising at the time when competition is scheduled [2]. It may also be advantageous to exercise at the time of day when the greatest effort can be generated, and this may change during Ramadan [4,5]. Finally, it is very important that the timing of training sessions coincide with the time when the athlete has ingested the proteins needed for synthesis of muscle tissue [8,31,32,45,51,53,62] and the glycogen that is important to expression of the genes involved in muscle hypertrophy [25]. This last aspect of timing becomes particularly important during the observance of Ramadan.

Maughan et al. [43] suggested a need to adjust the timing of conditioning sessions during Ramadan observance in order to optimize training responses. They argued that event organizers should also take account of the needs of Muslim athletes when scheduling the dates and timing of sports competitions; however, this is easier to arrange in Arab countries than in nations where the majority of athletes are not planning to observe Ramadan. Roy et al. [54] questioned 65 athletes who were observing Ramadan, finding a highly individualized pattern of coping to optimize training and competitive performance in various sports. The International Federation of Football Associations Medical Assessment and Research Centre also underlined that the best tactics for coping with Ramadan were those chosen by the individual athlete [69].

Roy et al. [54] suggested that in order to continue intensive training during Ramadan, athletes should shift their training time to either the early morning or the late evening. The customary mid-afternoon training time coincided with both a relatively long cumulative period of fasting (commonly 10–12 hours) and the hottest part of the day, although the fasting athlete could no longer ingest fluids to replace water losses during the daylight hours. Where possible, training should be shifted to the coolest part of the day in order to minimize fluid losses, and it should focus on quality (intensity) rather than quantity (duration).

Three potentially appropriate exercise times for those observing Ramadan are just before the evening meal, in the late evening, and in the morning, after a pre-dawn meal [16]. Burke [16] preferred the first of these options, because carbohydrate, protein and fluid were available immediately following training; however, the considerable dehydration developed over the day of fasting can sometimes impede motivation for maximal training [35,36]. Maughan et al. [43] and Aziz et al. [6] also proposed exercising close to or after sunset, taking into account the individual's training responses and the environmental conditions. Maughan et al. [43] pointed out that if training was taken late in the day, this allowed a meal to be eaten shortly after exercising, thus promoting an anabolic response.

The late evening and early morning are less convenient from a dietary point of view, as these are the times when athletes would have just consumed large amounts of food and fluids. If activity is undertaken in the evening, an hour or more after the evening meal [65,66], scheduling also becomes difficult (particularly if not all athletes are observing Ramadan). Furthermore, there is a strong likelihood that the late night exercise sessions will delay the circadian clock [3], with adverse effects upon both athletic performances and sleep patterns.

If the athlete trains early in the morning, he or she will have the psychological advantage of having consumed two meals since breaking the fast [35,36]. On the other hand, many competitors perceive that it is harder to carry out training early in the day [35,36,66]. Moreover, with such a plan, there is no longer a post-exercise infusion of protein and carbohydrate; rather, the body is attempting to undertake anabolic activity as blood levels of nutrients are waning.

There seem theoretical advantages and disadvantages to all three options, and a carefully controlled trial of their relative merits is needed. One comparison of daytime versus evening training during Ramadan in 34 athletes did not detect any major difference of response between these two approaches [37].

Practical Implications for Athletes

Elite athletes seem able to sustain their normal training load during Ramadan, without significant adverse effects upon health or performance [22,36,47]. Most studies show that if training is maintained, Ramadan observance has at most small effects upon physical performance. Practical and biological difficulties in maintaining training can generally be overcome by adjusting the timing and intensity of conditioning sessions, taking into account individual responses of the athletes to local conditions. The most frequent tactic is to move training sessions close to or after sunset. The training stimulus then coincides with a surge of amino acids and glucose that facilitates the anabolic process [30].

Maintenance of a normal training regimen is not easy during Ramadan, and some lower echelon competitors reduce the duration [66] and/or intensity of their training programme [20,21]. This adjustment can often be incorporated into a planned pre-competitive *tapering* of conditioning [46,63]. The optimal pattern of tapering has a maximum duration of about 2 weeks, with a 40%–60% decrease in the total training load [63]. Tapering yields an immediate gain in competitive performance, but if the reduced training continues, as much as 10% of previously achieved training adaptations may be lost [46].

Conclusions

In sedentary individuals, regular moderate physical activity plays an important role in reducing fat mass, conserving lean tissue and enhancing mood state. However, poor adherence remains a major challenge to programme organizers. An adequate ratio of total work to recovery times is important to achieving physiological adaptations and associated increases of performance with an athletic training programme. The intermittent fasting of Ramadan provides a physiological stimulus somewhat analogous to repeated bouts of exercise [59]. The metabolic (after training or competition) and nutritional recovery (after a day of fasting) should be sufficient to allow the athlete to undertake competition or a further training with maintained or even improved performance, and several reports have suggested that a normal training response can be achieved during Ramadan. The timing of training sessions should be adjusted during Ramadan so that they coincide with meal-related surges of nutrients and avoids the hottest periods of the day. The most popular option is currently to train immediately before the sunset meal, although there remains a need for a carefully controlled study of possible coping options.

Key Terms

Coping: Coping is the process whereby an individual reduces or counteracts the negative impact of an event or circumstance upon his or her physical or mental performance.

Fatigue: Fatigue can be defined as a reduction of physical or mental performance following exposure to a stressful situation (such as intense or prolonged exercise, prolonged dietary restriction, a disturbance of biological rhythm or illness). In the context of athlete assessment, it is often examined by having the competitor complete a profile of mood states questionnaire.

Overtraining: Overtraining is a condition that develops if an athlete engages in an intensity and/or duration of training that is excessive relative to current physical fitness, and/or the recovery interval following a training session is of inadequate duration. In its more moderate form of overreaching, the problem can be corrected by a few weeks reduction of training, but if fully developed, performance may remain impaired for many months. The only reliable indicators of overtraining are deterioration in athletic performance and an adverse score on the profile of mood states.

Tapering: Tapering denotes a planned reduction of training loads in the days immediately before competition; this maximizes recovery and optimizes an athlete's performance.

Training load: The training load reflects the combined stimulus to an improvement of physical condition, reflecting the intensity, frequency and duration of exercise, and the length of recovery periods used during training.

Key Points

1. Regular exercise is important to fat loss in sedentary subjects; careful programming is needed to maximize client programme adherence.
2. An adequate training and recovery ratio is important to the effective training of athletes, both when eating a normal diet and during periods of dietary restriction.

3. Training and fasting should be carefully graded to avoid fatigue, over-training and associated health problems.
4. Regular review and appropriate adjustments of both training and dietary restrictions (quality and quantity) should be undertaken, taking into account the physiological responses of the individual.
5. During Ramadan observance, the best option seems to move training sessions close to or immediately after sunset, although there remains a need for further study of possible options.
6. Elite athletes seem able to maintain a normal training regimen during Ramadan observance.
7. Further studies are needed to examine possible adaptations of training for athletes at lower levels of physical condition.

Questions for Discussion

1. What arguments would you advance to an obese person who was pre-pared to diet, but did not wish to increase their physical activity?
2. How would you determine the magnitude of the training stimulus in a given athlete, and how would you decide whether this was optimal?
3. What is the optimal training load to suggest to a fasting athlete?
4. How would you decide upon the optimal time to train during the obser-vance of Ramadan?
5. What considerations would guide your recommendation of tapering tac-tics to an athlete who wished to observe Ramadan?

References

1. Åstrand PO, Rodhal K. *Précis de physiologie de l'exercice musculaire*. Editions Masson, Paris, France, 1994.
2. Atkinson G, Reilly T. Circadian variation in athletic performance. *Sports Med* 1996;21:292–312.
3. Atkinson G, Edwards B, Reilly T et al. Exercise as a synchroniser of human circadian rhythms: An update and discussion of the methodological problems. *Eur J Appl Physiol* 2007;99:331–241.
4. Aziz AR, Slater GJ, Chiac MYH, Teh KC. Effects of Ramadan fasting on training induced adaptations to a seven-week high-intensity interval exercise programme. *Sci Sports* 2012;27:31–38.
5. Aziz AR, Chia MY, Low CY et al. Conducting an acute intense interval exercise session during the Ramadan fasting month: What is the optimal time of the day? *Chronobiol Int* 2012 Oct;29(8):1139–50.
6. Aziz AR, Png W, Che Muhamed A et al. Effects of Ramadan fasting on substrate oxi-dation, physiological and perceptual responses during submaximal intensity running in active men. *Sport Sci Health* 2014 Apr;10(1):1.
7. Banister EW. Modeling elite aerobic performance. In: Green H, McDougall J, Wenger H (eds.), *Physiological Testing of Elite Athletes*. Human Kinetics, Champaign, IL, 1991.
8. Beelen M, Burke LM, Gibala MJ et al. Nutritional strategies to promote post-exercise recovery. *Int J Sport Nutr Exerc Metab* 2010;20:515–532.

9. Borg G. The perception of physical performance. In: *Frontiers of Fitness*, Shephard RJ (ed.), Charles Thomas, Springfield, IL, 1971.

10. Bouhlel E, Salhi Z, Bouhlel H et al. Effect of Ramadan fasting on fuel oxidation during exercise in trained male rugby players. *Diabetes Metab* 2006;32:617–624.

11. Bouhlel E, Zaouali M, Miled A et al. Ramadan fasting and the GH/IGF-I axis of trained men during submaximal exercise. *Ann Nutr Metab* 2008;52:261–266.

12. Bouhlel H, Shephard RJ, Gmada N et al. Effect of Ramadan observance on maximal muscular performance of trained men. *Clin J Sport Med* 2013 May;23(3):222–227.

13. Bouhlel H, Shephard RJ, Adela H et al. Ramadan observance and aerobic exercise in male karatekas. *Health Fitness J Can* 2013;30:99–107.

14. Burgomaster KA, Cermak NM, Phillips SM et al. Divergent response of metabolite transport proteins in human skeletal muscle after sprint interval training and detraining. *Am J Physiol Regul Integr Comp Physiol* 2007 May;292(5):R1970–R1976.

15. Burgomaster KA, Howarth KR, Phillips SM et al. Similar metabolic adaptations during exercise after low volume sprint interval and traditional endurance training in humans. *J Physiol* 2008 Jan 1;586(1):151–160.

16. Burke L. Fasting and recovery from exercise. *Br J Sports Med* 2010;44(7):502–508.

17. Burke LM, King C. Ramadan fasting and the goals of sports nutrition around exercise. *J Sports Sci* 2012;30(Suppl. 1):S21–S31.

18. Chamari K, Haddad M, Wongdel P et al. Injury rates in professional soccer players during Ramadan. *J Sports Sci* 2012;30(Suppl. 1):S93–S102.

19. Chaouachi A, Chamari K, Roky R et al. Lipid profiles of judo athletes during Ramadan. *Int J Sports Med* 2008;29:282–288.

20. Chaouachi A, Leiper JB, Souissi N et al. Effects of Ramadan intermittent fasting on sports performance and training: A review. *Int J Sports Physiol Perform* 2009;4:419–434.

21. Chaouachi A, Coutts AJ, Chamari K et al. Effect of Ramadan intermittent fasting on aerobic and anaerobic performance and perception of fatigue in male elite judo athletes. *J Strength Condit Res* 2009;23:2702–2709.

22. Chaouachi A, Leiper JB, Chtourou H et al. The effects of Ramadan intermittent fasting on athletic performance: Recommendations for the maintenance of physical fitness. *J Sports Sci* 2012;30(Suppl. 1):S53–S73.

23. Chennaoui M, Desgorces F, Drogou C et al. Effects of Ramadan fasting on physical performance and metabolic, hormonal, and inflammatory parameters in middle-distance runners. *Appl Physiol Nutr Metab* 2009;34:587–594.

24. Chtourou H, Hammouda O, Chaouachi A et al. The effect of time of day and Ramadan fasting on anaerobic performances. *Int J Sports Med* 2012;33:142–147.

25. Churchley EG, Coffey VG, Pedersen DJ et al. Influence of preexercise muscle glycogen content on transcriptional activity of metabolic and myogenic genes in well-trained humans. *J Appl Physiol* 2007;102:1604–1611.

26. Damit NF, Lim VTW, Muhamed AMC et al. Exercise responses and training during daytime fasting in the month of Ramadan and its impact on training-induced adaptations. In: Chtourou H (ed.), *Effects of Ramadan Fasting on Health and Athletic Performance.* OMICS Group eBooks, Foster City, CA, 2013.

27. Dishman RK. *Exercise Adherence: Its Impact on Public Health.* Human Kinetics, Champaign, IL, 1988.

28. Edwards AM, Macfadyen AM, Clark N. Test performance indicators from a single soccer specific fitness test differentiate between highly trained and recreationally active soccer players. *J Sports Med Phys Fitness* 2003 Mar;43(1):14–20.

29. Eirale C, Tol JL, Smiley F et al. Does Ramadan affect the risk of injury in professional football? *Clin J Sport Med* 2013 Jul;23(4):261–266.

30. Godin G, Shephard RJ. Use of attitude-behaviour models in exercise promotion. *Sports Med* 1990;10:103–121.

31. Hartman JW, Tang JE, Wilkinson SB et al. Consumption of fat-free milk after resistance exercise promotes greater lean mass accretion than does consumption of soy or carbohydrate in young, novice, male weightlifters. *Am J Clin Nutr* 2007;86:373–381.

32. Hawley JA, Gibala MJ, Bermon S. Innovations in athletic preparation: Role of substrate availability to modify training adaptation and performance. *J Sports Sci* 2007;25(Suppl. 1): S115–S124.

33. Joyce D, Lewindon D. *High Performance Training for Sports*. Human Kinetics, Champaign, IL, 2014, p. 299.

34. Karli U, Güvenç A, Aslan A et al. Influence of Ramadan fasting on anaerobic performance and recovery from short high intensity exercise. *J Sport Sci Med* 2007;6:490–497.

35. Kirkendall DT, Leiper JB, Bartagi Z et al. The influence of Ramadan on physical performance measures in young Muslim footballers. *J Sports Sci* 2008;26(Suppl. 3):S15–S27.

36. Kirkendall DT, Chaouachi A, Aziz A-R et al. Strategies for maintaining fitness and performance during Ramadan. *J Sports Sci* 2012;30(Suppl. 1):S103–108.

37. Kordi R, Abdullahi M, Memari M-H et al. Investigating two different training time frames during Ramadan. *Asian J Sports Med* 2011;2:205–210.

38. Kreher JB, Schwartz JB. Overtraining syndrome. A practical guide. *Sports Health* 2012;4(2):128–138.

39. Leiper JB, Junge A, Maughan RJ et al. Alteration of subjective feelings in football players undertaking their usual training and match schedule during the Ramadan fast. *J Sports Sci* 2008;26(Suppl. 3):S55–S69.

40. Leiper JB, Watson P, Evans G, Dvorak J. Intensity of a training session during Ramadan in fasting and non-fasting Tunisian youth football players. *J Sports Sci* 2008 Dec;26(Suppl. 3): S71–S79.

41. Lim VTW, Damit NF, Aziz AR. In: Chtourou H (ed.), *Effects of Ramadan Fasting on Health and Athletic Performance*. OMICS Group eBooks, Foster City, CA, 2013.

42. Mackinnon LT, Hanrahan SJ, Hooper SL. *Over-Training and Recovery in Elite Athletes*. National Sports Training Research Centre, Belconnen, Australian Capital Territory, Australia, 1996.

43. Maughan RJ, Zerguini Y, Chalabi H, Dvorak J. Achieving optimum sports performance during Ramadan: Some practical recommendations. *J Sports Sci* 2012;30(Suppl. 1):S109–S117.

44. Meckel Y, Ismael A, Eliakim A. The effect of the Ramadan fast on physical performance and dietary habits in adolescent soccer players. *Eur J Appl Physiol* 2008;102:651–657.

45. Moore DR, Robinson MJ, Fry JL et al. Ingested protein dose response of muscle and albumin protein synthesis after resistance exercise in young men. *Am J Clin Nutr* 2009;89:161–168.

46. Mujika I, Padilla S, Pyne D. Swimming performance changes during the final 3 weeks of training leading to the Sydney 2000 Olympic Games. *Int J Sports Med* 2002 Nov; 23(8):582–587.

47. Mujika I, Chaouachi A, Chamari K. Precompetition taper and nutritional strategies: Special reference to training during Ramadan intermittent fast. *Br J Sports Med* 2010 Jun;44(7):495–501.

48. Onambele GN, Bruce SA, Woledge RC. Oestrogen status in relation to the early training responses in human thumb adductor muscles. *Acta Physiol* 2006;188(1):41–52.

49. Ramadan JM, Barac-Nieto M. Cardio-respiratory responses to moderately heavy aerobic exercise during the Ramadan fasts. *Saudi Med J* 2000 Mar;21(3):238–244.

50. Ramadan J. Does fasting during Ramadan alter body composition, blood constituents and physical performance? *Med Princ Pract* 2002;11(Suppl. 2):41–46.

51. Rasmussen BB, Tipton KD, Miller SL et al. An oral essential amino acid-carbohydrate supplement enhances muscle protein anabolism after resistance exercise. *J Appl Physiol* 2000;88:386–292.

52. Reilly T, Waterhouse J. Altered sleep-wake cycles and food intake: The Ramadan model. *Physiol Behav* 2007;90:219–228.

53. Rodriguez NR, Vislocky LM, Gaine PC. Dietary protein, endurance exercise, and human skeletal muscle protein turnover. *Curr Opin Clin Nutr Metab Care* 2007;10:40–45.
54. Roy J, Ooi CH, Singh R et al. Self-generated coping strategies among Muslim athletes during Ramadan fasting. *J Sports Sci Med* 2011;10:137–144.
55. Shephard RJ. *Physical Activity, Training and the Immune Response*. Cooper Publications, Carmel, IN, 1997.
56. Shephard RJ. Ramadan and sport: Minimizing effects upon the observant athlete. *Sports Med* 2013 Dec;43(12):1217–1241.
57. Spencer M, Bishop D, Dawson B, Goodman C. Physiological and metabolic responses of repeated-sprint activities: Specific to field-based team sports. *Sports Med* 2005;35(12):1025–1044.
58. Stannard SR, Thompson MW. The effect of participation in Ramadan on substrate selection during submaximal cycling exercise. *J Sci Med Sport* 2008 Sep;11(5):510–517.
59. Stannard SR. Ramadan and its effect on fuel selection during exercise and following exercise training. *Asian J Sports Med* 2011 Sep;2(3):127–133.
60. Sweileh NA. *The Effects of Ramadan Fasting on Maximum Oxygen Intake and Maximum Performance*. University of Alabama, Birmingham, U.K., 1988.
61. Sweileh N, Schnitzler A, Hunter GR et al. Body composition and energy metabolism in resting and exercising Muslims during Ramadan fast. *J Sports Med Phys Fitness* 1992;32:156–163.
62. Tipton KD, Elliot TA, Cree MG et al. Stimulation of net muscle protein synthesis by whey protein ingestion before and after exercise. *Am J Physiol* 2007;292:E71–E76.
63. Thomas L, Mujika I, Busso T. A model study of optimal training reduction during pre-event taper in elite swimmers. *J Sports Sci* 2008;26:643–652.
64. Vingren JL, Kraemer WJ, Ratamess NA et al. Testosterone physiology in resistance exercise and training: The up-stream regulatory elements. *Sports Med* 2010;40(12):1037–1053.
65. Waterhouse J. Effects of Ramadan on physical performance: Chronobiological considerations. *Br J Sports Med* 2010;44:509–515.
66. Wilson D, Drust B, Reilly T. Is diurnal lifestyle altered during Ramadan in professional Muslim athletes? *Biol Rhythm Res* 2009;40:385–397.
67. Zerguini Y, Kirkendall D, Junge A et al. Impact of Ramadan on physical performance in professional soccer players. *Br J Sports Med* 2007;41:398–400.
68. Zerguini Y, Dvorak J, Maughan RJ et al. Influence of Ramadan fasting on physiological and performance variables in football players: Summary of the F-MARC 2006 Ramadan fasting study. *J Sports Sci* 2008;26(Suppl. 3):S3–S6.
69. Zerguini Y, Ahmed QA, Dvorak J. The Muslim football player and Ramadan: Current challenges. *J Sports Sci* 2012;30(Suppl. 1):S3–S7.

Further Reading

Åstrand P-O, Rodahl K, Dahl H, Strømme SB. *Textbook of Work Physiology*, 4th edn. Human Kinetics, Champaign, IL, 2003.
Kreher JB, Schwartz JB. Overtraining syndrome. A practical guide. *Sports Health* 2012;4(2):128–138.
Mujika I. *Tapering and Peaking for Optimal Performance*. Human Kinetics, Champaign, IL, 2009.
Svedenhag J. Endurance conditioning. In: Shephard RJ, Åstrand P-O (eds.), *Endurance in Sport*, 2nd edn. Blackwell Scientific, Oxford, U.K., 2000, pp. 402–408.

12

Coping and Recovery Tactics during Fasting and Dietary Restriction

Ezdine Bouhlel, Roy J Shephard and Mohamed Dogui

Learning Objectives

1. To review some physiological mechanisms involved in recovery from exercise and to examine the likely impact of fasting and dietary restriction upon these mechanisms
2. To focus upon sleeping, napping, resting and mental preparation as important components of the recovery process
3. To learn some recovery tactics that can be recommended to athletes and coaches for use during the observance of Ramadan

Recovery Mechanisms Following an Exercise Bout

A full recovery following a bout of training is very important to continued effective conditioning and to the achievement of maximal exercise potential at the time when a competition is scheduled. An efficient training programme draws an appropriate balance between training loads and recovery intervals. Tactics for ensuring complete recovery in the period immediately before athletic competition include a tapering of conditioning [45], or if normal training is continued, appropriate nutrition, sleep and the use of relaxation techniques and mental preparation. Issues of tapering have been presented in Chapter 11.

The recovery processes include restoration of the initial metabolic status (oxygen and phosphagen stores, oxidation of accumulated lactate), the normalization of resting metabolism, the rebuilding of energy and fluid reserves and the repair of any tissue injury. We will examine each of these processes and will consider how they may be affected by fasting or dietary restriction.

Restoration of Initial Metabolic Status

Restoration of the initial metabolic status requires a rebuilding of energy stores and a full elimination of the metabolites accumulated during the preceding bout of exercise. An understanding of the time course of these processes is important both to the planning of interval training and to the design of training schedules that will not lead to overtraining and tissue injury.

Oxygen Stores

The lungs contain about 1000 mL of oxygen, and about a half of this can be used during activities such as a breath-hold dive. A normal oxygen concentration is restored with the first few breaths after completing a dive.

Some oxygen is also found in physical solution in the blood and tissues, but oxygenated haemoglobin and myoglobin provide the other main body stores of oxygen [63]. At full oxygen saturation, the haemoglobin in the blood has an oxygen content of some 200 mL/L, so that with a blood volume of 5 L, haemoglobin can carry a maximum of about 1000 mL of oxygen; in endurance athletes, the size of this potential store is augmented by an increase in the haemoglobin content of unit volume of blood and an expansion of the total blood volume. Under normal resting conditions, some 80% of the haemoglobin is in the venous part of the circulation, where the typical oxygen content is 140 mL/L, and most of the remaining 20% is in the arteries, where the oxygen content is normally about 190 mL/L. Thus, the typical resting oxygen store in the blood of a sedentary individual is around 750 mL.

The maximal oxygen content of myoglobin is about 11.2 mL/kg of muscle, and in a person with a body mass of 70 kg and a total muscle mass of 30 kg, this could provide a further store of up to 340 mL of oxygen. The magnitude of this oxygen store varies somewhat, depending on the individual's fibre composition, being greater in strength athletes than in endurance competitors. Myoglobin stores are also increased by both aerobic and muscular training.

Following a bout of exercise, oxygen stores are 75%–80% replenished in 10 s and fully replenished in 20–30 s. Thus, interval training commonly provides rest intervals of 10–30 s. Dehydration, whether for making weight or during Ramadan observance, could reduce a competitor's blood volume, but this should not change oxygen stores at least initially, because the haemoglobin concentration will increase.

Phosphagen Stores

The immediate source of energy for muscular contraction is found in the high-energy bonds of adenosine triphosphate (ATP) and creatine phosphate (CP) molecules within the active muscles. The total store of these molecules in a person with a muscle mass of 28 kg has been estimated at 193 mmol of ATP and 560 mmol of CP [63]. Depletion of the active muscles is relatively complete over as little as 5–6 seconds; replenishment is an exponential process, with a half-time that has been estimated at 20 seconds [63]; thus, at intervals of 30 s, 2 minutes and 4 minutes post exercise, restoration is 70%, 84% and 89%, and some 6–8 minutes is needed for full recovery [57].

Lactate Accumulation and Elimination

The lactate produced during intensive exercise reduces tissue pH, with a negative effect upon physical performance. The lactate is largely metabolized during the recovery process, although small amounts of lactate are also excreted in sweat and urine. Clearance proceeds in an approximately exponential fashion, although the speed of clearance is more rapid with active recovery (a continuation of moderate physical activity that maintains circulation to the muscles that have been exercised) than with passive recovery such as sitting on a cycle ergometer. The rate of lactate clearance is optimal if the continuing activity demands around 60% of the individual's maximal oxygen intake. Typical times to eliminate 50% of accumulated lactate are 6 minutes with active recovery compared with 10–15 minutes during passive recovery. The process is essentially complete with 20 minutes of active recovery, compared with up to 90 minutes during passive recovery [21].

There are two opinions about the main route of lactate metabolism during recovery. Brooks [8] argued that most of the lactate is oxidized to carbon dioxide and water in the muscles, myocardium and kidneys. In this context, Brooks [9,10] proposed the concept of a *lactate shuttle*; he argued that the lactate was transported via the blood stream to many parts of the body, particularly slow- and fast-twitch muscle fibres and the heart, where it was oxidized in place of alternative metabolites. Brooks emphasized that muscles were able not only to produce lactate but also to transport and to use it as a source of energy as soon as their oxygen supply was restored. The alternative fate of lactate is a resynthesis to glycogen in muscles, liver and kidneys, with the necessary energy for this process being derived from oxidation of perhaps 10% of the accumulated lactate [33]. This last process depends on levels of insulin and other anabolic hormones, and it may thus be slowed during fasting.

Normalization of Resting Metabolism

The resting metabolism remains elevated for a substantial time following a bout of vigorous exercise, sometimes as long as 24 hours. Many factors contribute to this delayed recovery, commonly described as excess post-exercise oxygen consumption (EPOC). Influences include the metabolism of lactate and the replenishment of fuel stores; a continuing increase of cardiac and respiratory energy expenditures; a persisting elevation of body temperature (which inevitably boosts the energy expenditure of all tissues); a continued circulation of stimulatory hormones, particularly the catecholamines; tissue repair; and hypertrophy. The magnitude of EPOC depends on both the intensity and the duration of the exercise session [39].

The post-exercise increase of oxygen consumption is an important consideration for people who are seeking to reduce body fat; this is one reason why the metabolic rate falls in those who rely simply upon dieting (Chapter 11), but remains at a normal level in those who combine dieting with a moderate exercise programme. There do not appear to have been any studies of EPOC during Ramadan, but to the extent that adrenaline levels are increased, it might last longer during Ramadan than at other times of the year.

Rebuilding of Energy and Fluid Reserves

Most bouts of physical activity deplete most of the body's glycogen reserves, and repeated exercise with inadequate recovery intervals (as in an event such as a cross-Canada run) or severe dietary restriction can also decrease fat stores and lead to the breakdown of tissue protein [46,62]. Water deficits can be made good within a few hours, the limiting factor being the gastric emptying rate of about 1 L/h. However, depending on diet and physical activity patterns, the restoration of protein and fat depots can take several months.

Glycogen Reserves

Glycogen depletion and lactate production can occur during submaximal exercise if activity continues for longer than 90 minutes. It develops much earlier during interval exercise, as high-intensity activity blocks local blood flow and forces the metabolism of carbohydrate rather than fat. With interval training, much thus depends on the intensity and duration of individual exercise bouts [59]. Glycogen usage is greater during intermittent exercise of 60 seconds duration with 120 seconds recovery intervals than it is in exercise of 10 or 20 seconds duration, with 20 and 40 seconds recovery intervals. During very short exercise bouts, much of the energy is provided from oxygen stores and phosphagen usage, rather than lactate production (see preceding text).

After a bout of exercise that induces glycogen depletion, resynthesis usually occurs in exponential fashion, although the speed of the recovery process depends on the extent of glycogen depletion, the physical fitness of the individual, and the dietary regimen that is followed. Resynthesis is usually 50% complete within about 5 hours [47], and the process is completed within about 2 days.

Carbohydrate Administration during the Recovery Period

Carbohydrate loading has beneficial effects, whether introduced before, during or after exercise. The glycogen depletion of prolonged exercise stimulates glycogen synthesis during recovery. The administration of carbohydrates augments activity of the enzyme glycogen synthase, with both an increase in the velocity of glycogen synthesis and an increase in the magnitude of final glycogen stores relative to initial values [58]. At least 50–100 g of carbohydrate should be consumed within 1–2 hours of ceasing exercise to maximize glycogen resynthesis [36], and in a person who is training hard, a total carbohydrate intake of 500–600 g may be needed to optimize glycogen stores [17]. Vigorous exercise can counter efforts at replenishment, but activities demanding less than 65% of maximal oxygen intake do not seem to have a negative effect [26]. The need for carbohydrate immediately following a training session is a factor that should be remembered when planning the times of conditioning during Ramadan observance.

The velocity of glycogen resynthesis depends on the nature of the carbohydrate that is ingested, in part because this modifies the rate of gastric emptying. Glucose and sucrose yield similar rates of muscle glycogen replenishment, both being more effective than complex carbohydrates or fructose, but fructose is the most effective carbohydrate for replenishing liver glycogen reserves [24]. Ingestion of a meal with a high glycaemic index speeds glycogen replenishment, but has the disadvantage that it also increases glycogen usage during a subsequent bout of physical activity [76,77]. A low glycaemic index meal taken 3 hours before exercise enhances endurance relative to a high glycaemic index meal of equal energy content [81]. The addition of protein to carbohydrate solutions also seems to extend the time to exhaustion, reduces markers of muscle damage and speeds post-exercise recovery, probably because of a synergistic action of carbohydrate and protein in stimulating insulin secretion [37]. On the other hand, damage to the muscle membrane induced by eccentric exercise can affect glucose transporters and thus reduce the rate of glycogen resynthesis [24].

Maximal glycogen storage is particularly important if an athlete must perform aerobic exercise on many days in succession, with inadequate time to replenish reserves. A sedentary person has a muscle glycogen store of some 400 g and a further 100 g of glycogen in the liver, but the peak glycogen stores of an endurance athlete can rise to at least 40 g/kg of body muscle, a total store of about 1.3 kg [60].

Recently, Che Muhamed et al. [13] reported that even mouth rinsing with either 25 mL carbohydrate solution or with 25 mL placebo for 5 seconds before exercise induced amelioration of 10 km time trial performance in Ramadan-fasted young subjects during endurance cycling in a heat stress environment (32°C and 75% relative humidity).

Some authors reported a large glycogen replenishment after ingesting a rich CHO diet (70% of CHO) consecutive to a significant decrease of glycogen stores. The decrease of CHO stores could be related to intense training and/or fasting [51,79]. Williams et al. [78] found aerobic performance enhancement after adopting a high-CHO diet. Exercise-induced glycogen depletion was more pronounced during fasting and was associated with enhanced glycogen synthesis during recovery periods.

Muscle Injuries

Sustained exercise appears to induce changes in the cell membranes of both skeletal and cardiac muscle, allowing the leakage of cellular contents into the blood stream. In the case of skeletal muscle, leakage is seen particularly after eccentric exercise; it gives rise to muscle soreness and is marked biochemically by increased concentrations of the enzyme creatine kinase in the plasma [4]. In the case of the heart, participation in ultramarathon and triathlon events is associated with a leakage of cardiac troponins into the plasma [61]. Potential factors influencing membrane permeability include mechanical stress, an increased production of oxidants (Chapter 8) and an altered acid–base balance.

Changes are usually short lived (1–3 days), and indeed, the increase in permeability of the cell membrane may be a necessary part of allowing entry of the additional amino acids required for tissue hypertrophy. Nevertheless, it seems unwise to undertake further very strenuous exercise until there is recovery from these changes. The speed of the recovery process is likely influenced by plasma concentrations of key amino acids. For this reason, it is important to ensure adequate protein intake during dietary restriction, and to arrange the timing of Ramadan training sessions so that they come shortly before or after the taking of high-protein meals.

Other Physical Recovery Techniques

The athlete may use a variety of personal techniques to cope with the immediate stresses of competition and speed physiological recovery. Options include active recovery techniques [22,25], warm baths and massage [19], contrast temperature water immersion [5,32], cryotherapy, oxygen therapy, compression garments, stretching and electromyostimulation. Such adjuvants are particularly important during dietary restriction, because training is then more difficult and there is a greater likelihood of minor muscle injury.

Hot baths and massage have much the same rationale as active recovery, speeding the local circulation, and facilitating the removal of lactate and oedema fluid. Heat, massage and stretching may also counter the delayed onset muscle soreness associated with minor muscle injuries. There is growing interest in post-exercise immersion in ice water or alternating cold and warm water [14,40], with several authors advocating either contrast immersion or immersion in cold water (10°C–15°C) for 5–15 minutes [49,73]. Contrast immersion induces periods of vasodilatation, followed by vasoconstriction, and it is argued that 3–6 sets of both treatments should stimulate the peripheral blood flow. Water immersion is claimed to minimize fatigue and to accelerate recovery, allowing greater training loads, and enhancing the effectiveness of a given training load [73]. Delextrat et al. [19] reported that both massage and cold-water immersion improved recovery processes and subsequent jump performance, although in their study of basketball players cold-water immersion seemed more effective than massage. Stretching also appeared to increase the efficacy of massage [20]. Cold-water immersion gave faster recovery than contrast water therapy in Australian football players who had undertaken repeated sprints [23].

Viitasalo et al. [74] suggested that underwater water-jet massage speeded recovery from intensive physical exercise. Hausswirth et al. [32] showed that after a track event causing muscle damage, whole body cryotherapy was more effective than far-infrared or passive recovery modalities. Bieuzen et al. [5] also found whole body cryotherapy was superior to passive recovery.

Psychological Recovery and Mental Preparation

Mental preparation and adequate relaxation are important tactics that can enhance recovery processes and thus the competitive performance of athletes [6,56]. Objectives are to enhance physical and mental activation, mood state, concentration, self-confidence and emotional control, sometimes described as psyching up for competition [6,31]. The development of positive attitudes is critical to competitive success [28]. Forms of mental imagery such as memorization of successful situations, positive self-talk and body language are techniques that have been used effectively by athletes both during and after competition [6,31,70]. Such positive thinking is particularly important during dietary restriction, when the temptation is to fear that competition with those who are not fasting is unlikely to be successful. The mental rehearsal of competitive skills can help performance, possibly as much as physical performance of the activities in question [35], and mental rehearsal is certainly a valuable early option when recovery is as yet insufficient to allow physical involvement.

Overactivity of the sympathetic nervous system is a characteristic of the athlete who has been overreaching or overtraining [30], and it may develop in response to the challenges of combining Ramadan observance with continued training and competition. Excessive arousal may be addressed by such techniques as meditation, listening to soothing music and the regulation of breathing. From a social perspective, distractions such as watching television, reading a book, sightseeing in a park, or joking with friends could diminish the stress arising from combined training and dietary restriction. In addition, those who are fasting may find comfort in daily prayers and in showing patience, self-control and a positive attitude toward others [56].

Rest, Napping and Sleeping during Fasting

Experimental Fasting

In general, those who are fasting tend to reduce their physical activity in order to minimize fatigue and avoid any associated health problems. The classical tactics of sleeping, napping and mental preparation can be helpful in coping with the constraints imposed by fasting. An empirical study of subjects with an initial normal body mass index [44] showed that at the end of 1 week of modified fasting (an energy intake 1.2 MJ/day) that reduced body mass by 3.5 kg, both the quality of sleep and daytime mental performance were improved. Following the modified fast, there were significantly fewer arousals, fewer leg movements, and a non-significant trend to an increase of rapid eye movement (REM) sleep. Daytime performance was also enhanced in terms of vigilance, vigor and emotional balance. The mechanisms of benefit have yet to be clarified; possible factors could include an increased nocturnal secretion of growth hormone and a lesser secretion of thyroid hormone.

Sleep Patterns

Sleep patterns can be investigated using such techniques as polysomnography and actigraphy or studying responses to standardized sleep questionnaires and daily journals. There are four main levels of sleep, identified by rapid eye movement (REM), are as follows:

- *NREM 1*: A stage between sleep and wakefulness, when the eyes roll slowly, opening and closing, and the electroencephalogram (EEG) shows alpha waves.
- *NREM2*: The EEG shows theta waves, and people are harder to awake.
- *NREM3*: Slow-wave sleep (SWS), with large delta waves in the EEG; many environmental stimuli no longer produce any reactions.
- *REM*: REM sleep is characterized by rapid eye movements. It is sometimes called paradoxical sleep, since the EEG waves are similar to those seen when waking, although the person is hardest to arouse at this stage in the sleep cycle.

Sleep proceeds through 4 or 5 cycles of some 90 minutes duration each night, usually in the sequence N1, N2, N3, N2, REM. Many people require 7–8 hours of good-quality sleep to restore all biological functions, but there are wide interindividual differences; sleep is relatively ineffective if it is taken at an inappropriate time in the individual's biological cycle. SWS (NREM3) comprises about 50% of a sleep cycle, and it makes the most important contribution to recovery processes. NREM3 sleep is most pronounced early during the night, and getting to sleep early is more reparative than remaining in bed in the morning. REM sleep is related to cognitive processes and learning; it is important later during the night. A combination of SWS and REM sleep permits both recovery and learning processes.

Disruption of sleep cycles during fasting could lead to fatigue and a reduction of both physical and cognitive performances.

Shlisky et al. [68] reviewed interactions between sleep deprivation and energy balance. Loss of sleep increased the secretion of ghrelin and decreased the output of leptin, increasing energy intake, and this problem was compounded by waking at night, with opportunities for additional snacking. Because of hormonal deregulation, there may also be a tendency to metabolize lean tissue rather than fat.

Most authors have observed that food intake is increased with severe sleep restriction [11,69], often with the development of obesity [15,16]. Provision of adequate sleep seems important to both the preservation of lean tissue and the avoidance of obesity.

Sleep and Recovery Processes

The quality and the quantity of sleep have a major impact upon the effectiveness of recovery processes, both in sedentary individuals and in athletes. Coaches should thus seek environmental conditions that favour adoption of good sleep patterns, while taking account of wide interindividual differences in the needs for both sleep and daytime naps and reactions to sleep deprivation [71].

Ramadan Observance and Sleep

Most studies of athletes observing Ramadan have shown some decrease in total sleep duration and a shift in the timing of sleep [55,65] (Table 12.1), although it has been less clear whether this reflected specific displacements of circadian rhythm, altered hormone secretion due to daytime abstinence from food and fluids, or simply the incidentals of Ramadan such as additional social and religious duties, late evening meals, training late at night and drinking additional fluids during the hours of darkness. In support of an incidental effect from the overall Ramadan environment, several authors have reported similar changes in observant and non-observant individuals [2,41,83]. Several authors have found that the sleep times of athletes were unchanged during Ramadan observance [7,29,38,43,67]. Güvenç [29] found unchanged sleeping time and daily energy of soccer players during Ramadan. Bouhlel et al. [7] also found unchanged sleep time in young karatekas. About a half of the athletes studied by Singh et al. [67] reported unchanged sleep patterns, but nevertheless, two-thirds of their group complained of increased daytime sleepiness. In contrast, Aziz et al. [1] found no increase of sleepiness during Ramadan observance in a small group of nine trained athletes. BaHammam et al. [3] also argued that despite some shifts in the timing and duration of sleep during Ramadan observance, there was no increase of sleepiness.

Any disturbances in sleep–wake behaviour during Ramadan are associated with a shortened total sleep time [34,65] and especially a loss of nocturnal sleep, with a deterioration of daytime vigilance [52,54,55] and increases in subjective and objective daytime sleepiness [53]. Roky et al. [52] attributed an increase in sleep latency and a decrease in SWS duration to the inversion of normal eating and drinking schedules. Any reduction in sleep time was often accompanied by negative effects on subjective well-being and athletic performance [53].

When Ramadan occurs during the winter, there is little reason why Ramadan observance should disrupt an athlete's sleep [65,66].

If Ramadan occurs in the summer, the situation is more difficult; the athlete should go to sleep as soon as possible after eating the evening meal and try to sleep through until the latest possible time for taking breakfast, supplementing this with daytime naps where possible.

TABLE 12.1 Changes of Sleep during Ramadan Observance in Sedentary and Athletic Individuals

Author	Subjects	Change during Ramadan Observance
Sedentary individuals		
BaHammam [2]	71 healthy non-athletes, 30 non-fasting	60–90 minutes delay in bedtime, no sleep loss. Sleep patterns also modified in controls
BaHammam et al. [3]	8 observant, 8 non-observant subjects	Start of work delayed 150 minutes for observant subjects, bedtime and waking times delayed, sleep time reduced by 60–70 minutes, no increase of daytime sleepiness, no change of reaction times
Roky et al. [52]	8 healthy males	Increase in sleep latency, decrease in slow-wave and REM sleep, 40 minutes shortening of sleep time
Roky et al. [53]	8 healthy males	Increase in subjective and objective daytime sleepiness
Athletes		
Aziz et al. [1]	9 trained athletes	No increase of daytime sleepiness, duration of sleep not reported
Bouhlel et al. [7]	15 karatekas	No change of sleeping time
Chennaoui et al. [12]	8 middle-distance runners	88 min/day of sleep loss during Ramadan
Güvenç [29]		No change of sleeping time or daily energy level
Herrera [34]	9 male soccer players	78 min/day less sleep in the fourth week of Ramadan compared with days before Ramadan
Karli et al. [38]	Male power athletes (2 wrestlers, 7 sprinters, 1 thrower)	No significant change of daily sleep time
Leiper et al. [41]	54 observant, 33 non-observant male soccer players	Loss of 60 minutes sleep/day throughout Ramadan in those fasting; those not fasting lost 105 min/day during the first week of Ramadan
Meckel et al. [43]	19 male adolescent soccer players	No change of daily sleep time
Singh et al. [67]	734 miscellaneous male and female junior athletes	No disturbance of sleep patterns
Waterhouse et al. [75]	20 male university sport students	Bedtime delayed 171 minutes, 126 min/day sleep loss
Wilson et al. [80]	20 male professional soccer players	Bedtime delayed 199 minutes, but total daily sleep increased 99 minutes
Zerguini et al. [83]	64 observant junior soccer players, 36 non-observant	Loss of 60 min/day sleep throughout Ramadan in those fasting; those not fasting lost 105 min/night during the first week of Ramadan (same group of subjects as Leiper)

Ramadan Observance and Napping

Any disruption of normal sleep patterns during Ramadan is likely to have negative effects upon both physical and cognitive performance [18,48,50,64,72]. Coaches should thus help athletes to plan their sleep patterns, adding daytime naps to compensate for any nighttime curtailment of sleep [55]. The quality and duration of nighttime sleep must be evaluated relative to the normal sleep patterns of the athlete, and any additional naps should be taken in a darkened room at a neutral temperature.

Wilson et al. [80] suggested that athletes should try to stay in bed until midafternoon, thus avoiding unnecessary incidental activities and conserving their energy reserves for competition. Others have found that light active recovery, for instance, swimming, playing volleyball or playing Frisbee in cold water, helped the recovery process. Certainly, the social components of Ramadan celebration should be minimized, and athletes should get to sleep as early as possible. They should also be encouraged to take afternoon naps if they feel sleepy during the daytime [56]. However, if naps are too prolonged, they can cause a loss of arousal in the central nervous system, with an increase of melatonin secretion that leaves the athlete feeling lethargic and dozy.

A varied combination of passive and active recovery seems the best approach to help the athlete recover metabolically, nervously and psychologically from intensive training.

Practical Implications for Athletes

A number of aspects of the recovery process are challenged by dietary restriction, but with careful management of lifestyle, successful competitive performance can be maintained. Rest and sleep are the most important coping tactics that can enhance recovery processes during fasting or dietary restriction, and every effort should be made to obtain adequate sleep throughout Ramadan. If sleep is inadequate, immune function is depressed [82], and even the healing of injuries is slowed [27]. The athlete should go to bed as early as possible; should take a nap in the afternoon in a calm, dark room at a neutral temperature, according to his or her needs; he or she should also minimize non-essential physical activities during the period of fasting. Periods of resting and sleeping can be interwoven with physiotherapeutic modalities that speed recovery, such as stretching, massage and water immersion. Contrast water immersion and/or cold water immersion are of special interest for athletes who are observing daytime water deprivation while living in hot countries, as they reduce the tendency to sweat. Individualized mental preparation supervised by a sports psychologist can also help the athlete to develop positive attitudes (calmness, concentration, self-control, determination and patience) despite the challenges imposed by dietary restriction.

Conclusions

Many studies show little disturbance of recovery patterns during the observance of Ramadan. Adequate sleep is the most important component of a full recovery, and unless great care is taken, the external concomitants of Ramadan such as late night meals and training can shift the hours of sleeping and the total time available for sleeping, with a negative impact upon the physical and mental performance of the athlete. If sleep is disturbed, it can have a much greater impact upon physical and cognitive performance than the intermittent hunger and thirst imposed by Ramadan. However, elite athletes have demonstrated that they can maintain their normal performance if physical training, food and fluid intake, and sleep are all appropriate and well controlled [42]. Coaches should plan sleep patterns for their athletes, taking into account essential activities, environmental conditions and individual differences in the need for sleep. Competitors should be advised to retire to bed early and to take an afternoon nap when necessary, under optimal conditions for relaxation. Nonessential physical activities should also be avoided to conserve energy reserves. Physiotherapeutic modalities such as massage, stretching and cold or contrast water immersions can be added to speed up the recovery; cold immersion is particularly helpful when observing Ramadan in a hot climate. Such tactics should be coupled with mental preparation to control emotions and to avoid the negative attitudes that can be caused by attempts to maintain training in the face of hunger and dehydration.

Key Terms

Cardiac troponin: There are two forms of troponin, one characteristic of skeletal muscle and the other of cardiac tissue. The appearance of cardiac troponin in the blood stream after prolonged and strenuous exercise is thought to indicate minor damage to the myocardial cells.

Contrast immersion: A technique used by some sports physiotherapists that involves immersing a limb in alternating warm and cold water following a bout of exercise. The expectation of those using this technique is that the warmth will produce vasodilatation, the cold vasoconstriction, and that the overall effect will be an increase of local circulation, removing oedema fluid and waste products.

Creatine kinase: The muscle damage associated with eccentric exercise is associated with the leakage of intracellular material into the blood stream. Plasma concentrations of the enzyme creatine kinase are commonly used as a biological marker of this process.

Cryotherapy: Cryotherapy is a physiotherapeutic modality based on the application of cold to the body or a part of the body; it may help the recovery process by decreasing inflammation.

Delayed-onset muscle soreness: Delayed onset muscle soreness is the discomfort and/or pain felt in muscles for hours to several days following a bout of severe physical activity, particularly eccentric exercise. It is thought to reflect microtrauma in the muscle fibres.

Electromyostimulation: Electromyostimulation involves the application of an electrical stimulus to muscle tissue (usually as square wave pulses of 50–100 Hz, lasting for 300–400 µs); one aim is to increase local blood flow and stimulate the repair of damaged tissue, but the contractions induced by the stimulus may also increase muscle strength and power.

Glycogen synthase: Glycogen synthase is the enzyme involved in the synthesis of glycogen; depletion of glycogen reserves stimulates the activity of this enzyme during the recovery process.

Haemoglobin: Haemoglobin is the red pigment in the red blood cells. It has a high affinity for oxygen, and if the blood is exposed to 100% oxygen, the oxygen content rises to around 200 mL/L.

Lactate shuttle: The lactate shuttle is a biochemical mechanism that transports lactate within and between cells; it plays an important role in eliminating lactate from the active muscle fibres following a bout of vigorous exercise.

Mental imagery: Athletes attempt to enhance their performance by mental imagery, where they imagine themselves as being successful in competition.

Myoglobin: Myoglobin is the red pigment found in muscle fibres, particularly fast-twitch muscle fibres. It has an even higher affinity for oxygen than haemoglobin, and oxygen is thus transferred from the blood stream to the muscles.

SWS: SWS is a deep form of sleep (stage 3 on the scale of the American Academy of Sleep Medicine). It is important for memory, learning and the recovery of brain function.

Stretching: Deliberate stretching of muscles is practised to develop flexibility as a means of warm-up, and to facilitate recovery after strenuous physical exercise.

Key Points

1. Adequate rest and sleep are more important than dehydration and hunger as determinants of physical and cognitive performance and recovery of function during the observance of Ramadan.
2. Coaches and athletes should control and respect individual sleep patterns and maximize opportunities for necessary sleep in order to permit efficient recovery between training sessions and events.
3. Rest and sleep can be supplemented by other sports physiotherapy modalities such as contrast water immersion and/or mental preparation to enhance recovery processes.

4. Taking an afternoon nap as needed and avoiding non-essential physical activities seem effective tactics to reduce fatigue during Ramadan observance.

5. Further studies are needed to determine how far Ramadan observance influences the recovery process and the optimal choice among many competing tactics for overcoming adverse influence of fasting and dietary restriction upon these processes.

Questions for Discussion

1. How would you determine whether an athlete was adopting optimal recovery tactics between training sessions?
2. Which components of sleep are most important to an athlete?
3. What advice about sleeping would you give to an athlete who was planning to observe Ramadan?
4. What sports physiotherapy modalities might be particularly helpful to recovery during Ramadan observance?

References

1. Aziz AR, Chia MY, Low CY et al. Conducting an acute intense interval exercise session during the Ramadan fasting month: What is the optimal time of the day? *Chronobiol Int* 2012 Oct;29(8):1139–1150.
2. BaHammam A. Assessment of sleep patterns, daytime sleepiness, and chronotype during Ramadan in fasting and nonfasting individuals. *Saudi Med J* 2005;26:616–622.
3. BaHammam AS, Alaseem AM, Alzakri AA, Sharif MM. The effects of Ramadan fasting on sleep patterns and daytime sleepiness: An objective assessment. *J Res Med Sci* 2013 Feb;18(2):127–131.
4. Baird MF, Graham SM, Baker JS et al. Creatine kinase and exercise-related muscle damage. Implications for muscle performance and recovery. *J Nutr Metab* 2012;ID 960363.
5. Bieuzen F, Bleakley CM, Costello JT. Contrast water therapy and exercise induced muscle damage: A systematic review and meta-analysis. *PLoS ONE* 2013 Apr 23;8(4):e62356.
6. Brody EB, Hatfield BD, Spalding TW et al. The effect of a psyching strategy on neuromuscular activation and force production in strength-trained men. *Res Q Exerc Sport* 2000 Jun;71(2):162–170.
7. Bouhlel H, Shephard RJ, Gmada N et al. Effect of Ramadan observance on maximal muscular performance of trained men. *Clin J Sport Med* 2013 May;23(3):222–227.
8. Brooks GA, Brauner KE, Cassens RG Glycogen synthesis and metabolism of lactic acid after exercise. *Am J Physiol* 1973 May;224(5):1162–1166.
9. Brooks GA. Anaerobic threshold: Review of the concept and directions for future research. *Med Sci Sports Exerc* 1985 Feb;17(1):22–34.
10. Brooks GA. Current concepts in lactate exchange. *Med Sci Sports Exerc* 1991;23(8):895–906.
11. Calvin AD, Carter RE, Adachi T et al. Effects of experimental sleep restriction on caloric intake and activity energy expenditure. *Chest* 2013 Jul;144(1):79–86.
12. Chennaoui M, Desgorces F, Drogou C et al. Effects of Ramadan fasting on physical performance and metabolic, hormonal, and inflammatory parameters in middle-distance runners. *Appl Physiol Nutr Metab* 2009;34:587–594.

13. Che Muhamed AM, Mohamed NG, Ismail N et al. Mouth rinsing improves cycling endurance performance during Ramadan fasting in a hot humid environment. *Appl Physiol Nutr Metab* 2014 Apr;39(4):458–464.
14. Cochrane DJ. Alternating hot and cold water immersion for athlete recovery: A review. *Phys Therap Sport* 2004;5:26–32.
15. Copinschi G. Metabolic and endocrine effects of sleep deprivation. *Essent Psychopharmacol* 2005;6(6):341–347.
16. Copinschi G, Leproult R, Spiegel K. The important role of sleep in metabolism. *Front Horm Res* 2014;42:59–72.
17. Coyle EF. Timing and method of increased carbohydrate intake to cope with heavy training, competition and recovery. *J Sports Sci* 1991;9:29–52.
18. Davis GM, Plyley MJ, Gottesman ST et al. Variations in cardiorespiratory and strength parameters during moderate exercise and sleep deprivation. *Can J Appl Sports Sci* 1982;7 236–237.
19. Delextrat A, Calleja-González J, Hippocrate A, Clarke ND. Effects of sports massage and intermittent cold-water immersion on recovery from matches by basketball players. *J Sports Sci* 2013;31(1):11–19.
20. Delextrat A, Hippocrate A, Leddington-Wright S, Clarke ND. Including stretches to a massage routine improves recovery from official matches in basketball players. *J Strength Cond Res* 2014 Mar;28(3):716–727.
21. di Prampero PE. Anaerobic capacity and power. In: Shephard RJ (ed.), *Frontiers of Fitness*. CV.C. Thomas, Springfield, IL, 1971.
22. Dodd S, Powers SK, Callender T, Brooks E. Blood lactate disappearance at various intensities of recovery exercise. *J Appl Physiol Respir Environ Exerc Physiol* 1984 Nov;57(5):1462–1465.
23. Elias GP, Varley MC, Wyckelsma VL et al. Effects of water immersion on posttraining recovery in Australian footballers. *Int J Sports Physiol Perform* 2012 Dec;7(4):357–366.
24. Friedman JE, Neufer PD, Dohm GL. Regulation of glycogen resynthesis following exercise. Dietary considerations. *Sports Med* 1991 Apr;11(4):232–243.
25. Gmada N, Bouhlel E, Mrizak I et al. Effect of combined active recovery from supramaximal exercise on blood lactate disappearance in trained and untrained man. *Int J Sports Med* 2005 Dec;26(10):874–879.
26. Goforth HD, Laurent W, Prusaczyk K et al. Effects of depletion exercise and light training on muscle glycogen supercompensation in men. *Am J Physiol* 2003;285:E1304–E1311.
27. Gümüştekín K, Seven B, Karabulut N et al. Effects of sleep deprivation, nicotine, and selenium on wound healing in rats. *Int J Neurosci* 2004;114(11):1433–1442.
28. Guthrie M. *Coaching Track and Field Successfully*. Human Kinetics, Champaign, IL, 2003.
29. Güvenç A. Effects of Ramadan fasting on body composition, aerobic performance and lactate, heart rate and perceptual responses in young soccer players. *J Hum Kinet* 2011 Sep;29:79–91.
30. Hahn AG. Training, recovery and overtraining—The role of the autonomic nervous system. *Sports Coach* 1994;29–30.
31. Hammoudi-Nassib S, Nassib S, Chtara M et al. Effects of psyching-up on sprint performance. *J Strength Cond Res* 2014 Jan 28. e-pubh. ahead of print.
32. Hausswirth C, Louis J, Bieuzen F et al. Effects of whole-body cryotherapy vs. far-infrared vs. passive modalities on recovery from exercise-induced muscle damage in highly-trained runners. *PLoS ONE* 2011;6(12):e27749.
33. Hermansen L. Effect of metabolic changes on force generation in skeletal muscle during maximal exercise. In: CFS 82 (ed.), *Human Muscle Fatigue: Physiological Mechanisms*. Pitman Medical, London, U.K., 1981.
34. Herrera CP. Total sleep time in Muslim football players is reduced during Ramadan: A pilot study on the standardized assessment of subjective sleep-wake patterns in athletes. *J Sports Sci* 2012;30(Suppl. 1):S85–S91.

35. Holmes PS, Collins DJ. The PETTLEP approach to motor imagery: A functional equivalence model for sport psychologists. *J Appl Sport Psychol* 2001;13:60–83.
36. Ivy JL, Katz AL, Cutler CL et al. Muscle glycogen synthesis after exercise: Effects of time of carbohydrate ingestion. *J Appl Physiol* 1988;65:1480–1485.
37. Jenkins DJA, Wolever TMS, Jenkins AL et al. The glycaemia response to carbohydrate foods. *Lancet* 1984;2:388–391.
38. Karli U, Güvenç, A, Aslan A et al. Influence of Ramadan fasting on anaerobic performance and recovery from short high intensity exercise. *J Sport Sci Med* 2007;6:490–497.
39. La Forgia J, Withers RT, Gore CJ. Effects of exercise intensity and duration on the excess post exercise oxygen consumption. *J Sports Sci* 2006;24(12):1247–1264.
40. Lateef F. Post exercise ice water immersion: Is it a form of active recovery? *J Energ Trauma Shock* 2010;3(3):302–310.
41. Leiper JB, Junge A, Maughan RJ et al. Alteration of subjective feelings in football players undertaking their usual training and match schedule during the Ramadan fast. *J Sports Sci* 2008;26(Suppl. 3):S55–S69.
42. Maughan RJ, Zerguini Y, Chalabi H, Dvorak J. Achieving optimum sports performance during Ramadan: Some practical recommendations. *J Sports Sci* 2012;30 (Suppl. 1): S109–S117.
43. Meckel Y, Ismael A, Eliakim A. The effect of the Ramadan fast on physical performance and dietary habits in adolescent soccer players. *Eur J Appl Physiol* 2008;102:651–657.
44. Michalsen A, Schlegel F, Rodenbeck A et al. Effects of short-term modified fasting on sleep patterns and daytime vigilance in non-obese subjects: Results of a pilot study. *Ann Nutr Metab* 2003;47(5):194–200.
45. Mujika I, Chaouachi A, Chamari K. Precompetition taper and nutritional strategies: Special reference to training during Ramadan intermittent fast. *Br J Sports Med* 2010 Jun;44(7):495–501.
46. O'Hara WJ, Allen C, Shephard RJ et al. La Tulippe: A case study of a one hundred and sixty kilometre runner. *Br J Sports Med* 1977;11:83–87.
47. Piehl K. Time course for refilling of glycogen stores in human muscle fibres following exercise-induced glycogen depletion. *Acta Physiol Scand* 1974 February;90(2):297–302.
48. Plyley MJ, Shephard RJ, Davis GM, Goode RC. Sleep deprivation and cardiorespiratory function. Influence of intermittent sub-maximal exercise. *Eur J Appl Physiol* 1987;56:388–344.
49. Pournot H, Bieuzen F, Duffield R et al. Short term effects of various water immersions on recovery from exhaustive intermittent exercise. *Eur J Appl Physiol* 2011 Jul;111(7):1287–1295.
50. Reilly T, Waterhouse J. Altered sleep-wake cycles and food intake: The Ramadan model. *Physiol Behav* 2007 Feb 28;90(2–3):219–228.
51. Riché D. *Guide nutritionnel des sports d'endurance*. Editions Vigot, Paris, France, 1998, p. 369.
52. Roky R, Chapotot F, Hakkou F et al. Sleep during Ramadan intermittent fasting. *J Sleep Res* 2001 Dec;10(4):319–327.
53. Roky R, Chapotot F, Benchekroun MT et al. Daytime sleepiness during Ramadan intermittent fasting: Polysomnographic and quantitative waking EEG study. *J Sleep Res* 2003 Jun;12(2):95–101.
54. Roky R, Houti I, Moussamih S et al. Physiological and chronobiological changes during Ramadan intermittent fasting. *Ann Nutr Metab* 2004;48(4):296–303.
55. Roky R, Herrera CP, Ahmed Q. Sleep in athletes and the effects of Ramadan. *J Sports Sci* 2012;30(Suppl. 1):S75–S84.
56. Roy J, Hwa OC, Singh R et al. Self-generated coping strategies among Muslim athletes during Ramadan fasting. *J Sports Sci Med* 2011;10:137–144.
57. Sahlin K, Harris RC, Hultman E. Resynthesis of creatine phosphate in human muscle after exercise in relation to intramuscular pH and availability of oxygen. *Scand J Clin Lab Invest* 1979 Oct;39(6):551–558.

58. Saitoh S, Tasaki Y, Tagami K et al. Muscle glycogen repletion and pre-exercise glycogen content: Effect of carbohydrate loading in rats previously fed a high fat diet. *Eur J Appl Physiol* 1994;68:483–488.
59. Saltin B, Karlson J. Muscle glycogen utilization during work of different intensities. In: Pernow B, Saltin B (eds.), *Muscle Metabolism during Exercise*. Plenum, New York, 1971, pp. 289–300.
60. Saltin B, Hermansen L. Glycogen stores and prolonged severe exercise. In: Blix G (ed.), *Nutrition and Physical Activity*. Almqvist and Wiksell, Uppsala, Sweden, 1967.
61. Shave R, Baggish A, George K et al. Exercise induced cardiac troponin elevation: Evidence, mechanisms and implications. *J Am Coll Cardiol* 2010;56(3):169–176.
62. Shephard RJ, Conway DS, Thomson M et al. Nutritional demands of sub-maximum work: Marathon and Trans-Canada events. In: Pavluk J (ed.), *International Symposium on Athletic Nutrition*. Polska Federacja Sportu, Warsaw, Poland, 1977.
63. Shephard RJ. *Physiology and Biochemistry of Exercise*. Praeger Publications, New York, 1982.
64. Shephard RJ. Sleep, biorhythms and human performance. *Sports Med* 1984;1:11–37.
65. Shephard RJ. The impact of Ramadan observance upon athletic performance. *Nutrients* 2012 Jun;4(6):491–505.
66. Shephard RJ. Ramadan and sport: Minimizing effects upon the observant athlete. *Sports Med* 2013 Dec;43(12):1217–1241.
67. Singh R, Hwa OC, Roy J et al. Subjective perception of sports performance, training, sleep and dietary patterns of Malaysian junior Muslim athletes during Ramadan intermittent fasting. *Asian J Sports Med* 2011 Sep;2(3):167–176.
68. Shlisky JD, Hartman TJ, Kris-Etherton PM et al. Partial sleep deprivation and energy balance in adults: An emerging issue for consideration by dietetics practitioners. *J Acad Nutr Diet* 2012 Nov;112(11):1785–1797.
69. St-Onge MP. The role of sleep duration in the regulation of energy balance: Effects on energy intakes and expenditure. *J Clin Sleep Med* 2013 Jan 15;9(1):73–80.
70. Tod D, Iredale F, Gill N. 'Psyching-up' and muscular force production. *Sports Med* 2003;33(1):47–58.
71. Van Dongen HPA, Baynard MD, Maislin G et al. Systematic interindividual differences in neurobehavioral impairment from sleep loss: Evidence of trait-like differential vulnerability. *Sleep* 2004;27(3):423–433.
72. Van Dongen HP, Dinges DF. Sleep, circadian rhythms, and psychomotor vigilance. *Clin Sports Med* 2005 Apr;24(2):237–249, vii–viii.
73. Versey NG, Halson SL, Dawson BT. Water immersion recovery for athletes: Effect on exercise performance and practical recommendations. *Sports Med* 2013 Nov;43(11):1101–1130.
74. Viitasalo JT, Niemelä K, Kaappola R et al. Warm underwater water-jet massage improves recovery from intense physical exercise. *Eur J Appl Physiol Occup Physiol* 1995;71(5):431–438.
75. Waterhouse J, Alabed H, Edwards B et al. Changes in sleep, mood and subjective and objective responses to physical performance during the daytime in Ramadan. *Biol Rhythm Res* 2009;40:367–383.
76. Wee S-L, Williams C, Gray S et al. Influence of high and low glycemic index meals on endurance running capacity. *Med Sci Sports Exerc* 1999;31(3):393–399.
77. Wee S-L, Williams C, Tsintzas K et al. Ingestion of a high-glycemic index meal increases glycogen storage at rest but augments its utilization during subsequent exercise. *J Appl Physiol* 2005;99(2):707–714.
78. Williams C, Brewer J, Walker M. The effect of a high carbohydrate diet on running performance during a 30-km treadmill time trial. *Eur J Appl Physiol Occup Physiol* 1992;65(1):18–24.
79. Williams MH. *Nutrition for Health, Fitness & Sport*. McGraw Hill, Boston, MA, 1999, 500pp.

80. Wilson D, Drust B, Reilly T. Is diurnal lifestyle altered during Ramadan in professional Muslim athletes? *Biol Rhythm Res* 2009;40:385–397.
81. Wu CL, Williams C. A low glycemic index meal before exercise improves endurance running capacity in men. *Int J Sport Nutr Exerc Metab* 2006;16(5):510–527.
82. Zager A, Andersen ML, Ruiz FS et al. Effects of acute and chronic sleep loss on immune modulation of rats. *Am J Physiol* 2007;293 (1):R504–R509.
83. Zerguini Y, Dvorak J, Maughan RJ et al. Influence of Ramadan fasting on physiological and performance variables in football players: Summary of the F-MARC 2006 Ramadan fasting study. *J Sports Sci* 2008;26(Suppl. 3):S3–S6.

Further Reading

Barnett A. Using recovery modalities between training sessions in elite athletes: Does it help? *Sports Med* 2006;36(9):781–796.
Hausswirth C, Mujika I. *Recovery for Performance in Sport*. Human Kinetics, Champaign, IL, 2013.
Hussain TP. *Sports Physiotherapy*. Pinnacle Technology, Lawrence, KS, 2011.
Minett GM, Duffield R. Is recovery driven by central or peripheral factors? A role for the brain in recovery following intermittent-sprint exercise. *Front Physiol* 2014 February 3;5:24.
Shephard, RJ. *Physiology and Biochemistry of Exercise*. Praeger Publications, New York, 1982.
Wilcock IM, Cronin JB, Hing WA. Physiological response to water immersion: A method for sport recovery? *Sports Med* 2006;36(9):747–765.
Zuluaga M. *Sports Physiotherapy: Applied Science and Practice*. Churchill-Livingstone, Melbourne, Victoria, Australia, 1995.

13

Miscellaneous Medical Issues during Dietary and Fluid Restriction

Roy J Shephard

Learning Objectives

1. To learn the implications of dietary and fluid restrictions for those involved in doping control
2. To understand the impact of dietary and fluid restrictions upon the use of prescribed medications
3. To evaluate the impact of a combination of vigorous exercise and repeated fasting upon long-term health
4. To assess the risk of athletic injuries during Ramadan and other forms of dietary and fluid restriction
5. To understand the implications of Ramadan observance and other forms of fluid restriction for the regulation of body temperature
6. To learn ways in which athletes who observe dietary and fluid restrictions can be helped during international competitions

Dietary and Fluid Restrictions and Doping Control Measures

Current Regulations

The commonest form of doping control applied by the World Anti-Doping Agency (WADA) is to test urine specimens for the presence of drugs on a list of prohibited substances. *In competition* tests are conducted on the winners and other randomly selected competitors. *Out of competition* tests are also conducted at various times

257

during the year, without advance warning; the athlete must provide details of his or her whereabouts on a continuous basis in order to allow such testing when required by the regulators.

Case of Christian Negouai

Christian Negouai was a member of the Manchester City professional soccer team. In the year 2002, he had been fined £2000 (about $3000) after missing a required drug test. He was again selected for a random drug test in 2003, following a routine training session. He was not very cooperative, and (in conjunction with the team manager) he claimed that he had been forced to break his fast and drink water in order to provide the required volume of urine [65]. However, after an inquiry into this allegation, U.K. Sport's chief executive officer denied this report; doping control officers had been willing to wait until nightfall, if necessary, for the required sample, thus allowing Negouai to rehydrate within the framework of Ramadan. U.K. Sport further noted that test candidates 'are always provided with sealed, non-alcoholic, caffeine-free drinks to aid them in producing a sample, but the use of these is no more than a recommendation'.

Urine specimens are collected in the presence of a chaperone from the agency and also an athlete's representative (if so desired). The specific gravity (SG) of the urine must meet a minimum value; with the most accurate method of measurement (a refractometer [62]), the threshold SG is 1.05, and if the determination is made with the much less reliable reagent strips, the requirement is an SG of 1.010; no threshold has been specified for use of a hydrometer, and no maximum SG is specified. The volume of the urine sample should be at least 90 mL. If this volume cannot be produced, the sample is declared a partial sample, and the athlete must wait under supervision until a further specimen can be produced.

Problems in Providing the Minimum Required Volume of Urine

Difficulty in producing the required minimum volume of urine is possible with any type of severe dehydration, but has been documented particularly in those observing Ramadan. Such athletes, if required to produce a urine sample immediately following an event, may be sufficiently dehydrated that they cannot produce a 90 mL specimen. The problem is most likely to arise after endurance events and team games. In the London Olympics of August 2012, two of the Morocco men's soccer team were asked to provide urine samples for doping control. They were contacted immediately after their match, and had not drunk any fluid for about 12 hours, so they experienced difficulty in producing the required specimens. In accordance with the WADA and International Olympic Committee rules, they agreed to remain in the stadium in the presence of the antidoping officers, until they were finally able to produce small samples of urine about 150 minutes after competition [70].

Waiting under supervision for 150 minutes after an event is plainly unpopular, and it has occasionally led to charges of religious discrimination, as in the case of Christian Negouai, a British national league soccer player [4,66]. Officials commonly offer test candidate non-alcoholic, caffeine-free drinks to help them in urinating. However, the immediate use of such a beverage is not compulsory. In the case of Negouai, the stated policy of U.K. Sport was to wait with the player until nightfall, if necessary, in order to obtain the required sample of urine [69].

Problems in Analysing Concentrated Urine Specimens

Competitors are allowed to use some substances, but only in small amounts as monitored by specific upper limits that are set for urinary concentrations. In theory, this might pose problems for athletes who produce a highly concentrated urinary specimen because of the dehydration associated with Ramadan observance or other types of dehydration.

Caffeine is one such restricted drug. Urinary concentrations of up to 12 mg/L are considered as representing a normal daily consumption of caffeine-containing beverages, but concentrations >12 mg/L are seen as evidence of deliberate doping. About 1000 mg of caffeine, equivalent to eight cups of coffee, is required to exceed the 12 mg/L limit in a normally hydrated athlete, but this threshold could be surpassed much more readily in a seriously dehydrated competitor.

The inhaled bronchodilator salbutamol is another substance where urinary concentrations have been used to monitor deliberate overdosing. A peak urinary concentration of 1000 ng/mL is permitted, and in one of eight individuals who were tested, the urinary concentration reached 904 ng/mL following a dose of 800 µg of salbutamol [60]. The normal therapeutic dose is 200 µg, but some individuals require larger amounts to control exercise-induced bronchospasm, and indeed the current WADA rules allow the use of 1600 µg of salbutamol over a 24-hour period, so that problems could arise from the detection of excessive concentrations of salbutamol and permitted analogues in concentrated urine [26]. However, as yet, there have been no reports of conflict with antidoping regulations attributable to Ramadan-related dehydration.

One issue that merits future inquiry is whether the tendency to a loss of muscle during Ramadan increases the temptation to abuse anabolic steroids during and following the fast. Again, there is no published information on this question.

Finally, it should be underlined that the detection of diuretics in a urine specimen would breach doping rules, mainly because the use of such agents has been used to mask other doping agents [19].

Dietary Restrictions and Prescribed Medication

Many common medications are taken immediately before or after meals, and this can create problems with the altered meal schedules that are necessary during Ramadan. The swallowing of pills may also be hampered by thirst due to any form of dehydration. Failure to continue with the prescribed regimen is an all-too-frequent problem among those observing Ramadan, and the efficacy of some medications depends on their dose and timing at a specific point in the circadian cycle, which tends to be modified during Ramadan.

A survey of 81 Kuwaitis found that 42% adhered to their drug schedules during Ramadan, but 58% did not. Among the latter group, 35 stopped taking their medication altogether, and four took all of their daily requirement as a single dose [11]. A second study of 325 patients by the same authors found rather similar patterns of behaviour; 64% of this group changed their routine during Ramadan, and 18% took their medications as a single dose [12]. In a third group of 124 individuals with idiopathic epilepsy, 27 developed seizures during Ramadan; 20 of these 27 admitted that during Ramadan they had not taken their medication during daylight hours [31]. Others have pointed out that altered pharmacokinetics, fasting, and tiredness could all contribute to an increased frequency of epileptic seizures during Ramadan [36]. Garcia-Bunuel discussed the specific case of a person who normally controlled his epilepsy by taking 100 mg of phenytoin three times per day; however, he omitted the second and third doses of his medication during Ramadan. In consequence, he sustained a seizure while driving his car. Garcia-Bunuel argued that this problem could have been avoided by taking a 300 mg slow-release preparation of phenytoin at night while observing Ramadan [34].

In terms of circadian rhythm, changes to the cyclic variation in gastric pH can modify the absorption of some drugs, such as theophylline [35,39], and the plasma half-life of many medications is also modified during Ramadan [1].

Where possible, medication that is normally taken several times per day should be replaced by slow-release drugs, and anyone taking medication on a regular basis would be wise to discuss the implications of Ramadan fasting with their physician [2].

Dietary Restrictions and General Health

Acute Health Problems

General dietary restriction to reduce body fat content is generally beneficial rather than harmful to health, provided that the precautions noted in Chapter 2 are followed, particularly the avoidance of an excessive energy deficit and the provision of appropriate vitamins and micronutrients. Excessive restriction of food intake, however, could lead to the female athletic triad and anorexia nervosa (Chapter 2).

In general, the observance of Ramadan has little influence upon either the incidence or the course of acute health problems, and athletes face few serious risks to their health, provided that they continue to take any prescribed medications appropriately [47]. A study of records for a hospital emergency department found no differences in admissions for 10 common medical conditions between Ramadan and other times of the year. However, consultations for hypertension and uncomplicated headache were more frequent during Ramadan, and admissions for diabetes mellitus were also more frequent [68]. The most likely source of difficulty is in the handling of diabetes mellitus. Particularly in the case of athletes with type I diabetes mellitus, the wisest course is to seek an exemption from the requirement of fasting on medical grounds [6]. Ramadan fasting is technically quite possible for sedentary individuals with well-balanced type 2 diabetes mellitus, although such patients should have a careful preliminary discussion with their physician covering possible changes of insulin dosage and an appropriate night-time diet; they must also be prepared to monitor their blood glucose, food, and drug intake closely [5,7,13–15,24,29,41,43–45,49,52,53,62]. There have been occasional episodes of biochemical hypoglycaemia among diabetic children who were observing Ramadan [54], but acute complications from either hypo- or hyperglycaemia are extremely rare [25,62]. Problems seem most likely if patients opt not to take hypoglyacemic agents during daylight hours [64]. Sedentary individuals with type I diabetes who wish to engage in daytime fasting should monitor their blood glucose four to six times a day and keep in close contact with their physician; they may find it possible to keep glucose levels within acceptable limits by the use of fast-absorption insulin instead of carrying an emergency supply of carbohydrates [25], but they should be prepared to abandon their fast (and know what emergency measures to take) if blood glucose levels drop below 4.4 mmol/L or rises above 16.7 mmol/L [30].

Involvement in heavy training or endurance competition increases an individual's vulnerability to upper respiratory infections [18], and indeed respiratory ailments are among the most common complaints made by those attending medical facilities at international competitions [59]. There has as yet been little study of how Ramadan and other types of dietary restriction influence an athlete's risk of upper respiratory infections. Nevertheless, the combination of disturbed sleep, stress, and a negative energy balance seem likely to have a negative effect upon the immune system [17], thus increasing the likelihood of developing an upper respiratory infection. Preventive measures include assuring an adequate intake of key amino acids, carbohydrates, antioxidants, and micronutrients [58].

A further possible concern is an exacerbation of the female athletic triad [48] by Ramadan fasting. Again, there has been no formal scientific study of this question, but the average loss of body mass over the month of intermittent fasting is such (Chapter 2) that Ramadan observance may not do very much to exacerbate the condition of a woman with this syndrome.

Chronic Health Issues

Ramadan may have a favourable impact upon the long-term course of chronic diseases such as diabetes and atherosclerosis in sedentary individuals, particularly if opportunity is taken to reduce the body mass during Ramadan [51]. However, any benefit only persists for as long as the reduction in body mass is maintained.

An improvement of lipid profile is probable during Ramadan fasting, and there may also be a reduction of lipid peroxidation [10] and changes of apolipoprotein fractions [3], both of which could have a favourable influence upon the course of atherosclerosis. For sedentary individuals, the incidence of sudden cardiac arrest and myocardial infarction remains unchanged during Ramadan [66], but because of the altered timing of meals and sleep, the normal morning peak of heart attacks [9] and strokes [28] is not seen. Ramadan observance has a minimal impact upon the course of chronic congestive heart disease [21]. There seems no published information concerning the possible influence of Ramadan fasting upon the risk of sudden cardiac death in athletes.

Dietary Restrictions and the Risk of Injury

Does the observance of Ramadan or other forms of dieting leave a person more vulnerable to injury on the road, on the playing field, in the factory, and at home? And is there evidence of a greater prevalence of overreaching and overtraining among Muslim athletes at this season? Irritability is likely enhanced by a low blood sugar, and in those observing Ramadan, this is exacerbated by a combination of sleep loss, dehydration, and resulting fatigue, leading to a loss of vigilance that might predispose to accidents. Failure to take prescribed medications might be a further adverse factor with either dietary or fluid restriction.

A number of newspaper reports have suggested that there is indeed a high incidence of road traffic accidents during Ramadan. However, the empirical evidence is conflicting (Table 13.1).

Where comparisons are made between Ramadan and other times of the year, the analysis may be complicated by increased travel to festive gatherings during Ramadan and, in some countries, by a reduced consumption of alcohol, which leads to a month-long closure of liquor stores in some countries such as Morocco [38] and shorter working hours in many Arab countries. Some people certainly report feeling more irritable during Ramadan [30,40,50]. However, one author has argued that the spiritual atmosphere of the season counters the irritability and nervousness that would normally be associated with a low blood sugar [42], and that this makes motorists more courteous and less vulnerable to accidents.

In terms of empirical data, one study from Saudi Arabia noted that the maximum number of road accident victims was seen during the month of Ramadan [57]; however, another study from Saudi Arabia found no difference of traumatic injuries in children (commonly from traffic accidents) during Ramadan [8]. A study from the United Arab Emirates also commented that the risk was 'slightly higher' during Ramadan [16], and in Pakistan values for Ramadan (August) were slightly higher than for the previous 8 months [63].

In England, there was a significant increase in the proportion of hospital emergency department consultations attributable to Muslims during Ramadan (5.1% vs. 3.6%); consultations related to traffic accidents appeared to show a similar trend, but because of smaller absolute numbers, the difference in traffic accidents was not statistically significant [46]. In contrast, studies from Jordan [42] and Morocco [52] noted that motor vehicle accident rates were lower during Ramadan than at other times during the year. A recent study from Kazakhstan (a state with

TABLE 13.1 Studies Showing the Influence of Ramadan on the Frequency of Admissions to Hospital Emergency Departments for Automobile Accidents

Country	Sample Size	Study Duration	Findings	Authors
United Arab Emirates	1,197 injuries with hospital	1 year	Risk 'slightly higher' during Ramadan	Bener et al. [16]
Jordan	228	2 months	Decreased by 27% during Ramadan	Khammash et al. [42]
Morocco	250–500 accidents/day	1 year	'Significantly decreased'	Herrag et al. [38]
Saudi Arabia	361	1 year	'Maximum number of patients seen during Ramadan'	Shanks et al. [57]
Saudi Arabia	3,766 cases of pediatric trauma	8 years	No difference in child trauma injuries during Ramadan	Alnasser et al. [8]
United Kingdom	386 Muslims vs. 8,893 non-Muslims		Proportion of Muslims attending outpatients increased from 3.6% to 5.1% during Ramadan; rise in accidents similar but not statistically significant	Langford et al. [46]
Kazakhstan	6,065 injuries	3 years	Non-significant trend to less injuries during Ramadan	Tiemissov et al. [67]
Pakistan	12,969 road traffic crashes	8-month average, 11,523	Small increase in Ramadan (August) compared with 8-month average	Tahir et al. [63]

a large and growing proportion of Muslims) examined injury rates in those over the age of 60 years [67]; this also showed a non-significant trend to fewer injuries both in men (−10.7%) and women (−2.7%).

At the *First Consensus Conference on Ramadan and Football* held in Qatar, in November 2011, Nadir Belhadj, an Algerian professional soccer player, declared '*I feel there are for sure more injuries during fasting*'. [32]. However, there have as yet been only two formal studies of injury rates in athletes. The first seemed to suggest an effect from changes of nutrition, with altered inflammatory and immune responses [22], rather than from mood disturbances of vigilance and mood state. Observations on 42 top Tunisian soccer players were continued over two seasons. Overuse and non-contact injuries were more frequent during Ramadan, but there was no increase in the number of contact injuries [20]. A second report from Qatar compared observant and non-observant first division male soccer players both during Ramadan and at other times of the year. It found that those who did not observe Ramadan had a higher incidence of injuries than those who did engage in intermittent fasting, and the observant players showed no increase in their injury rates during the month of Ramadan [27]; however, there were some limitations to the comparison. The non-observant players were younger, and often foreign and unaccustomed to the heat of Qatar, thus increasing their risk of injury. Moreover, the observant players may have reduced the intensity of their training, making them less susceptible to injury. There thus remains scope for further study of this important question.

Other forms of severe dieting are likely to predispose to various types of injury, in part because of a low blood glucose and associated irritability and in part from a loss of lean tissue that reduces the potential to correct errors of movement and leaves the bone more exposed to direct trauma.

Restriction of Fluid Intake and Heat Stress

Risk

The prohibition of daytime fluid intake leaves those observing Ramadan vulnerable to hypohydration, with a danger of resulting heat stress, whether they are engaged in a prolonged athletic event (Chapter 5) or performing heavy work in a hot factory [56]. Loss of fluids during the 'making of weight' also influences both performance and heat tolerance (Chapter 2). When performing a sedentary task, a 2% decrease of body water is sufficient to cause impairment in various measures of mental performance [33,37]. However, the margin is somewhat larger for an endurance athlete, as exercise may liberate some 2 L of water from the breakdown of glycogen and metabolism in general (Chapter 5). Thus, a 2% decrease of body mass induced by running on a treadmill in impermeable clothing had negligible effects on neuromuscular function [55]. However, with a 5% decrease of body mass, the elevation of core temperature for a given bout of exercise is about 1°C greater, often enough to make the difference between an acceptable and a dangerous increase of body temperature [55].

The limits of an acceptable increase of body core temperature are progressively being reduced by those concerned with safety in sport and in industry. At one time, it was fairly common to find endurance athletes with post-race rectal temperatures of 41°C, and the aim of industrial hygienists was to keep the body core temperature of employees below a ceiling of 39.2°C, but now the Department of Occupational Health and Safety in Ontario requires employers to limit the body temperature of their workers to 38°C.

To date, there have been no measurements of core temperatures in athletes who are observing Ramadan, and no published studies have shown decreases of body mass as large as 5%. However, the danger of heat stress cannot be entirely dismissed, since there is little or no information on responses in the most vulnerable group of athletes, those who engage in endurance and ultraendurance activities.

Potential Preventive Measures

Part of the loss of performance during fluid deprivation is psychological, and performance can thus be enhanced by periodic 5 seconds rinsing of the mouth with glucose-containing solutions; this practice is allowed during Ramadan, provided that the fluid is subsequently spat from the mouth [23]. Possible measures to reduce the risk of heat stress for those who are incurring a fluid deficit, particularly those observing Ramadan, include the maximization of fluid intake during the hours of darkness, remaining in cool areas as much as possible prior to competition, and further conserving sweat by wetting the clothing immediately before an event, particularly if the exercise is to be performed out of doors during the daytime.

Warning Symptoms

In addition to dryness of the mouth and thirst, warning signs of severe dehydration include difficulty in urinating, a dry skin under conditions where sweating would normally be anticipated, fatigue, light-headedness, dizziness, and/or confusion, with an increase of pulse and breathing rates. Because sweating is impaired by dehydration, the body temperature can rise to dangerously high levels. In heat stress, the symptoms of headache, sluggishness, poorly coordinated movements, hallucinations, seizures, and a loss of consciousness are added to the symptoms already seen with dehydration.

Treatment

Heat stress is potentially fatal, and treatment is urgently needed to prevent permanent brain damage. The affected individual should be moved indoors to the coolest room available, clothing removed, and cool water applied to the skin, with fanning to encourage evaporation. The feet should also be slightly elevated, to maximize blood flow to the brain. Transfusion of saline may be required to restore the plasma volume.

General Medical Advice

The sports physician is in a position to offer general support to athletes who have for any reason decided to restrict the intake of food and/or fluid in the face of international competition, and medical officers should be prepared to offer informed professional advice on risks and appropriate countermeasures, taking due account of the competitor's age, sex, and experience, the type of athletic event, and the challenges posed by the local environment. The competitor should be guided in developing optimal tactics to meet the needs for energy, fluids, and training despite the restrictions that have been adopted. If possible, event organizers should also consider rescheduling both training times and competition events to the night hours or even to a different time of the year in order to avoid long daylight hours of exposure to summer heat.

Conclusions

Severe dietary and/or fluid restriction raises several medical issues for athletes and sports physicians. Can normal measures of doping control be applied when an athlete is severely dehydrated and has difficulty in urinating? Do the altered meal times of Ramadan conflict with the use of previously prescribed medication? Does the combination of vigorous exercise with a month of intermittent fasting have any adverse effect on health? Do the combined effects of sleep loss, general irritability, and cognitive disturbance associated with hypoglycaemia increase the risk of injury? And can dehydration during an event develop to such an extent that it predisposes to dangerous levels of heat stress? Overzealous reduction of body mass by severe dietary restriction and artificial depletion of body fluids is to be discouraged, but available information suggests that with the possible exception of type I diabetes mellitus, none of these issues present sufficient health concerns to advise a devout Muslim athlete against Ramadan observance.

Key Terms

Female athletic triad: The female athlete triad is encountered mainly in athletic disciplines where scores are influenced by appearance, such as gymnastics. Excessive weight loss due to an inadequate food intake is associated with a cessation of menstruation and a decrease of bone density.

Half-life: The time required for the concentration of a substance (such as a blood stream medication) to decrease to a half of its initial value.

Hyperglycaemia: An increase of serum glucose concentration above an arbitrary normal limit, for example, 16.7 mmol/L.

Hypoglycaemia: A decrease of serum glucose concentration below an arbitrary normal limit, for example, 4.4 mmol/L.

Overreaching: An excessive accumulation of training and other stressors leading to a short-term decrease in an athlete's performance.

Overtraining: A more serious consequence of excessive training, with a long-term deterioration in the athlete's performance.

Peroxidation: Peroxidation is a process that leads to the oxidative degradation of lipids; it can have serious effects, as free radicals 'steal' electrons from the lipids in cell membranes.

pH: The pH is a measure of the acidity of a substance; a low pH indicates a strong acid medium.

Phenytoin: Phenytoin is a depressant medication, commonly used in the suppression of epileptic seizures.

Refractometer: A refractometer is a device that can be used to determine the SG of urine; measurements are based on the degree to which a light beam is refracted.

Salbutamol: Salbutamol is a short-acting drug that acts on beta-2 adrenergic receptors, relieving exercise-induced bronchospasm. Antidoping regulations permit athletes with exercise-induced bronchospasm to take small quantities of salbutamol by inhalation.

Specific gravity: The SG is the density of a substance relative to that of water at a specified temperature.

Key Points

1. Athletes who are restricting fluid intake due to making weight or observing Ramadan may have difficulty in producing urine for doping control immediately after competition. However, they are permitted to wait with a doping control official until fluid balance has been restored.
2. Urinary concentration due to dehydration could in theory cause a legitimate intake of caffeine or inhaled salbutamol to reach a prohibited concentration in the urine.
3. Problems can arise from forgetting to take medication or altered pharmacokinetics with altered meal schedules during Ramadan and other forms of dieting. Several authors have commented on an increased incidence of epileptic seizures among those prone to epilepsy. Where possible, repeated daily doses of a medication should be replaced by once daily use of a slow-release preparation.
4. Sedentary individuals with well-controlled diabetes mellitus can observe Ramadan and other moderate forms of dieting safely, but they must monitor their blood sugar levels frequently and must be prepared to abandon their fast and take appropriate corrective actions if blood glucose levels fall outside the range 4.4–16.7 mmol/L. Athletes should generally accept a medical exemption from fasting.
5. There is as yet no consensus as to whether a restriction of food or fluid intake increases the risk of athletic injuries.
6. In the groups of athletes studied to date, dehydration during Ramadan seems insufficient to cause a dangerous heat stress, but there is a need to study responses in endurance and ultraendurance competitors.

Questions for Discussion

1. When monitoring for the possible abuse of prohibited drugs in an athlete who is observing Ramadan or other types of restricted fluid intake, what special issues should be considered?

2. What measures might avoid problems when taking prescribed medications during Ramadan and other types of food restriction?
3. Should an athletic competitor with type I diabetes mellitus be allowed to observe Ramadan or other types of dietary restriction? If so, what precautions should be observed?
4. Do you think athletes who claim an increased susceptibility to injury during Ramadan are correct in their opinion? What measures could you suggest to mitigate this risk?
5. How would you minimize the rise of body temperature in an athlete who is competing in a distance race while restricting the intake of fluids?

References

1. Aadil N, Fassi-Fihri A, Houti I et al. Influence of Ramadan on the pharmacokinetics of a single oral dose of valproic acid administered at two different times. *Methods Find Exp Clin Pharmacol* 2000;22:109–114.
2. Aadil N, Houti IE, Moussamih S. Drug intake during Ramadan. *Br Med J* 2004;329:778–782.
3. Adlouni A, Ghalim N, Saile R et al. Beneficial effect on serum apo AI, apo B and Lp AI levels of Ramadan fasting. *Clin Chim Acta* 1998;271:179–189.
4. World-Wide Religious News. Anti-doping officials accused of pressuring player to break Ramadan fast 2003. http://wwrn.org/articles/14540/? (Accessed April 15, 2015).
5. Al-Jewari MMM, Mohammed KLA, Al-Hakim SAG. Effect of Ramadan fasting on clinical, biochemical and immunological parameters in healthy fasting and type 2 diabetes mellitus patients. *Iraqi Postgrad Med J* 2007;6:272–275 (Accessed April 15, 2015).
6. Alkandari JR, Maughan RJ, Roky R et al. The implications of Ramadan fasting for human health and well-being. *J Sports Sci* 2012;30(Suppl. 1):S9–S19.
7. Al Nakhi A, Al Arouj M, Kandari A, Morad M (eds.). Multiple insulin injection during fasting Ramadan in IDDM patients. In: *Proceeding of the Second International Congress on Health and Ramadan*, Istanbul, Turkey, December 1–3, 1997. FRSMR (Hassan II Foundation for Scientific and Medical Research on Ramadan), Morocco, Africa, 1997.
8. Alnasser M, AlSelaim N, Aldhukair S et al. Patterns of pediatric trauma in Ramadan: An observational study. *Ann Pediatr Surg* 2012;8(1):9–11.
9. Al Suwaidi J, Bener A, Gehani AA et al. Does the circadian pattern for acute cardiac events presentation vary with fasting? *J Postgrad Med* 2006;252:30–33.
10. Asgary S, Aghaei F, Naderi GA et al. Peroxidation, serum lipids and fasting blood sugar. *Med J Islamic Acad Med Sci* 2000;13:35–38.
11. Aslam M, Healy MA. Compliance and drug therapy in fasting Moslem patients. *J Clin Hosp Pharm* 1986;11:321–325.
12. Aslam M, Assad A. Drug regimens and fasting during Ramadan: A survey in Kuwait. *Public Health* 1986;100:49–53.
13. Athar S, Habib M (eds.). Management of stable type II diabetes NIDDM during Ramadan fasting. In: *Proceeding of the First International Congress on Health and Ramadan*. FRSMR (Hassan II Foundation for Scientific and Medical Research on Ramadan), Morocco, Africa, 1994.
14. Azizi F, Rasouli HA. Serum glucose, bilirubin, calcium, phosphorus, protein and albumin concentrations during Ramadan. *Med J Islamic Repub Iran* 1987;1:38–41.
15. Benaji B, Mounib N, Roky R et al. Diabetes and Ramadan: Review of the literature. *Diabetes Res Clin Pract* 2006;73:117–125.

16. Bener A, Absood GH, Achan NV, Sankaran-Kutty M. Road traffic injuries in Al-Ain City, United Arab Emirates. *J R Soc Health* 1992;112:273–276.
17. Bragazzi NL. Ramadan fasting and immunity system. In: Chtourou H (ed.), *Effects of Ramadan Fasting on Health and Athletic Performance*. Omics Book Group, New York, 2013.
18. Brenner IKM, Shephard RJ. Infection in athletes. *Sports Med* 1994;17:86–107.
19. Cadwallader A, de la Torre X, Tieri A et al. The abuse of diuretics as performance-enhancing drugs and masking agents in sport doping: Pharmacology, toxicology and analysis. *Br J Pharmacol* 2010;161(1):1–16.
20. Chamari BK, Haddad M, Wong DP et al. Injury rates in professional soccer players during Ramadan. *J Sports Sci* 2012;30(Suppl. 1):S93–S102.
21. Chamsi-Pasha H, Ahmed WH. The effect of fasting in Ramadan on patients with heart disease. *Saudi Med J* 2004;25:47–51.
22. Chaouachi A, Coutts AJ, Wong dP et al. Haematological, inflammatory, and immuno-logical responses in elite judo athletes maintaining high training loads during Ramadan. *Appl Physiol Nutr Metab* 2009;34:907–915.
23. Che Muhamed AMC, Mohammed NG, Ismail N et al. Mouth rinsing improves cycling endurance during Ramadan fasting in a hot humid environment. *Appl Physiol Nutr Metab* 2014;39:458–464.
24. Das R. Diabetes mellitus and Ramadan. A narrative review of literature. *Ital J Publ Health* 2011;8:247–254.
25. Davidson JC. Muslims, Ramadan and diabetes mellitus. *Br Med J* 1979;ii:1511–1512.
26. Dickinson J, Hu J, Chester N et al. Impact of ethnicity, gender and dehydration on the urinary excretion of inhaled salbutamol with respect to doping control. *Clin J Sports Med* 2014;24(6):482–489.
27. Eirale C, Tol JL, Smiley F et al. Does Ramadan affect the risk of injury in professional football? *Clin J Sports Med* 2013;23(4):261–266.
28. El-Mitwalli A, Zaher AA, El Menshawi E. Circadian rhythm of stroke onset during the month of Ramadan. *Acta Neurol Scand* 2010;122:97–101.
29. Elnasri H, Ahmed AM. Effects of Ramadan fasting on blood levels of glucose, triglyceride and cholesterol among type II diabetic patients. *Sudanese J Publ Health* 2006;1:203–206.
30. Ennigrou S, Zenaidi M, Ben Slama F et al. Ramadan and customs of life: Investigation with 84 adult residents in the district of Tunis. *Tunis Méd* 2001;79:508–514.
31. Etemadyfar M. Effect of Ramadan on frequency of seizures. *Iran J Endocrinol Metab* 2001; Abstract book, Congress on Health and Ramadan, October 2001:32.
32. FIFA. Muslim players asking scientists for help 2012. http://www.fifa.com/aboutfifa/footballdevelopment/medical/news/newsid=1552131/ (Accessed February 20, 2013).
33. Ftaiti F, Grélot L, Coudreuse JM, Nicol C. Combined effect of heat stress, dehydration and exercise on neuromuscular function in humans. *Eur J Appl Physiol* 2001;84:87–94.
34. Garcia-Bunuel L. Clinical problems during the fast of Ramadan. *Lancet* 1989;i:1396.
35. Gay JP, Cherrah Y, Aadil N et al. Influence of Ramadan on the pharmacokinetics of a SR preparation of theophylline and cortisol cycle. *J Interdisc Cycle Res* 1990;21:190–192.
36. Gomceli YB, Kutlu G, Cavdar L, Inan LE. Does the seizure frequency increase in Ramadan? *Seizure* 2008;17:671–676.
37. Gopinathan PM, Pichan G, Sharma VM. Role of dehydration in heat-stress induced varia-tions in mental performance. *Arch Environ Health* 1988;43:15–17.
38. Herrag M, Lahmiti S, Alaoui Yazidi A. Ramadan: A different side of the emergencies? *Afr Health Sci* 2010;10:215–216.
39. Iraki L, Bogdan A, Hakkou F et al. Ramadan diet restrictions modify the circadian time structure in humans: A study on plasma gastrin, insulin, glucose, and calcium and on gastric pH. *J Clin Endocrinol Metab* 1997;82:1261–1273.
40. Kadri N, Tilane A, El Batal M et al. Irritability during the month of Ramadan. *Psychosom Med* 2000;62:280–285.

41. Katibi IA, Akande AA, Bojuwoye BJ, Okesina AB. Blood sugar among fasting Muslims with type 2 diabetes mellitus in Ilorin. *Niger J Med* 2001;10:132–134.
42. Khammash MR, Al-Shouha TF. Do road traffic accidents increase during the fasting month of Ramadan? *Neuroscience (Riyadh)* 2006;11:21–23.
43. Klocker N, Belkhadir J, El Ghomari H et al. (eds.). Effects of extreme chrono-biological diet alternations during Ramadan on metabolism in NIDDM diabetes with oral treatment. In: *Proceeding of the Second International Congress on Health and Ramadan*, Istanbul, Turkey, December 1–3, 1997. FRSMR (Hassan II Foundation for Scientific and Medical Research on Ramadan), Morocco, Africa, 1997.
44. Kobeissy A, Zantout MS, Azar ST. Suggested insulin regimens for patients with type 1 diabetes mellitus who wish to fast during the month of Ramadan. *Clin Ther* 2008;30:1408–1415.
45. Laajam MA. Ramadan fasting and non-insulin-dependent diabetes: Effect on metabolic control. *East Afr Med J* 1990;67:732–736.
46. Langford EJ, Ishaque MA, Fothergill J, Touquet R. The effect of the fast of Ramadan on accident and emergency attendances. *J R Soc Med* 1994;87:517–518.
47. Leiper JB, Molla AM, Molla AM. Effects on health of fluid restriction during fasting in Ramadan. *Eur J Clin Nutr* 2003;57(Suppl. 2):S30–S38.
48. Loucks AB. The endocrine system: Integrated influences on metabolism, growth and reproduction. In: Tipton CM, Sawka MN, Tate CA, Terjung RL (eds.), *ACSM's Advanced Exercise Physiology*. Lippincott, Williams & Wilkins, Philadelphia, PA, 2006.
49. Mafauzy M, Mohammed WB, Anum MY et al. A study of the fasting diabetic patients during the month of Ramadan. *Med J Malaysia* 1990;45:14–17.
50. Maughan RJ, Bartagi Z, Dvorak J, Zerguini Y. Dietary intake and body composition of football players during the holy month of Ramadan. *J Sports Sci* 2008;26(Suppl. 3): S20–S38.
51. Nematy M, Alinnezhad-Namaghi M, Rashed MM et al. Effects of Ramadan fasting on cardiovascular risk factors: A prospective observational study. *Nutr J* 2012;11:69–75.
52. Omar M, Motala A. Fasting in Ramadan and the diabetic patient. *Diabetes Care* 1997;20:1925–1926.
53. Rashed H. The fast of Ramadan: No problem for the well: The sick should avoid fasting. *Br Med J* 1992;304:521–522.
54. Salman H, Abdallah MA, Al Howasi M. Ramadan fasting in diabetic children in Riyadh. *Diabetes Med* 1992;9:583–584.
55. Sawka MN, Montain SJ. Fluid and electrolyte supplementation for exercise heat stress. *Am J Clin Nutr* 2000;72(Suppl. 2):564S–572S.
56. Schmahl FW, Metzler B, Born M, Elmadfa I. Ramadan, Gesundheitsgefährdung während des Fastenmonats (Ramadan: Health risk during the month of fasting). *Dtsch Ärzteblatte* 1988;85:B842–B844.
57. Shanks NJ, Ansari M, Al-Kalai D. Road traffic accidents in Saudi Arabia. *Publ Health* 1994;108:27–34.
58. Shephard RJ. *Physical Activity, Training and the Immune Response*. Cooper Publishing, Carmel, IN, 1997.
59. Shephard RJ. *Medical Surveillance of Endurance Sport*. In: Shephard RJ, Åstrand P-O (eds.), *Endurance in Sport*. Blackwell Scientific, Oxford, U.K., 2000, pp. 653–666.
60. Sporer BC, Sheel AW, Taunton J, Rupert JL, McKenzie DC. Inhaled salbutamol and doping control effects of dose on urine concentrations. *Clin J Sports Med* 2008;18:282–285.
61. Stuempfle KJ, Drury DG. Comparison of 3 methods to assess urine specific gravity in collegiate wrestlers. *J Athl Train* 2003;38:315–319.
62. Sulimani RA. Ramadan fasting: Medical aspects in health and disease. *Ann Saudi Med* 1991;11:637–641.
63. Tahir MN, Macassa G, Akbar AH et al. Road traffic crashes in Ramadan: An observational study. *East Mediterr Health J* 2014;19(Suppl. 3):S147–S151.
64. Tang C, Rolfe M. Clinical problems during fast of Ramadan. *Lancet* 1989;i:1396.

65. Taylor D, MacKay D. City say Negouai drug test 'violated' Ramadan 2003. *Manchester Guardian*. http://www.theguardian.com/football/2003/nov/06/newsstory.sport7 (Accessed February 12, 2013).
66. Temizhan A, Donderici O, Ouz D, Demirbas B. Is there any effect of Ramadan fasting on acute coronary heart disease events? *Int J Cardiol* 1999;70:149–153.
67. Tiemissov A. Does the number of injuries among the elderly increase during Ramadan? In: *IEA World Congress of Epidemiology*, Anchorage, AK, August 2014.
68. Topacoglu H, Kaqrcioglu O, Yuruktumen A et al. Impact of Ramadan on demographics and frequencies of disease-related visits in the emergency department. *Int J Clin Pract* 2005;59:900–905.
69. Wallace S. Keegan's test claim rejected 2003. *The Telegraph*. http://www.telegraph.co.uk/sport/football/2424842/Keegans-test-claim-rejected.html (Accessed February 12, 2013).
70. White J. Doping control presents unique challenge for 2 Ramadan-fasting Moroccan footballers 2012 (Accessed February 12, 2013).

14

Conclusions

Ezdine Bouhlel

For many decades, several methods of dietary restriction have been used to make changes in body composition. These methods have been adopted by various categories of people (sedentary and athletic individuals, both healthy and clinical patients). Total fasting, dietary restriction and/or Ramadan observance are the most commonly used options to induce changes in body mass and particularly of body fat in overweight or obese subjects. Body mass reductions may also be sought by weight-categorized athletes and others who wish to induce changes in body composition, particularly reductions in body fat and gains in fat-free mass to optimize muscle performance.

Irrespective of the category of individual concerned, whether a sedentary obese person or an active athlete, such dietary manipulations should be undertaken with appropriate precautions to ensure beneficial changes in body composition. If the total dietary intake is reduced, minimum dietetic requirements for protein, essential fatty acids and micronutrients should be respected. Moreover, dieting should be combined with aerobic exercise to maximize fat oxidation and conserve lean tissue. The injection of high-intensity exercise into a training programme may facilitate anaerobic metabolism and thus enhance gains in muscle mass. A combination of fasting or dietary restriction with graduated aerobic and anaerobic training is a valuable tactic to promote fat loss and to maintain fat-free mass, both in the obese and in athletes.

During total fasting or severe dietary restriction, a reduction in body glycogen stores offers a major problem when undertaking sustained endurance activity. In athletes who continue to train or who must participate in prolonged endurance competitions, an important objective is to conserve these glycogen stores despite the dietary modification.

If the decrease in glycogen caused by a combination of fasting and continued training is followed by a high-carbohydrate diet, the replenishment of glycogen stores is optimized; athletes who have fasted should thus elect high-carbohydrate meals during refeeding, in order to compensate for the losses induced by fasting and training. However, some reports suggest that short periods of fasting and the intermittent fasting of Ramadan observance have little effect upon muscle glycogen levels and aerobic performance. Hormonal changes and the resulting modulation of metabolism likely play a major role in augmenting fat metabolism during fasting. If adaptations to fasting are well managed, they can induce substantial reductions in fat mass.

Short-term fasting in healthy subjects has little adverse effect upon protein metabolism, overall body composition, the training response or competitive performance. Glycogenolysis is the main source of the body's glucose needs during the first 24 hours of fasting. However, if the fast is of longer duration, gluconeogenesis and lipolysis account for a progressively increasing proportion of total energy usage. With total fasting, or a reduced protein intake, gluconeogenesis leads to a progressive loss of lean tissue, with adverse effects upon strength and resistance performance. Protein supplementation is important to the conservation of lean tissue and resistance performance during severe dietary restriction. The issue is particularly acute for athletes who are engaged in competitions lasting longer than 90 minutes, since there is then a tendency to catabolize muscle during an event, even if glycogen stores are initially well filled. More research is needed in situations where the protein supply is challenged (prolonged fasting, participants in ultraendurance events, those from low-level socioeconomic categories, and those following vegetarian diets).

Fasting or dietary restriction without ingestion of water will probably compromise fluid balance, particularly if prolonged exercise must be performed under warm conditions. Even during the intermittent fasting of Ramadan, reports show decreases of plasma volumes in athletes during the afternoon. Often, the color of the urine offers a simple indication of hydration status. Training and competition in hot ambient conditions exacerbate this issue, and coaches must encourage athletes to compensate by an increased fluid intake during the hours of darkness, in order to avoid a cumulative dehydration, with associated health problems and impairments of performance.

Although a large proportion of athletes currently take antioxidant supplements such as vitamins C and E in the hope of reducing muscle damage from free radicals produced during the training process, beneficial effects have yet to be confirmed. Nevertheless, there does not seem any great harm in a prudent use of antioxidant supplements as an insurance against the combined demands of dietary restriction and heavy physical exercise. Nutrients rich in minerals such as iron, zinc, and selenium and vitamins C and E could serve to enhance the individual's total antioxidant status.

Some authors have argued that fasting or dietary restriction can enhance the antioxidant system. Likewise, an appropriate training programme, with a well-chosen ratio of training loads to recovery intervals can improve antioxidant defenses. However, further studies are needed to clarify relationships between training, dietary intake and athletic performance in relation to antioxidant requirements.

A combination of central and muscular factors can limit physical work during fasting, including changes in motivation and sleep patterns, a reduction of glycogen stores, dehydration and in some cases a reduction of training loads. The relative importance of these parameters to impairments of physical performance and cognitive function as yet remains unclear. In general, the effects of short-term fasting upon physical performance and cognitive function appear to be relatively small, but nevertheless they may be sufficient to influence competitive standing. The impact of dietary restriction varies with the type, duration and intensity of competition. Short-term fasting usually has no detrimental effect upon single bouts of short-term intensive exercise (for example, hand grip, vertical jumping, short sprints or throwing). However, if the short-term exercise must be repeated, as when training or competing in heats, a small deterioration of performance is often observed. Effects are greatest in prolonged events that place greater demands on reserves of glycogen and fluid; the greatest deterioration of performance is observed when prolonged aerobic exercise must be performed using a large muscle mass.

Recovery tactics play a major role in limiting the negative effects of short-term and intermittent fasting. Appropriate tactics should aim at restoring muscle and liver glycogen stores, replacing fluid and electrolytes losses, and assuring adequate supplies of protein for anabolic repair, anabolic responses to training and health of the immune and antioxidant systems.

Individualized control of training loads and lifestyle should help the athlete to maintain aerobic performance during short-term and intermittent fasting. Metabolic recovery (elimination of metabolites after training or competition) and nutritional recovery (for example, ensuring a high-carbohydrate diet after a fasting day) should allow an athlete to compete effectively once again. However, there is no evidence of benefit from fasting during competition. During Ramadan observance, the timing of training sessions will probably need adjustment; ideally, they should be undertaken before or shortly after feeding, so that plasma amino acid levels are optimal for anabolism. Training late in the evening probably has some physiological advantages, including probably sufficient replenishment of carbohydrates, although further comparisons of the various options are required.

Adequate sleep is important to athletic performance. Indeed, the impact of sleep disturbances on the physical and cognitive performance of athletes during Ramadan observance could be more important than the issues of intermittent hunger or thirst. Many studies have shown changes in sleep patterns and shifts in the times of sleeping during Ramadan. These changes should be countered by recovery tactics such as napping that take into account the individual's sleep needs, the activities to be performed and the provision of environmental conditions conducive to sleep.

Coaches should plan the sleep patterns of their athletes, advising them to retire early and to take a nap when necessary, under optimal environmental conditions. Nonessential physical activities should be avoided during fasting, in order to spare both energy and fluid reserves. Resting and sleeping could be combined with other physiotherapeutic recovery modalities, such as massage, stretching, cold or contrast water immersion and mental preparation to control emotions and avoid negative attitudes. Coaches can educate athletes to understand, plan and use recovery tactics effectively. The athlete can learn to optimize training loads, to increase performance, to reduce training-induced injuries and illnesses, and to develop appropriate, self-directed recovery tactics that take into account the individual's sleep–wake cycle, physiological responses to training, emotional status and environmental conditions.

If the attention is paid to recovery processes, fasting or dietary restriction could have negative effects on health and performance. Dehydration could predispose to dangerous levels of heat stress. The combined effects of sleep loss and circadian rhythm disturbance could increase the risk of injury. Abstinence from food and/or fluid could also conflict with the use of previously prescribed medications. However, available information suggests that with the possible exception of diabetes mellitus, none of these issues raises sufficient health concerns to advise an athlete against short-term fasting or Ramadan observance if he or she so desires.

Much research has been undertaken on fasting, particularly in relation to Ramadan observance, in recent years. In general, it seems that by dint of considerable self-discipline, athletic performance can be sustained. However, there remain some areas still to be explored, particularly the impact of reduced glycogen stores on endurance and ultraendurance performance, the optimization of training and recovery processes, and a possible increase in the prevalence of injuries. Further, most of the research to date has been in young athletic men. There remains a need to explore the effects of age, sex, physical fitness level and environmental conditions such as temperature and humidity conditions upon both metabolism and performance during fasting and/or dietary restriction.

Index